PHARMACO VIGILANCE

FROM   A   TO   Z

ADVERSE DRUG EVENT SURVEILLANCE

PHARMACO-VIGILANCE

FROM A TO Z

ADVERSE DRUG
EVENT SURVEILLANCE

BARTON L. COBERT, MD • PIERRE BIRON, MD

Senior Director
Medical and Safety Services
Schering-Plough Research Institute

Professor of Pharmacology
Faculty of Medicine
Université de Montréal

b

**Blackwell
Science**

©2002 by Blackwell Science, Inc.

Editorial Offices:

Commerce Place, 350 Main Street, Malden, Massachusetts 02148, USA

Osney Mead, Oxford OX2 0EL, England

25 John Street, London WC1N 2BS, England

23 Ainslie Place, Edinburgh EH3 6AJ, Scotland

54 University Street, Carlton, Victoria 3053, Australia

Other Editorial Offices:

Blackwell Wissenschafts-Verlag GmbH, Kurfürstendamm 57, 10707 Berlin, Germany

Blackwell Science KK, MG Kodenmacho Building, 7-10 Kodenmacho Nihombashi, Chuo-ku, Tokyo 104, Japan

Iowa State University Press, A Blackwell Science Company, 2121 S. State Avenue, Ames, Iowa 50014-8300, USA

Distributors:

The Americas

Blackwell Publishing

c/o AIDC

P.O. Box 20

50 Winter Sport Lane

Williston, VT 05495-0020

(Telephone orders: 800-216-2522; fax orders: 802-864-7626)

Australia

Blackwell Science Pty, Ltd.

54 University Street

Carlton, Victoria 3053

(Telephone orders: 03-9347-0300; fax orders: 03-9349-3016)

Outside The Americas and Australia

Blackwell Science, Ltd.

c/o Marston Book Services, Ltd.

P.O. Box 269

Abingdon

Oxon OX14 4YN

England

(Telephone orders: 44-01235-465500; fax orders: 44-01235-465555)

Acquisitions: Laura DeYoung

Development: Julia Casson

Production: Shawn Girsberger

Manufacturing: Lisa Flanagan

Marketing Manager: Toni Fournier

Printed and bound by Capital City Press

Printed in the United States of America

01 02 03 04 5 4 3 2 1

The Blackwell Science logo is a trade mark of Blackwell Science Ltd., registered at the United Kingdom Trade Marks Registry

Library of Congress Cataloging-in-Publication Data

Cobert, Barton L.

Pharmacovigilance from A to Z / by Barton L. Cobert and Pierre Biron.

p. ; cm.

Includes bibliographical references.

ISBN 0-632-04586-8

1. Pharmacoepidemiology—Encyclopedias. 2. Drugs—Side effects—Encyclopedias. I. Biron, Pierre. II. Title.

[DNLM: 1. Pharmacoepidemiology—Handbooks. 2. Product Surveillance, Postmarketing—Handbooks. 3. Pharmaceutical preparations—adverse effects—handbooks. 4. Risk Assessment—handbooks. QZ 39 C655p 2001]

RM302.5 .C63 2001

615'.704—dc21

00-140126

Alphabetical listing

FOREWORD

It is a pleasure to be able to introduce this compendium to those with an interest in pharmacovigilance. Books like this should be mandatory in all technical fields and kept up to date by knowledgeable and dedicated individuals, such as the two authors. Dr. Pierre Biron in particular has been working in a scholarly fashion for many years, producing the French version, and now with the help of Dr. Barton Cobert, has given us this English edition.

The work is immense to keep abreast of the developments in the field, and the authors have had to select from all kinds of information and to make interpretations for us. This work covers information and opinion on subjects as diverse as: the acceptability of an ADR (clinical); to CAST: a brief summary of the importance of a cohort study (epidemiology); to ICH E2B (jargon); to organization of pharmacovigilance (regulation); to seriousness (philosophical and scientific); and even Uppsala reports (a newsletter). Such is the broad nature of pharmacovigilance that one is full of admiration for people who keep up with a rapidly developing field and produce balanced commentary.

The book is intended for new entrants into the field: it will certainly be valuable for them to have a copy to refer to as they tackle such important issues as the time relationships between drug and adverse reaction in assessing causality. Indeed, they will find a good deal on case causality assessment. They will also find it interesting to look at the legal part if this section to start to consider the difficulties of interacting with the legal professionals over such matters.

Although the intention is to provide some starting material for the pharmacovigilance field, there are many items which will be useful to "old hands" in pharmacovigilance. The coverage of the book is international, and even for those who believe they know the field well, the availability of a handy "aide memoire," with such breadth, is a major benefit.

The world of drug safety and benefit–risk analysis and the impact of both on public health and good therapeutics have many huge challenges, scientific and clinical. I have been greatly concerned as to whether we communicate effectively about these important issues. This book is an undoubted aid to communication because it presents many explanations of terms, and web site and literature references.

There are inescapable doubts about many points relating to pharmacovigilance and particularly to new and rare adverse events/adverse drug reactions. The authors cannot be expected to provide all the answers to the many continuing and new debates in and around pharmacovigilance. What they do is to provide information which allows us all to enter the debates in a more informed way.

We do not have many educational tools to help us in pharmacovigilance, or is it that we have far too many? It is assumed that those interested in the subject will somehow pick up the necessary knowledge in clinical medicine, pharmacology, pharmacy, toxicology, epidemiology, law, politics, public health, economics, and perhaps a few others. If you are, quite reasonably, overwhelmed by the prospect of accessing key knowledge in pharmacovigilance, then this is a most valuable book for you.

Prof. I. Ralph Edwards
Uppsala Monitoring Centre
WHO Collaborating Centre for International Drug Monitoring
Stora Torget 3
S-75320 Uppsala, Sweden

INTRODUCTION

Pharmacovigilance, the last phase in drug development, is the postmarketing surveillance and study of adverse drug reactions, with the ultimate goal of preventing or minimizing their occurrence. New prescription drugs are only marketed after carefully controlled clinical trials have shown them to be sufficiently safe and effective, but this system does not have the sensitivity for the detection of adverse events that appear only after the "uncontrolled" use of the marketed drug in large numbers of heterogeneous patients, in contrast to the carefully controlled use in limited numbers of relatively homogeneous patients enrolled in trials. The major source of signals of new unlabeled serious adverse reactions is the spontaneous reporting system, a system unfortunately endowed with much uncertainty. Pharmacoepidemiology methods allow more scientifically rigorous evaluations of drugs in the postmarketing setting, but its potential has yet to be exploited fully.

The conduct of pharmacovigilance by both industry and health authorities, which nowadays costs billions of dollars annually, includes the collection, compilation, quality control, and analysis of the spontaneous reports. Their evaluation must bear on the validity of reports, the causality assessment of the cases, the adverse events' severity and outcome, the signaling value (newness) of the cases, and its impact on the benefit/risk ratio of the drug. When an important drug safety signal is detected, it may lead to a pharmacovigilance investigation that could—and often does—result in regulatory actions ranging from changes in labeling to restrictions on the drug's use or even withdrawal from the market.

As for estimates of frequencies of marketed drugs' adverse drug reactions (ADRs) in the entire exposed populations and particularly in their more vulnerable subsets, we are lagging far behind the first-rate information obtained during clinical trials. Yet the availability of such information to clinicians could make them better and safer prescribers.

Pharmacovigilance is a necessary interface between therapeutics and clinical epidemiology. Although it is the "poor relative" of pharmacology and the "bogeyman" of the sellers of new drugs, pharmacovigilance is, nevertheless, of premier importance to those who are charged with developing guidelines and labeling for the rational use of these products. This is not an easy task since there is great uncertainty inherent in the assessment of case reports and in the interpretation of results from pharmacoviglance investigations, all done under industry pressures for the continued use of a successful drug on one side, and governmental pressures on the other side to protect the health of patients exposed to increasingly powerful medications.

The development of "applied pharmacovigilance" came about to study subgroups particularly vulnerable to drug risks. The subsets exposed vary from the defenseless fetus in utero to the fragile octogenarian exposed to excessive and prolonged polypharmacy. The suspected drugs may extend from the simple over-the-counter analgesic to the most toxic of prescribed antineoplastic chemotherapies.

This work is aimed at

- newcomers to drug safety and its regulations, both in drug industries and in health agencies, who wish to—or who are obliged to—learn the basics of the business on their own
- hospital clinicians, pharmacists, and nurses, who are often the "privileged" witnesses of the most serious adverse reactions

- lawyers faced with the complex process of determining responsibilities when drugs are associated with adverse events
- medical educators, for whom it is time to recognize the importance of offering graduate courses and undergraduate courses in drug safety for future prescribers
- anyone who has just begun to show an interest in the safety aspect of drug development

We hope to raise their interest in this fascinating field, where activities are often run "behind the scene," and to ease their first experiences when going through references or handling real-life case reports. This is an introductory handbook, a primer, presenting in alphabetical order the main terms, concepts, issues, backgrounds, and tools—printed or on the Web—needed for understanding this field and preparing oneself to assume responsibilities in drug safety. Specific and supporting examples are provided.

ABOUT REFERENCES

Journal articles are included in the text and abbreviated by last name of first author, journal abbreviation in italics, year, volume, and first page. Example:

Edwards, *Drug Saf* 1994;10:93.

Frequently quoted books and documents are abbreviated as follows:

Bénichou 1994
Bénichou C, Editor. Adverse drug reactions: a practical guide to diagnosis and management. New York: Wiley, 1994.

FDA. *Desk Guide* 1996
FDA/CDER. The FDA desk guide for adverse event and product problem reporting. Rockville, MD: FDA, 1996.

CIOMS I 1990
Final Report of CIOMS I Working Group. International reporting of adverse drug reactions. Geneva: CIOMS, 1990.

CIOMS II 1992
Final Report of CIOMS Working Group II. International reporting of periodic drug: safety update summaries. Geneva: CIOMS, 1992.

CIOMS III 1995
Report of CIOMS Working Group III. Guidelines for preparing core clinical-safety information on drugs. Geneva: CIOMS, 1995.

CIOMS IV 1998
Report of CIOMS Working Group IV. Benefit-risk balance for marketed drugs: evaluating safety signals. Geneva: CIOMS, 1998.

PEDS
Pharmacoepidemiology and Drug Safety.

Stephens 1999
Stephens MDB, Talbot JCC, and Routledge PA, Editors. Detection of new adverse drug reactions, 4th edition. London: Macmillan, 1999.

Strom 2000
Strom BL, Editor. Pharmacoepidemiology, 3nd edition. Chichester: Wiley, 2000.

ABBREVIATIONS

Selected abbreviations used in this book in the text or in websites. For a more comprehensive list of abbreviations, see Stephens 1999.

AAPP	American Association of Pharmaceutical Physicians
ACE	Angiotensin converting enzyme
ADE	Adverse drug event, experience
ADME	Administration, distribution, metabolism and excretion
ADR	Adverse drug reaction
ADRAC	Australian Drug Reactions Advisory Committee
ADROIT	Adverse Drug Reactions On-Line Information Tracking (UK)
AE	Adverse event or experience
AERS	Adverse Event Reporting System (FDA)
AFSSPS	Agence Française de Securité Sanitaire de Produits de Santé (France); formerly Agence du Médicament
ALT	Alanine aminotransferase (formerly SGPT)
AMA	American Medical Association
ARME-P	Association pour la recherche méthodologique en pharmacovigilance (France)
ASA	Acetylsalicyclic acid
ASAP	ADR Signals Analysis Project (WHO)
ASPP	Anonymised Single Patient Printout (UK)
AST	Aspartate aminotransferase (formerly SGOT)
ATC	Anatomical-Therapeutic-Chemical (WHO)
BCDSP	Boston Collaborative Drug Study Program
BfArM	Bundesinstitut für Arzneimittel und Medizinprodukte (Germany); German Drug Agency
BGA	Bundesgesundheitsampt (Germany) ; former name for BfArM
BNF	British National Formulary
BMA	British Medical Association
CBER	Center for Biologics Evaluation and Research of the FDA (USA)
CCDS	Company Core Data Sheet
CCSI	Company Core Safety Information
CDC	Center for Disease Control (USA)
CDER	Center for Drug Evaluation and Research of the FDA (USA)
CIOMS	Council for International Organizations of Medical Sciences
COSTART	Coding Symbols for Thesaurus of Adverse Reaction Terms (USA)
CPMP	Committee for Proprietary Medicinal Products (EU)
CPS	*Compendium of Pharmaceuticals and Specialties* (Canada)
CRO	Clinical Research Organization; Contract Research Organization
CSM	Committee on Safety of Medicines (UK)
DDD	Defined daily dose
DES	Diethylstilbestrol
DIA	Drug Information Association
DURG	Drug Utilization Research Group
EC	European Community

EMEA	European Medicinal Evaluation Agency
ESOP	European Society for Pharmacovigilance
ESTRI	Electronic Standards for the Transfer of Regulatory Information
EU	European Union
EUDRANET	European Union Drug Regulatory Authority Network
FDA	Food and Drug Administration (USA)
FOI	Freedom of Information (USA)
GMP	Good Manufacturing Practice
GPRD	General Practice Research Data Base (UK)
HLGT	High Level Group Term (MedDRA)
HLT	High Level Term (MedDRA)
HMO	Health maintenance organization (USA)
HRG	Health Research Group (USA)
IAAAS	International Agranulocytosis and Aplastic Anemia Study
IB	Investigator's Brochure
IBD	International Birth Date
ICCPTT	International Journal of Clinical Pharmacology, Therapy and Toxicology
ICD	International Classification of Disease
ICH	International Conference on Harmonization of Technical Requirements for Registration of Pharmaceuticals for Human Use
ICH E2A	Definitions and Standards for Expedited Reporting
ICH E2B	Data Elements for Transmission of Individual ADR Reports
ICH E2C	Content and Format for Periodic Safety Update Reports for Marketed Drugs
IFPMA	International Federation of Pharmaceutical Manufacturers Association
IMS	IMS Health Inc.
IMT	*International Medical Terminology* (now called *MedDRA*)
INDA	Investigational New Drug Application (USA)
INN	International Non-Proprietary Name
INTDIS	International Drug Information System (WHO)
IPEC	International Pharmaceutical Excipients Council
IRB	Institutional Review Board (USA) ; Ethics Committee
ISDB	International Society of Drug Bulletins
ISPE	International Society for Pharmacoepidemiology
ISS	Integrated Summary of Safety (US)
J-ART	Japanese Adverse Reaction Terminology
JAMA	*Journal of the American Medical Association*
LLT	Low Level Term (MedDRA, *WHO-ART*, *COSTART*)
M1	Medical Terminology Expert MedDRA Working Group
M2	Electronic Standards for the Transfer of Regulatory Information (ESTRI Working Group)
MA	Marketing Authorization
MAH	Marketing Authorization Holder
MAR	Monitored Adverse Reaction (USA)
MCA	Medicines Control Agency (UK)
MEDDRA	*Medical Dictionary for Drug Regulatory Affairs* (UK)
MedDRA	*Medical Dictionary for Regulatory Activities* (ICH)
MHW	Ministry of Health and Welfare (Koseisho – Japan)

MIMS	*Monthly Index of Medical Specialties* (Australia)
MMWR	*Morbidity and Mortality Weekly Report* (USA)
MSSO	Maintenance Services and Support Organization
NCE	New Chemical Entity
NDA	New Drug Application (USA)
NDS	New Drug Submission (Canada)
NIH	National Institutes of Health (USA)
NME	New Medical Entity
NNH	Number Needed to Harm
NNT	Number Needed to Treat
NSAID	Nonsteroidal Anti-inflammatory Drug
OPDRA	Office of Post-Marketing Drug Risk Assessment of the FDA (USA)
OTC	Over the counter
PC/HRG	Public Citizen/Health Research Group (USA)
PDR	*Physician's Desk Reference* (USA)
PEDS	*Pharmacoepidemiology and Drug Safety*
PEM	Prescription Event Monitoring (UK)
PERI	Pharmaceutical Education and Research Institute (USA)
PhRMA	Pharmaceutical Research and Manufacturers of America (formerly PMA)
PhVWP	Pharmacovigilance Working Party of the CPMP
PMA	Pharmaceutical Manufacturers of American (now PhRMA)
PMS	Post-Marketing Surveillance
PMSB	Pharmaceutical and Medical Safety Bureau (JAP)
PSUR	Periodic Safety Update Report
PT	Preferred Term (MedDRA, *WHO-ART, COSTART*)
RUCAM	Roussel Uclaf Causality Assessment Method
SADRAC	Swedish Adverse Drug Reaction Advisory Committee
SAE	Serious Adverse Event
SAMS	Safety Assessment of Marketed Medicines (UK)
SAR	Serious Adverse Reaction
SED	*Side Effects of Drugs, Meyler's*
SEDA	*Side Effects of Drugs Annual*
SIGAR	Special Interest Group on Adverse Reactions
SMON	Subacute myelooptic neuropathy
SmPC	Summary of Product Characteristics
SNIP	Syndicat National de l'Industrie Pharmaceutique (France)
SOC	System Organ Class
SOS	System Organ System
SPC	Summary of Product Characteristics
SRS	Spontaneous Reporting System
TEN	Toxic epidermal necrolysis
UK	United Kingdom
UMC	Uppsala Monitoring Center
VAERS	Vaccine Adverse Event Reporting System (USA)
VAMP	Value Added Medicinal Products Database (See GPRD)
WHO	World Health Organization
WHO-ART	*WHO Adverse Reaction Terminology*
WHODD	*WHO Drug Dictionary*

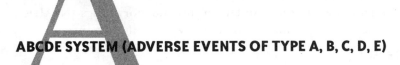

ABCDE SYSTEM (ADVERSE EVENTS OF TYPE A, B, C, D, E)

HISTORY

Hurwitz and Wade proposed many years ago four categories of AEs (*Br Med J* 1969; Mar 1(643):531). The first two mechanisms have been combined under category A and the second two mechanisms under category B.

- Side effect
- Excess effect
- Allergy (hypersensitivity)
- Idiosyncrasy

DeSwarte classified ADRs into eight categories (*Arch Intern Med* 1986;146:649):

- Overdose
- Side effect
- Secondary, indirect effect
- Interaction
- Intolerance
- Idiosyncrasy (primary toxicity)
- Allergy
- Pseudoallergy (anaphylactoid)

Note that overdose and interaction are risk factors and the indirect or secondary effect is a physiologic consequence. Further information can be found in Meyboom (*PEDS* 1997;16:355) and in Royer (*PEDS* 1997;6:S43).

TYPE A ADVERSE EVENT

Rawlins and Thompson of Newcastle, Great Britain, have classified AEs into type A and type B on the basis of the mechanism of action. A type A event is one that is due to an extension of the active pharmacologic properties of the drug (*A* indicates *augmented*). They are also called *predictable* or *anticipated events*. They are generally less severe and more frequent than type B events. This augmented pharmacologic action may occur at the targeted receptors or at other nontargeted receptors producing *lateral effects*, *parallel effects*, or *side effects*. They are usually detected during the clinical trials done before marketing. There are two subclasses:

▶ Exaggerated Desired Effect

The undesirable exaggeration of a desired pharmacologic effect after a normal dose in a susceptible subject or after a higher than normal dose. This results from the excess stimulation of targeted receptors by the therapeutic agent. Orthostatic hypotension with an antihypertensive, daytime somnolence after a sedative-hypnotic taken for sleep, and hypoglycemic shock after insulin are examples of this phenomenon.

▶ Undesired Effect

The appearance of an undesired pharmacologic effect, known as *lateral or parallel stimulation*, can be seen after a normal dose or a higher than normal dose in a susceptible subject; it is due to *the stimulation of untargeted receptors* by the therapeutic agent. Examples include constipation due to morphine, gastrointestinal irritation with nonsteroidal antiinflammatory drugs (NSAIDs), hair loss from chemotherapy, and loss of libido with antidepressants.

TYPE B ADVERSE EVENT

A type B reaction is one that is not due to an extension of the active pharmacologic properties of the drug; the *B* indicates *bizarre*. They are called *pharmacologically unexpected, unpredictable,* or *idiosyncratic adverse reactions.*

There are two subclasses:

▶ **Immunologic**

An *allergic* or *hypersensitivity* reaction occurs as a result of an immunologic mechanism.

A *pseudoallergy* or *anaphylactoid* reaction is the result of a mechanism involving the release of the same mediators released during an immunologic reaction due to immunoglobobulin E (IgE). Such reactions can occur with radiocontrast agents, NSAIDs, for example (see ALLERGY, DRUG).

▶ **Idiosyncratic**

The term *idiosyncratic* is often used in a broad sense to designate qualitatively abnormal adverse reactions that occur in a given individual and whose mechanism is not yet understood. These reactions are usually quite rare and in some cases may be due to a genetic or acquired enzyme abnormality with the formation of toxic metabolites. This is also known as *primary toxicity.*

Congenital enzyme abnormalities may produce adverse reactions such as the hemolytic anemia due to glucose-6-phosphate dehydrogenase (G6PD) deficiency.

Acquired enzyme abnormalities result from a drug effect that produces enzyme inhibition or induction.

Types C, D, and E are not mechanisms but characteristics of their manifestations; they are not referred to frequently in the literature. The letter *C* refers to *continuous, chronic.* Type D refers to *delayed* in appearance, making them difficult to diagnose. Type E refers to *end of use.*

ABUSE POTENTIAL (see PHARMACODEPENDENCE)

ACCEPTABILITY (OF AN ADVERSE DRUG REACTION)

In drug surveillance, an ADR is deemed acceptable when its frequency and severity are sufficiently compensated for by the frequency and magnitude of the therapeutic benefit of the drug. This is necessarily a value judgment. Similar to the risk/benefit judgment made in clinical therapeutics for an individual patient, a risk/benefit judgment can be made in pharmacovigilance from a population point of view. When an ADR that is clearly greater than the drug benefit expected occurs (e.g., severe gastrointestinal (GI) bleeding with a mild analgesic), the ADR is referred to as *alarming.* On the other hand, a headache, for example, seen with an acquired immunodeficiency syndrome (AIDS) or cancer medication would be deemed acceptable.

In pharmacotherapy, whenever a product is incorrectly prescribed or used, the benefit expected is considered to be zero for the calculation of the risk/benefit ratio. An example would be the prescription of an antibiotic for a simple cold of viral origin, in which case no ADR would be acceptable since there is no pharmacologic benefit to be expected.

Note also that in the pharmaceutic sciences, the term *acceptability* is used in another sense, namely, that of the quality of the galenic form in regard to ease of administration (timing, mode of administration, volume of the tablet, taste of the suspension, packaging, etc.).

IN CLINICAL PRACTICE

In the course of pharmacologic therapy, the clinician makes a decision in regard to the acceptability of an ADR and decides whether or not to modify the treatment in a given patient. Here are four examples.

Before the occurrence of an ADR: In a patient with newly diagnosed hypertension, the practician may hesitate between prescribing a thiazide diuretic and a beta-blocker. However, the presence of asthma in the patient makes the beta-blocker unacceptable. The thiazide is thus chosen in order to prevent the risk of possible bronchospasm with the beta-blocker.

After the occurrence of an ADR: A hypertensive patient has an acute episode of gout after having started treatment with a thiazide, which now makes this treatment unacceptable. The clinician substitutes a beta-blocker.

After the occurrence of an ADR but before the occurrence of the desired beneficial effect: A patient suffering from prostatitis has been taking an antibiotic. There is no improvement in his symptoms and he is now complaining of daily abdominal discomfort associated with his medication. The prescriber would be more likely to stop the drug, deeming the ADR unacceptable, because the prostatitis was not improving.

After the occurrence of an ADR and after the occurrence of the desired beneficial effect: A hypertensive patient tolerates neither thiazides nor beta-blockers. Her blood pressure is well controlled with an angiotensin converting enzyme (ACE) inhibitor, but she has an occasional mild dry cough. After a discussion between the prescriber and the patient, the two agree that the mild cough is acceptable since good pharmacologic control of her blood pressure has been obtained.

ON A POPULATION LEVEL

Health authorities perform their duties of drug surveillance during the two periods of development of a new product:

Before marketing authorization: The authorities responsible for the approval of a new drug must examine the dossier submitted and may refuse to approve the drug if the risks observed during clinical development outweigh the degree of therapeutic innovation, especially when safer alternative therapies are already available.

After marketing authorization: After the marketing of a drug, health authorities may take various regulatory measures, ranging from restrictions on the use of the drug to its complete withdrawal from the market. These measures are taken when the risk, first seen in the spontaneous AE reports, is confirmed by a pharmacovigilance evaluation and when this risk clearly outweighs the expected pharmacologic benefit.

ABOUT BENEFITS

Since the comparison of risk to benefit is used during safety investigations and during the selection of regulatory measures, let us review the various types of benefits attainable from a medication:

Overdose correction: antidotes, antagonists.

Diagnostic: contrast agents, radioisotopes, allergens.

Cure: antibiotics, antivirals, gene therapies.

Prophylaxis: prevention of cerebrovascular or cardiovascular accidents by hyperlipidemics, antihypertensives, platelet antiaggregants, and anti-arrhythmics. In prophylactic pharmacotherapy one must always make the distinction between a *pharmacologic effect*, which serves as an intermediate measure or end point (surrogate marker) used in many clinical trials, and a therapeutic (clinical) benefit, which can often be found only in large, long-term, costly, and relatively rarely performed clinical trials. For instance, the measurement of cholesterol levels in a short-term trial using a new cholesterol lowering agent is a surrogate end point, whereas the measurement of myocardial infarcts, cerebrovascular accidents, and death in a long-term survival study represents the clinical benefit.

Replacement therapy: hormones (e.g., insulin), electrolytes (e.g., potassium), metabolites (e.g., glucose), blood products, vitamins (e.g., B_{12}), and others.

Symptomatic treatments: analgesics, antiemetics, others.

Treatment of side effect: use of antihistamines to counter neuroleptic induced ADRs.

ACCEPTABLE RISK

The risk of an ADR becomes acceptable when the expected benefit is greater than the likelihood that the ADR will occur. This is a medical judgment made by the regulatory authorities when approving a new drug, by the physician when prescribing the drug, and by the patient when taking it. It is based on the frequency and severity of the ADR(s), the frequency and magnitude of expected benefit, and the severity of the disease.

ACCOUNTABILITY

In the context of pharmacovigilance, *accountability* refers to the responsibility of each person in the development, research, and use of drugs to ensure that they are used in a rational, efficacious, benevolent, and safe manner. There are complex and multiple interdependencies and responsibilities in this chain affecting all parties involved to varying degrees: pharmaceutical companies, legislators, health authorities, medical educators, editors of medical journals, prescribers, sellers, dispensers, and users. The goal of all of the people and organizations involved is to prevent ADRs due to negligence, imprudence, errors, or "irregularities," as these ADRs are preventable (see CAUSALITY, Legal).

A textbook covering this area is useful to those in pharmacovigilance and especially those with medicolegal issues (Dukes M, Mildred M, and Swartz B. Responsibility for drug-induced injury. Amsterdam: IOS Press, 1998). Another interesting book, written by a layman whose wife suffered an ADR, is Stephen Fried's *Bitter Pills* (New York: Bantam Books, 1998).

ACKNOWLEDGMENT LETTER

All pharmacovigilance centers (governmental, industrial, or academic) should reply promptly to every person who notifies them of an AE. This reply may be a personalized letter but can be a phone call, fax, or e-mail; it should thank the sender for the information, acknowledge its receipt, and ask for further information if needed to clarify the case. If the acknowledgment letter does not produce a response, it is necessary to send a follow-up letter (see this term).

The acknowledgment letter should be sent by a reliable system (such as certified mail) and should contain the following:

■ A postal return receipt should be enclosed if sent by mail; this may not be necessary if sent by a private courier that maintains a website capable of tracking all letters and packages sent.
■ A statement of appreciation for the report and a request for additional medical information if needed should be included. A standardized form may used (some use a blank CIOMS I form; others use a customized form).
■ A postage-paid business reply envelope should be included.

Some centers may also send information about similar AEs already in the database.

Additional information should be requested when

■ The information is insufficient or certain lab tests are needed for validation of the event (e.g., cardiograms, radiograph or scan reports).
■ The case represents a particularly important signal.
■ The event is very severe medically and that severity may alter the risk/benefit ratio if confirmed.

ACTIONS (MEASURES) TAKEN

When a signal is felt to be confirmed after a pharmacovigilance investigation, the governmental health authorities and the manufacturer take various measures to reduce inevitable and unacceptable risk in order to make continued use of the product safer.

REGULATORY MEASURES; REGULATORY ACTIONS TAKEN

Regulatory measures or actions taken represent changes in the status of the drug that are made during or after a pharmacovigilance investigation with the goal of preventing further ADRs that are judged unacceptable with respect to public health. Such measures can be taken either separately or together by the manufacturer and the health authorities. Actions taken by the manufacturer may be either voluntary or obligatory. In most cases, action is taken only after a signal is confirmed. However, if a new ADR appears to be clearly unacceptable and/or too frequent to allow the risk of waiting for confirmation from a request for intensified adverse effect reporting or from clinical trials, urgent temporary regulatory measures can be taken.

TRANSMISSION OF INFORMATION: LABEL CHANGES

Changes in medical information are usually included not only in the Product Monograph (labeling) but also in the medical information for the health care professional as well as for the patient (Patient Information Leaflet). Sometimes information is even added to the packaging, for example, by attaching a sticker to the bottle.

If the label changes are significant, they are often referred to as *health authority required* or *regulatory changes* as they are usually governed by the drug laws and regulations of each country, at least in developed countries. These changes are often the result of a negotiation between the health authorities and the manufacturer (voluntary changes) but may be imposed by the health agency (mandatory or obligatory changes). In many countries, if there is a compelling safety issue, the manufacturer is permitted to make a safety change without prior notification or approval of the authorities if the change is related only to safety and makes the label more restrictive.

These changes produce alterations in the package insert (official labeling) and possibly on the packaging or bottle. These changes can include the following:

- A reduction in the recommended dose
- The removal of one or more indications
- An absolute or relative restriction on the population being treated
- A new contraindication for patients with certain medical conditions or diseases (concomitant morbidity)
- A restriction, contraindication, or warning regarding use with other specific drugs or classes of drugs (drug interaction)
- Use of the product as a secondary or tertiary treatment rather than a primary treatment
- Recommendation of concomitant treatment with another drug to prevent or correct the problem produced by the drug
- Recommendation of periodic lab testing or clinical follow-up (e.g., alanine aminotransferase (ALT) for hepatotoxic products, electrocardiograms for cardiotoxic products)

The changes are sometimes printed in bold letters or presented in a black box to underline the importance of the changes and to note that they are recent additions to the label. Sometimes a "Dear Doctor" (or "Dear Health Care Professional") letter is sent as well as a press release and a note on the health authority's website.

LIMITATION OF ACCESS TO THE DRUG

- Alteration of availability (e.g., changing of its *listedness* or addition of an *annex*): narcotic, controlled drug, limited prescription, "exceptional medication," temporary use authorization
- Limitation on the prescribers (e.g., reserved only to specialists) for the initial prescription or for renewals
- Limitation on methods of prescription (e.g., no automatic renewals, no telephone prescriptions, limitation of number of tablets dispensed)
- Limitation to hospital dispensation (e.g., new and/or renewals)
- Limitation to place of dispensation: over the counter (OTC) (unrestricted sale in pharmacies) or "behind-the-counter" (requiring pharmacist consultation) or permit for sale anywhere (e.g., supermarkets): that is, potential change of OTC product to behind the counter or prescription-only status
- Obligatory laboratory testing (e.g., negative pregnancy test result before, during, and for some months after stopping of treatment)
- Written justification of the indication by the prescriber
- Informed consent signed by the patient and possibly the prescriber or pharmacist
- Withdrawal of patients under treatment
- Requirement of other measures while taking the drug (e.g., two methods of contraception for teratogenic medications)

MODIFICATION OF THE PRODUCT ITSELF

▶ **Change in the Active Ingredient**

Removal or substitution of one of the active ingredients in a combination product

Removal of one of the dosage strengths available (e.g., usually the highest dose, though in rare cases it might be the weakest dose if it is judged to be ineffective and only the higher dose has the appropriate risk/benefit ratio); for example, after a pharmacovigilance investigation, removal of the 100-mg dosage form of an antibiotic and retention of the 200-mg form on the market.

▶ **Change in the Galenic Form**

Change or removal of excipients

Modification of the quantity in the bottle or box

Change in packaging

Change in an accompanying device: for example, when a parenteral product for a chronic infection produces injection site reactions and a different needle is packaged with the product and used for the injection

▶ **Change in Storage or Preparation**

For example, a refrigerated injectable product that produced pain and burning on injection; marked improvement resulted after the label was changed to indicate that it should be at room temperature before injection.

WITHDRAWAL FROM MARKET

- Withdrawal of a particular active ingredient, a specific product, a specific formulation
- Temporary or definitive suspension of sales
- Cessation of manufacture and distribution
- Withdrawal of stocks from the wholesaler, pharmacist, or patient, depending upon the severity of the problem
- Withdrawal (weaning) of the drug from individual patients under medical care

CHOICE OF COMMUNICATION CHANNELS

- The labeling in the official monograph (labeling, package insert, summary of product characteristics, etc.)
- The labeling in the packaging documentation (annex)
- The labeling on the sticker of the box or bottle
- A Dear Doctor, Dear Pharmacist, or Dear Health Care Professional letter (soon likely to be e-mail)
- Direct notification of the prescribing physicians by the manufacturer's sales representatives (usually limited to drugs prescribed by limited numbers of specialists)
- A pharmacovigilance bulletin either in writing or on the Internet or in both
- An article in a scientific or professional periodical
- A press release to the media and on the Internet
- An alert notification from one health authority or nongovernmental organization (WHO) to another (e.g., WHO Uppsala alert to worldwide health agencies)
- In rare instances, direct use of mass media to alert the general public of a critical safety issue

ACTIVE INGREDIENT; ACTIVE MOIETY

The principal medicinal ingredient of a pharmaceutical product that is responsible for its pharmacodynamic effects, in contrast to an *excipient* which is (supposedly) inactive but is capable of occasionally producing allergic or toxic ADRs themselves or of modifying the kinetics of the active ingredient.

The actions of the active ingredient can be modified by confidence that the product has a positive effect (placebo effect) and by confidence that the product has a negative effect (nocebo effect).

ADDICTION

Addiction to a pharmaceutical product taken in a "medical" context can be referred to as *pharmacodependence* (see PHARMACODEPENDENCE), to prevent confusion with "street drug" addiction.

ADMINISTRATION SITE REACTION

One of the nontemporal characteristics of an AE is its location, its "human body topography," when the reactions occur at the administration site, the transit site, or the concentration site (see TRANSIT SITE REACTION and CONCENTRATION SITE REACTION). Not all "site of administration reactions" are injections (see INJECTION SITE REACTION). Sometimes an ADR is associated with an error of administration, as in the following example:

> *Nonoxynol 9:* This spermicide can be formulated as a vaginal ovule and used as a contraceptive. The first case (index case) of hemorrhagic cystitis due to erroneous insertion into the urethra was published in 1980. Other cases followed. This "site" ADR was obviously not detectable before the commercialization of the product. Only after the first cases were noted could prescribers be informed on how to prevent future cases and how to treat the reaction should it occur. Preventive measures described the precautions needed during insertion of the ovule to prevent urethral penetration (Gottesman, *N Engl J Med* 1980;302:633; Cattolica, *Urology* 1982;20:293; Meyersak, *J Urol* 1993;149:835).

"Site" reactions sometimes stem from nonprescription products. Indeed certain mouthwashes or liquid iron supplements taken without a straw may darken teeth.

ADVERSE DRUG REACTION (ADR)

The term *adverse drug reaction* is not specifically defined in the Food and Drug Administration regulations but the FDA has indicated it accepts the ICH definitions.

In the European Medicinal Evaluation Agency (EMEA) regulations, the International Conference on Harmonization (ICH) definition is essentially used (CMPM/ICH/377/95):

> In the *pre-approval clinical experience* with a new medicinal product or new uses of an old drug, particularly as the therapeutic dose(s) may not be established: *all noxious and unintended responses to a medicinal product related to any dose should be considered ADRs.*

> The phrase "responses to a medicinal products" means that a causal relationship between a medicinal product and an AE is at least a reasonable possibility, i.e., the relationship cannot be ruled out.

Regarding *marketed medicinal products,* a well-accepted definition of an ADR in the post-marketing setting is found in WHO Technical Report 498(1972) and reads as follows:

A response to a drug which is noxious and unintended and which occurs at doses normally used in man for prophylaxis, diagnosis, or therapy of disease or for modification of physiologic function.

This definition has been agreed to by the International Conference on Harmonization (see this term) and has been adopted by many health authorities around the world and the WHO Monitoring Centre (which played a major role in its creation). A copy of the ICH E2B document containing this and other definitions is available (www.ifpma.org/pdfifpma/e2a.pdf).

In summary, an adverse effect that is suspected of being related to the drug is an ADR.

ADVERSE DRUG REACTION CASE REPORT

Sometimes referred to simply as a *case report* or, to use the ICH E2B terminology, *individual case safety report* (ICSR). This report consists of the details of a published or spontaneously reported AE or reaction. Information should include full details of the case to allow proper assessment of causality and seriousness.

ADVERSE DRUG REACTIONS ON-LINE INFORMATION TRACKING (ADROIT)

The software and database of the Committee on Safety of Medicines (CSM), the official pharmacovigilance structure of the United Kingdom.

ADVERSE EVENT OR EXPERIENCE (AE)

U.S. Food and Drug Administration definition (21CFR310.305) is as follows:

Adverse drug experience: Any AE associated with the use of a drug in humans, whether or not considered drug related, including the following: an AE occurring in the course of the use of a drug product in professional practice; an AE occurring from drug overdose whether accidental or intentional; any AE occurring from drug abuse; an AE occurring from drug withdrawal; and any failure of expected pharmacological action.

The European Medicinal Evaluation Agency (EMEA) definition (CMPM/ICH/ 377/95) is as follows:

Any untoward medical occurrence in a patient or clinical investigation subject administered a pharmaceutical product and which does not necessarily have to have a causal relationship with this treatment. An AE can therefore be any unfavorable and unintended sign (including an abnormal laboratory finding, for example), symptom, or disease temporally associated with the use of a medicinal product, whether or not considered related to the medicinal product.

Note that in some countries (United States and the European Union), the lack of efficacy of a marketed drug is also, by regulatory definition, an AE such that this concept is included in the definition of an AE.

Older definitions exist for this term and, in the past, distinguished between marketed and clinical trial events. Some are mentioned in the following for historical interest.

FOR A MARKETED PRODUCT

Any clinically undesirable occurrence in a person exposed to a drug whether or not there is a causal link with the drug:

- Even if the drug is not suspected (e.g., a concomitant medication)
- Even if the drug was suspected and exonerated after validation and causality assessment

It is defined by the World Health Organization (WHO) and the International Conference on Harmonization (ICH) as "*any untoward medical occurrence in a patient administered a pharmaceutical product and which does not necessarily have to have a causal relationship with this treatment.*" (Edwards, *Drug Saf* 1994;10:93; ICH E2A 1994.)

According to CIOMS I (1990:14) spontaneous alert reports are not supposed to report undesirable events for which causality has not been evaluated. An event becomes a reaction when a physician or other health professional has concluded that there is a "reasonable possibility" or suspicion of a causal link between the undesirable occurrence and the drug.

As soon as there is the slightest suspicion by a clinician, whether or not a formal causality assessment has been done, the *event* becomes a *reaction*. If the causality assessment has ruled out the drug as a cause of the problem, the *reaction* becomes an *event*. Logically then, this case should be removed from the pharmacovigilance database (whether governmental or corporate). However, in many countries, regulations require that AEs be kept in the database as if they were ADRs.

In practice, most pharmaceutical companies do not perform causality assessments on spontaneously reported occurrences from health care practitioners since the very fact that a practitioner thinks enough to report the occurrence at all renders it "possibly related" to the drug and thus a reportable ADR. Many countries (United States, European Union, Canada) consider all spontaneously reported AEs to be, by definition, ADRs.

DURING A CLINICAL TRIAL

According to ICH, an AE is "*any untoward medical occurrence in a clinical investigation subject administered a pharmaceutical product and which does not necessarily have to have a causal relationship with this treatment*" (ICH E2A 1994).

According to CIOMS (1;1990:14), "Events are completely and routinely recorded during a study and the rates of these events for different study groups are compared. Only those study events which a physician has judged it reasonable to suspect . . . should be considered as possible subjects of CIOMS reports."

It is clear that during clinical trials two types of causality analyses are possible:

- Group causality assessment: an unbiased statistical analysis comparing the frequency of AEs between or among the treatment groups
- Case causality assessment: an assessment of causality of individual cases done on a case by case basis

IN PHARMACOEPIDEMIOLOGY

During cohort and case-control trials the frequency of AEs is counted for each group. The AEs become ADRs for the exposed group of patients if an unbiased statistical association is demonstrated between the exposure to the suspect drug and the occurrence of the undesirable events.

SUMMARY

The standardized term (ICH/CIOMS) is *AE* or less frequently *adverse experience* when an untoward incident occurs whether or not the drug is suspected to be the cause. When a drug cause is indeed suspected or proved to any extent, the preferred term is *ADR* or *adverse reaction* (AR).

In other words, an untoward event that occurs in a patient on a drug is an AE unless there is a suspicion that the event is possibly or probably related to the drug, in which case it becomes an ADR. This terminology is arcane and complicated but nonetheless, when used correctly, makes useful distinctions between such problems.

ADVERSE EVENT DICTIONARY

A dictionary of synonyms (thesaurus) of medical terms for describing AEs and reactions. These dictionaries are used for the coding of adverse effects in computerized databases. The *WHO-ART* (WHO) and *COSTART* (FDA) are the most well known, but a new dictionary *MedDRA* is likely to supplant the other AE dictionaries in the next few years (see *MedDRA*).

ADVERSE EXPERIENCE (see ADVERSE EVENT OR EXPERIENCE)

ADVERSE REACTION AND MEDICATION ERROR ASSESSMENT DIVISION

The official Canadian bureau responsible for pharmacovigilance within the Therapeutic Products Program (the national authority that evaluates and monitors drugs, devices, and other products for safety and efficacy), which itself is a part of Health Canada. It corresponds to the Committee for Safety of Medicines in the United Kingdom, to the Adverse Drug Reaction Advisory Committee in Australia, and to the Office of Postmarketing Drug Risk Assessment (OPDRA) of the Center for Drug Evaluation and Research (CDER) and the Office of Biostatistics and Epidemiology of Center for Biologics Evaluation and Research (CBER) in the U.S. FDA. See the website of the Health Protection Branch (www.hc-sc.gc.ca/hpb/index_e.html).

AGE

The age of the patient must be taken into account when completing an AE/ADR report form because it facilitates the identification of the patient and the assessment of causality. However, even if the number of serious ADRs in a population is greater among the elderly, this does not, in and of itself, prove that advanced age constitutes a major risk factor for the occurrence of ADRs. One must also take into account cofactors such as body weight, renal function, prior history of an ADR, comorbidity, and comedications.

Age must also be considered by the clinician when prescribing, especially in children and the elderly, in whom supratherapeutic doses are to be avoided. In the course of daily practice, prescribers too often forget about age by using "adult" doses; if a patient is exposed to polypharmacy, he or she is put at risk for unsafe blood levels of the drug in question.

AGENCE FRANÇAISE DE SÉCURITÉ SANITAIRE DES PRODUITS DE SANTÉ (AFSSPS)

The name for the official agency in France for the evaluation, authorization, and surveillance of medications (The Agency for Safety of Healthcare Products, AFSSPS, pronounced "afspas"). Equivalent agencies in other countries include the Medicines Control Agency (MCA) in Great Britain, the Food and

Drug Administration in the United States and the Therapeutic Products Programme in Canada. The agency stands out among others in making the use of a causality assessment compulsory. The French method contains six questions presented as a decision table.

ALANINE AMINOTRANSFERASE (ALT)

An enzyme found in hepatocytes and elsewhere. In hepatovigilance, the elevated serum level of this transaminase, if it is of hepatic origin, suggests a cytolytic process. Formerly serum glutamic-pyruvic transaminase (SGPT) (see ALT/AP RATIO).

ALERT, ADVERSE DRUG REACTION (ADR)

Regulatory actions aiming at prevention of further cases of a newly discovered ADR, usually started with the public announcement of measures being taken to reduce the risk of an ADR judged to be unacceptable. This includes measures such as the addition of safety information to the product monograph and labeling, restrictions on usage, and even withdrawal from the market.

The regulatory measures taken after the confirmation of a signal are usually definitive and irreversible although sometimes they can be provisional if the new signal has not been confirmed but is still judged to be unacceptable and avoidable. In these cases it is deemed too risky to await the results of the ongoing pharmacovigilance inquiry.

In general, if such an announcement turns out to be premature and the drug is ultimately found to be "innocent," the stigma of the alert remains and may reduce usage or even "kill" the drug.

ALERT REPORT (see EXPEDITED REPORT)

ALLERGY, DRUG

Drug allergy is also called *hypersensitivity*; it represents a type B adverse reaction due to an immunologic reaction of the host. A classification scheme proposed by Gell and Coombs has been in use since 1975:

TYPE 1 IMMEDIATE, MAST CELL MEDIATED
The antigen attaches to a specific immunoglobulin (IgE) antibody on the surface of the mast cell, producing the release of inflammatory mediators. There are several types: *atopic* reactions such as atopic asthma, atopic dermatitis, serum sickness, *urticarial* reactions, *angioedema,* and *anaphylaxis,* of which *anaphylactic* shock is the most severe, as bronchospasm and/or circulatory shock may prove fatal.

> ▌ **Note on Anaphylactoid Reactions**
> An ADR is said to be anaphylactoid or *pseudoallergic* when its mechanism of action does not involve the antibodies of the host but nevertheless does involve the direct liberation of inflammatory mediators from mast cells (histamine and others). The clinical presentation is that of an immunoallergic reaction. It can be localized or generalized. Urticaria, angioedema, nasal congestion, asthma, and fatal anaphylactoid shock can occur and rarely can be fatal. Its mechanism makes it a type A reaction, but the clinical picture is similar to that of a true type B allergic reaction.

■ Iodinated contrast agents (causing the release of histamine) and nonsteroidal anti-inflammatory drugs (NSAIDs) (causing the release of leukotrienes)—in particular acetylsalicylic acid (ASA)—are most often involved.

■ Morphine, curare, polymyxin B also can cause the release of histamine.

■ Vancomycin is an intravenous antibiotic capable of producing the "red neck syndrome," which is associated with high-dose therapy and with rapid infusion rates.

TYPE 2 CYTOTOXIC

A circulating immunoglobulin (Ig) antibody reacts with a cell membrane bound antigen. The cytotoxic reaction is a frequent one in hematovigilance literature. Examples include hemolytic anemia due to penicillin and methyldopa and thrombocytopenia due to quinidine.

TYPE 3 IMMUNE COMPLEX

Complement is activated, and vascular damage occurs. Examples include serum sickness. It may be induced by penicillamine or gold salts.

TYPE 4 T-CELL MEDIATED

Also called *delayed type reaction*, such as contact dermatitis.

VAN ARSDEL CLASSIFICATION

Stephens (1999;429) finds the Van Arsdel classification more useful. It contains seven classes: mast-cell mediated, T-cell mediated, phototodermatitis, skin reactions of unknown mechanism, drug fever, systemic lupus erythematosus and related autoimmune disorders, and others, by organ classes.

ALLERGY, SURVEILLANCE OF DRUG

The surveillance of immunologic and allergic ADRs. Sometimes referred to as *allergovigilance.*

ALT/AP RATIO

In hepatovigilance, it has been suggested that when the alanine aminotransferase/alkaline phosphatase ratio (ALT/AP or ALT/AlkPhos ratio) is greater than 5, the hepatic lesion can be considered to be hepatocellular (cytolytic). When the ratio is less than 2, the hepatic lesion is considered to be cholestatic. If the ratio is between 2 and 5, the picture may considered to be mixed. If ALT is not available, the aspartase aminotransferase (AST) value may be used in the calculation (Danan, in Benichou 1994:3)

ANATOMIC, THERAPEUTIC, CHEMICAL CLASSIFICATION (ATC, NORDIC ATC)

A drug classification developed in Oslo, Norway, by the WHO Collaborating Centre for Drug Statistics Methodology which was also responsible for developing the defined daily dose (DDD) (see DEFINED DAILY DOSE).

ANECDOTE

The term *anecdote* refers to a case report of an ADR that is single in number (or a very small number) and may only be weakly associated with the drug (i.e., causality is not strong). The inability to ascribe a strong causality may be due to confounding factors (e.g., comedications or concomitant diseases), insufficient information (quite common), uncertain plausibility, or unreliable medical information. When the case is convincing, it is sometimes called an orphan AE (see ORPHAN ADVERSE EVENT). The reader should be aware that pharmacovigilance has its detractors, who may use this term—incorrectly and pejoratively—to downgrade valid isolated spontaneous reports or publications of ADRs and minimize their potential value as signals.

ANGIOEDEMA

Angioedema is localized edema found in the deep layers of the skin and is indicative of a severe stage of an immediate type of drug allergy. This term is frequently used in dermatovigilance and allergy surveillance. Its seriousness depends on its anatomic site. There is an immediate, life-threatening risk of airway obstruction when the larynx or glottis are involved. Angioedema may be due to an anaphylactic reaction, in which bronchospasm and shock can be life-threatening if untreated. The face, the eyes, and the lips are most often involved.

For example, visceral angioedema associated with angiotensin converting enzyme (ACE) inhibitors can be difficult to diagnose for two reasons: The site is rare, the intestine is not an expected location for angioedema, and a high level of suspicion is needed along with confirmation by abdominal scanning. Second, the time to onset (during ongoing treatment) of the ADR is quite variable and is often very long—sometimes measurable in years (Mullins, *Med J Aust* 1996;165:319; Gregory, *N Engl J Med* 1996;334:1641).

ANIMAL TOXICOLOGY: WHY IT IS NOT SUFFICIENT

Animal toxicology cannot replace pharmacovigilance; nor does it seem likely that it ever will. These studies are conducted on animal models and preparations of organs, cells, microsomal fractions, and nuclear constituents such as deoxyribonucleic acid (DNA), etc. and represent one of the major areas in the development of a drug.

OVERVIEW
Acute toxicity may be studied by giving a single dose, usually to rodents (e.g., rats, mice) and nonrodents (e.g., dogs).

Subacute (also called *subchronic*) toxicity may be studied after 7 to 14 days of dosing at three levels.

Chronic toxicity may be studied after longer-term treatment usually from 2 to 52 weeks. If longer term treatment is ultimately expected in humans, then the animal chronic toxicity studies can be prolonged. The rat is often used as well as the beagle.

Pharmacokinetics may be studied in animals by using radioisotopes and autoradiography. Microsomal preparations from animals and humans are also used.

Special studies, individualized to each drug, may be used if a specific area is suspected of being particularly susceptible to toxicity.

GENOTOXICITY
This examination is done rather early in the preclinical phase of development of a new molecule; should mutagenicity be found, further development usually stops. A drug may be mutagenic if it interacts with DNA in somatic cells. Genetic mutations, chromosomal abnormalities, and DNA damage are examined.

CARCINOGENICITY

The potential for the production of cancers may be usually examined for 6 to 12 or even 24 months in the rat and mouse.

REPRODUCTION

The studies of possible drug interference with reproduction proceed in three segments:

Segment I: The drug product is administered before mating to examine the effect on fertility. For example, if a product is to be used in men, it would be administered for 70 days (i.e., the length of spermatogenesis) in male rats.

Segment II: The drug product is administered during pregnancy to the female to examine its teratogenic potential (rat and rabbit).

Segment III: The drug product is administered during the perinatal and postnatal periods (rat).

THE PROBLEM

During the early phase I clinical trials, all of the potential toxicity of the new molecular entity is not yet known. Why?

Animals do not react 100% of the time in the same way that humans do. The parallel animal = human is not always true. Thus the absence of teratogenicity in the animal does not guarantee its absence in human males and females.

Subjective ADRs seen in animals cannot be evaluated. A rat cannot be asked whether it has a headache.

Many drug-induced pathologic conditions in humans do not have a counterpart in animals.

The number of animal species evaluated for a drug is limited—usually to several rodents (useful and inexpensive) and a few nonrodents. Otherwise the cost and time would become prohibitive.

History has shown us that although we may have felt secure about a particular class of drugs, a new molecule that is minimally different in structure can produce severe and previously unseen ADRs.

Hence, animal studies are useful and necessary but are not sufficient in drug development. Nonetheless, such studies may point the way to areas of human toxicity and, of course, may help in the development of drugs for animals.

ANONYMIZED SINGLE-PATIENT CASE REPORT (ASPP)

A document available from a pharmacovigilance center after the receipt and entry into a computerized database of an ADR report. It contains a summary of the event in which the patient and the reporter (usually a health care professional) are anonymous. This information is usually available only from governmental health authorities and not from pharmaceutical company pharmacovigilance units.

As an example, in the United States, under the Freedom of Information (FOI) act, MedWatch forms are available at nominal cost from the Food and Drug Administration. Usually the adverse effects reported for a specific drug are requested. As there are over 1 million reports in the FDA's databases, care should be taken in carefully defining the cases desired. See FDA's FOI website (www.fda.gov/foi/foia2.htm).

ANOREXICS: PULMONARY HYPERTENSION

From the withdrawal of Aminorex in Switzerland in the 1970s to the worldwide withdrawal of dexfenfluramine and fenfluramine on 15 September 1997, primary pulmonary hypertension has haunted the world of anorexics.

The anorexic Aminorex was launched in Switzerland before 1970. Within 9 months of commercialization, symptoms of primary pulmonary hypertension began to appear in up to 10% of the subjects treated for more than 1 year. After 18 months of treatment, nearly 1% of obese patients had died. A pharmacovigilance inquiry was done because the risk/benefit ratio seemed to be unacceptable. This "epidemic" led to the withdrawal of the product from the market and a decrease in the incidence of pulmonary hypertension. In epidemiologic jargon this is a *positive population dechallenge*. Other products were the object of case-control studies. The prolongation of treatment with some newer anorexics (now voluntarily withdrawn) may increase the relative risk of developing pulmonary hypertension, an ADR that is very rare but nonetheless serious and sometimes fatal.

ANTAGONIST RESPONSE: DIAGNOSTIC USEFULNESS

When a medication is administered after the start of an AE/ADR to treat and correct the reaction, the clinician should note this point in the report of the AE/ADR in order to give complete information. He or she should indicate whether the treatment was or was not effective in order to aid in the evaluation of the causality of the AE. The level of the corrective treatment employed by the clinician is usually a function of the severity of the event. Although often required medically, the simultaneous administration of a treatment of the AE and the dechallenge (stopping) of the suspect drug make the interpretation of a positive dechallenge difficult if not impossible.

TREATMENT SPECIFIC TO A DRUG PRODUCT

A positive response to a specific treatment, separate from the dechallenge, is a point in favor of a drug causality for an AE (i.e., it is likely an ADR).

Digitalis: The cessation of an arrhythmia in a patient on digitalis, after treatment with antibodies specific to digoxin, is evidence in favor of digoxin being the cause of the arrhythmia.

TREATMENT SPECIFIC TO A CLASS OF DRUGS

Positive responses to such a treatment must be interpreted with caution. However, when it is clear that the patient was exposed to *only one* drug of this class, then the treatment is considered specific to the drug and is no longer a class treatment.

Naloxone: This antagonist is used to treat opiate overdoses or to counteract the effects of opiates when used for sedation or anesthesia (e.g., in endoscopy). It is helpful in the differential diagnosis in a case of coma in a drug addict or after a suicide attempt. Coma or respiratory depression that is rapidly corrected by naloxone weighs strongly in favor of an opiate cause of the coma. The presence of only a single opiate in the patient with multiple other suspect drugs makes the naloxone a specific treatment rather than a class treatment.

Flumazenil: If a comatose patient who is a drug addict or who has made a suicide attempt arrives in the emergency room with no clear cause of coma, the rapid correction by use of this benzodiazepine antagonist strongly suggests that the cause of the coma is a benzodiazepine. If only a single benzodiazepine was ingested, then this treatment is a specific one.

ANTIMICROBIAL (BACTERIAL) RESISTANCE: AN ECOLOGIC ADVERSE DRUG REACTION

Microorganisms can become resistant to antibiotics or antibacterials in the same patient or, more frequently, in other persons who are infected with the same microorganism. This phenomenon is reaching disquieting levels and is producing major public health problems (e.g., resistant tuberculosis). The prescriber's weapons are limited to using antibiotics only when truly indicated (Kunin, *Ann Intern Med* 1993;118:557; O'Brien, *Clin Infect Dis* 1997;24(S-1):S-2; Virk, *Mayo Clinic Proc* 2000;75(2):200; Lavin, *Infect Control Hosp Epidemiol* 2000;suppl 1:S32–S35). The latter article is a view from the pharmaceutical industry.

One of the solutions proposed for this vexing problem is the continuing education of health care professionals. A program in Finland and Iceland reduced the approved daily dose from 2.4 per 1000 inhabitants to 1.4 per 1000 inhabitants. Rate of resistance by group A streptococci in throat swabs to erythromycin fell from 16.5% in 1992 to 8.6% in 1996 (Seppala, *N Engl J Med* 1997;337:441).

APPLIED PHARMACOVIGILANCE

There are certain tools available for special reactions, patients, and products.

REACTIONS

▶ The Benichou Guidebook

This work is a textbook of *applied pharmacovigilance* aimed at helping the clinician who is attempting to assess case causality. It contains different categories of ADRs grouped according to the body system affected and the type of reaction as well as by the diagnosis. Definitions and causality criteria for specific clinical events worked out at expert consensus conferences are given. This book is useful to clinical pharmacists and nurses who wish to understand the approach of the physician (differential diagnosis) better and to exclude the various alternative (non-drug) causes systematically (Benichou C, Editor, *Adverse Drug Reactions: a practical guide to diagnosis and management.* New York: Wiley, 1994).

The first section concerns the diagnosis and approach to various types of reactions: hepatic, hematologic, cutaneous, anaphylactic, renal, digestive, respiratory, hyper- and hypoglycemic, neuromuscular, hypertensive, cardiac, and pediatric. Also discussed are patients undergoing chemotherapy, patients with acquired immunodeficiciency syndrome (AIDS) and those participating in clinical trials. The second section deals with the harmonization of laws and regulations and of terminology. A "universal data collection form" is proposed as well as body system–specific forms for hepatic, hemolytic, renal, thrombocytopenic, neutropenic, and dermatologic ADRs. In addition, two questionnaires are provided; one is universal and the other is for hepatic reactions.

CAUSALITY ALGORITHMS

Specific tools have been developed to aid in the determination of causality of hepatic, hematologic, dermatologic, and other AEs/ADRs (Danan G, *J Clin Epidemiol* 1993;46:1323; Benichou C, *J Clin Epidemiol* 1993;46:1331).

DEFINITIONS

Definitions of certain ADRs involving the liver, the blood, the kidney, the skin, and other systems have been the subject of consensus conferences aiming to establish precise criteria to use to distinguish between two different pathologic conditions and to define the levels of severity (see DEFINITIONS BY CONSENSUS).

PATIENTS

▶ Embryo, Fetus, Newborn

Teratovigilance in its broad sense studies the risks from conception to the neonatal period as well as fetal toxicity, neonatal surveillance, withdrawal effects seen after birth, and risks of drugs transmitted during breast-feeding.

▶ Pediatrics and Geriatrics

Patients at either end of the age spectrum present particular problems. In children the recommended dose of a drug is rarely established before marketing approval because infants are rarely the subject of clinical trials. Children are also uniquely at risk of ADRs that affect growth and development.

Elderly persons are exposed to the risks of drug interactions, polypharmacy, and slowing of drug metabolism as well as other kinetic alterations. It is also sometimes difficult to determine whether a drug is truly the cause of an AE in an elderly patient with multiple diseases. Surveillance in the elderly, which is a growing area of interest as the population in the industrialized nations ages, is known as *gerontovigilance.*

▶ AIDS Patients

In 1997, because of the gravity and newness of AIDS and AIDS medication ADRs, the United Kingdom created a national program for the spontaneous reporting of AEs/ADRs associated with anti–human immunodeficiency virus (anti-HIV) medications (the HIV ADR Reporting Scheme), which is the equivalent of "intensified reporting" in standard pharmacovigilance. A specialized data collection form and periodical were developed. In addition, the confidentiality of the data was reaffirmed (MCA/CSM, *Curr Probl Phamacovigil* 1998;24:3). Similarly, in the United States, various pharmaceutical companies, in cooperation with the FDA, created AIDS-specific registries for AE/ADR information reported with their products.

PRODUCTS

▶ Excipients

Additives, vehicles, fillers, and other so-called inactive ingredients may be allergenic or toxic. Excipients present a significant problem for those involved in pharmacovigilance. Rarely are excipients considered by the reporting health care practitioner or those involved in pharmacovigilance as a cause of AEs/ADRs since most people think only about the "active" ingredients. Excipients are sometimes changed if the drug's manufacturing process is changed and, although duly reported to the governmental authorities under good manufacturing processes (GMPs), are rarely reported to the pharmacovigilance units of the company or government. For example, an excipient that can produce significant gastrointestinal symptoms is lactose, which is frequently used as a bulk filler in capsules or tablets.

▶ Blood Products Surveillance (Hemovigilance)

Surveillance of the risks associated with the use of blood products. This task is usually confided to a separate agency or division within governmental pharmacovigilance systems. The scandals seen with HIV-contaminated blood have demonstrated the importance of this public function—if such a demonstration is still needed. Blood products safety surveillance and recalls in the United States are described on the FDA website (http://www.fda.gov/cber/recalls.htm).

▶ Device Surveillance (Materiovigilance)

The surveillance of medical and dental devices as well as their material defects. In the United States, the FDA has included device reporting in the same form that is used for drug reporting (the MedWatch form).

▶ Oncovigilance

The surveillance of ADRs from antineoplastic therapy is a particularly tricky area of pharmacovigilance and is generally the domain of oncologists, who are best able to determine the risk/benefit ratio. There is unfortunately a tendency for oncologists to underreport AEs/ADRs as they argue, not unreasonably, that their patients are almost always very ill and the chemotherapy drugs are all very toxic. Thus all patients have AEs and ADRs, and some practical judiciousness in what is reported is necessary.

▶ Phytovigilance

The surveillance of medicinal plants is becoming more and more important in the West as the level of usage of these products increases. (See PHYTOVIGILANCE.)

▶ Vaccinovigilance

The surveillance of vaccines is almost always conducted separately from surveillance of drugs and biologics by a separate governmental agency. For the United States see the FDA's website on vaccines (http://www.fda.gov/cber/vaers/vaers.htm).

APPROVAL PROCEDURES – EUROPE

There are three types of approval procedures:

▶ The Centralized Procedure

This term refers to the approval process in the European Union in which a drug dossier is submitted to the EMEA (see EUROPEAN MEDICINALS EVALUATION AGENCY) for review and approval. It began in January 1995 with the creation of the EMEA. If approved, a Marketing Authorization (see MARKETING AUTHORIZATION) is granted by the European Commission for sale in all of the countries of the European Union (plus any other affiliated countries that agree to abide by the EMEA's decisions). The procedure takes, in theory, about a year and, like the FDA fee for NDA submissions, costs the applicant about $200,000 per application.

▶ The Mutual Recognition Procedure

The alternative route for drug approval is the "mutual recognition procedure" in which the application is made to one of the EU member states as selected by the application. The procedure operates by the acceptance by some or all of the other members states ("mutual recognition") of the single national approval.

▶ Single Country Procedure

This procedure is used if the applicant desires marketing authorization in only one country of the EU.

The choice of which route to use is complex. The EU is moving to the single centralized procedure that is obligatory for all biologics and is expected to become the route of choice (if not obligation) in Europe.

ARSENIC

In 1922 arsenic was noted to produce jaundice when used for the treatment of syphilis. This miniepidemic contributed to the formation of the first Council on Pharmacy and Chemistry by the American Medical Association in 1929.

ASPARTATE AMINOTRANSFERASE (AST)

A term widely used in hepatovigilance. It is an enzyme found in hepatocytes and elsewhere and formerly called serum glutamic-oxaloacetic transaminase (SGOT). It can be used in place of alanine aminotransferase (ALT) in determining the ALT/Alkaline Phosphatase (ALT/AP) ratio, which may be used to distinguish hepatocellular, cholestatic, and mixed hepatic drug reactions (see ALT/AP RATIO)

ASSOCIATION FOR METHODOLOGY RESEARCH IN PHARMACOVIGILANCE (ARME-P)

Created for "the research and transmission of new methodologic approaches for the surveillance and the detection of adverse reactions associated with marketed medications," this nonprofit organization was begun by the pharmaco-epidemiology group in Bordeaux directed by Prof. Bernard Begaud. They have explored the statistical approach in the assessment of series of case reports in ARME-P *Methodological Approaches in Pharmaco-Epidemiology: Application to Spontaneous Reporting* (Amsterdam: Elsevier, 1993).

Their methodology was also published by Van Boxtel CJ, (Van Boxtel CJ, Editor, ARME-P, Co-editor, *Post Marketing Surveillance* 1993:7(1,2):1–171). When looking at the bibliographic listings, note that this journal has been taken over by *Pharmacoepidemiology and Drug Safety (PEDS)*.

ATTRIBUTABLE BENEFIT

By analogy to *attributable risk*, the *attributable benefit* is equal to the level of cure (i.e., benefit sought) in those exposed to a medication minus the level of cure in those who did not receive the medication. For example, if 80% of ulcer patients treated with a histamine receptor H_2 blocker are found to be ulcer-free by endoscopy after 4 weeks, and 60% of ulcer patients treated with a placebo are also ulcer-free at 4 weeks, then the attributable benefit is 20%. It would thus follow that 80% (100% - attributable benefit) (or 0.8) did not benefit from the pharmacologic effect of the H_2 blocker treatment.

A very useful and clinically meaningful way of looking at this concept is to calculate the number of patients needed to be treated in order to get a cure (i.e., attain the benefit) in one patient (often called *number needed to treat*). In this example that would be $1/0.2 = 5$. Thus five patients need to be treated in order to obtain one pharmacologic benefit. Stated more pessimistically, four of five patients did not obtain pharmacologic benefit from this treatment.

ATTRIBUTABILITY (see CAUSALITY: THREE TYPES)

ATTRIBUTABLE RISK; EXCESS RISK (see RISK ATTRIBUTABLE TO A DRUG)

In pharmacovigilance this epidemiologic term is equivalent to the rate of an AE in patients exposed to a suspect drug minus the baseline, reference rate (in similar patients unexposed to the suspect drug).

AUDITS (see REGULATORY REPORTING REQUIREMENTS)

AUSTRALIAN ADVERSE DRUG REACTIONS BULLETIN

National bulletin of Australian pharmacovigilance prepared by the Australian Drug Reactions Advisory Committee (ADRAC). It is available on the Internet at http://www.health.gov.au/hfs/tga/docs/html/aadrbltn/aadrbidx.htm and is regularly reviewed in *Reactions Weekly* published by Adis. Back issues have been computerized since vol. 14, no. 1 (February 1995). Several important signals first appeared in this very well thought of bulletin.

AUSTRALIAN DRUG REACTIONS ADVISORY COMMITTEE (ADRAC)

A subcommittee of the Australian Drug Evaluation Committee consisting of physicians reporting to the Therapeutic Goods Administration of the Ministry of Health. They edit the *Australian Adverse Drug Reactions Bulletin*.

AUSTRALIAN PRESCRIBER

An independently published quarterly on pharmacotherapy distributed without charge. Although it is subsidized by the health authority, its editors have consistently maintained an independent point of view. It is a member of the *International Society of Drug Bulletins* whose editors are known for their uprightness. It is now available on the Internet (*Australian Prescriber*, POB 100, WODEN ACT 2606, Australia, www.australianprescriber.com).

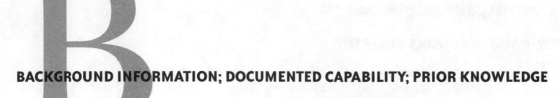

BACKGROUND INFORMATION; DOCUMENTED CAPABILITY; PRIOR KNOWLEDGE

IN CASE CAUSALITY ASSESSMENT

An important characteristic of a spontaneous report answering the question, Does this product have a history of being able to cause this adverse effect? In other words, can it? This suspicion that the product can indeed cause the type of AE in question is based on the product monograph, other reports of similar AEs, and other information supplied by the sponsor or manufacturer.

In the Bayesian model this background information is used as a preliminary step to create a list of suspect drugs that might have caused the AE in question and therefore deserve to be formally assessed for causality by comparing them with alternative nondrug causes (Lane, *Drug Inf J* 1986;20:445).

IN PHARMACOTHERAPY

When faced with an AE that could be associated with a drug, the health care professional (physician, pharmacist, nurse, etc.) consults his or her national compendium (*Physician's Drug Reference* (PDR) in the United States, the *Vidal* in France, the *Compendium of Pharmaceuticals and Specialties* (CPS) in Canada, the *Rote Liste* in Germany, etc.) to find out whether the event is mentioned (labeled) or not (unlabeled). If not labeled, the product can be assumed, at least for now, not to be capable of producing this type of AE. In general, type A reactions are picked up during the phase III clinical trials, which "tell us whether the drug can cause a particular event" (Stephens, *Drug Inf J* 1984;18:307).

Clinical trials are generally held to be the gold standard for proof of drug causality of an ADR (usually of type A) if they occur more frequently than in control, especially placebo control, groups. Type B reactions, being much rarer, are usually not unearthed in the clinical trials and are only discovered after marketing, when, unfortunately, causality becomes harder to determine.

BACKGROUND RISK; BASELINE RISK

In pharmacoepidemiology these terms refer to the incidence of an adverse effect in individuals not exposed to the drug and who may be considered comparable to those exposed to the drug. This risk is not necessarily that of the entire population but only that of the patients with the indication for the drug in question. Incidence implies the concept of time (occurrence over a specified time period). The baseline risk is used in the Bayesian model of case causality assessment for determining the *general prior odds* (Lane, *Drug Inf J* 1986;20:445). Two examples are presented:

> According to a study of computerized patient charts in the General Practice Research Database (formerly called VAMP) in the U.K., covering 4.3 million person-years from January 1988 to August 1992, the incidence (baseline risk) of diffuse pulmonary infiltrates was estimated at 1.2 cases per 10,000 person-years. Many factors other than drugs were felt to produce this problem (Martinez, *PEDS* 1997;6(suppl 2):S115).

In Sweden a study showed a baseline risk of the Guillain-Barré Syndrome of 20 cases per million patient-years (Kaitin, *Clin Pharmacol Ther* 1989;46:121). These figures are useful when this syndrome is associated with a new drug or vaccine.

BAYESIAN APPLICATIONS TO CASE REPORTS

The Bayesian probabilistic approach has occasionally been used by industry, government, and academe.

- Zimeldine: Guillain Barre (acute polyradiculopathy syndrome) (Naranjo, *J Clin Pharmacol* 1990;30:174)
- Sulfonamide: hypersensitivity (Ghajar, *Semin Dermatol* 1989;8:213)
- Benzodiazepines: withdrawal syndrome (Nida, *Res Monog Ser* 1992;119:424)
- Gentamicin: acute renal insufficiency (Hutchinson, *Drug Information J* 1986;20:475)
- Zomepirac: fatal anaphylaxis (Kramer, *Drug Information J* 1986;20:505)
- Minoxidil: Stevens-Johnson syndrome (Jones, *Drug Information J* 1986;20:487)
- Lithium: exfoliative dermatitis (Kramer, *Drug Information J* 1986;20:523)
- Chlorpromazine: cholestatic jaundice (Naranjo, *Drug Information J* 1986;20:465). The same case is reexamined by a modified approach that uses educated clinical guesses for determining the ratios rather than hard epidemiologic data (Hoskins, *PEDS* 1992;1:235)

BAYESIAN CAUSALITY ASSESSMENT (see also CASE CAUSALITY ASSESSMENT)

This model for analysis of the causality of an ADR uses conditional probabilities which are, in turn, modified with each new piece of information obtained, successively altering the preceding probabilities in order to come up with a final causality. It is also called *probabilistic causality*. This approach has also been applied to the differential diagnosis of medical conditions. Thomas Bayes (1702–1761), a Protestant minister and amateur mathematician, developed a theorem on conditional probabilities that supplied the theoretical basis for this approach. However, it was two centuries later when this concept was actually applied to medical diagnosis in general and ADRs in particular (Bayes T, An essay towards solving a problem in the doctrine of chances. *Philos Trans R Soc Lond (Biol)* 1763;53:370–375 (reprinted in *Biometrika* 1958;45:296–315)).

It represents one model for diagnostic reasoning; others are multiple regression and various expert systems. Its rigorous use is occasionally possible, however, only in the context of a pharmacoepidemiology study or trial or a pharmacovigilance investigation. A formidable problem is the lack of literature containing AE rates in exposed and unexposed populations, from which it becomes much easier to derive relative risks and attributable risks of ADRs. It is more useful to consider this approach as a conceptual method of clinical reasoning (Davidoff, *Med Care* 1989;29:45).

Each judgment takes the form of a ratio whose numerator represents the *drug etiology hypothesis* and whose denominator represents the *alternative, nondrug etiology*. The clinician must therefore start by choosing the most suspect drug among those possibly taken by the patient, and the most likely alternative explanation in terms of the patient's medical condition.

Then the relevant information is broken down into four categories of criteria:

▶ **Prior, predictive**

General prior odds (drug's background knowledge)

Case-specific prior odds, modified by history (risk factors)

▶ **Likelihood ratios of AE characteristics**

Temporal (timing, rechallenge, etc.)

Nontemporal (site of application, etc.)

Those criteria are presented in the entry CASE CAUSALITY ASSESSMENT.

THE USE OF THE BAYESIAN APPROACH IN CAUSALITY

After the first use of the equation by M. Auriche (*Thérapie* 1985;40:301) for the purpose of ADR causality assessment, this approach was applied to several specific situations (Jones J and Herman R, Editors, *Drug Inf J* 1986;20(4, special issue):383). Especially enlightening is the paper by Lane (*Drug Inf J* 1986;20:455). Other publications have attempted to promote this approach (Lane, *Pharmaceut Med* 1987;2:265; Hutchinson, *J Clin Epidemiol* 1989;42:5) with little success.

A COMPROMISE

Two Swiss pharmacoepidemiologists have proposed an approach that may represent a useful operational compromise. This method uses ratios based on the opinion of an acknowledged clinical expert rather than calculated from hard epidemiologic data, which are often unavailable or difficult to find (Hoskins, *PEDS* 1992;1:235).

BAYESIAN CONFIDENCE PROPAGATION NEURAL NETWORK (BCPNN)

Methodology developed by the World Health Organization (WHO) Monitoring Centre in Uppsala to improve the detection of signals found in their spontaneous pharmacovigilance database (Bate, *Eur J Clin Pharmacol* 1998;54:315). According to the authors, some of the signals that led to the withdrawal of certain medications from the Swedish market would have been detected 4 to 6 months sooner had this new methodology been used (see UPPSALA MONTEREY CENTRE).

BEHIND THE COUNTER DRUG

A product that is dispensed by the pharmacist (without a physician's prescription), as opposed to an *over the counter* product, which the patient can choose freely from the shelves of the pharmacy (or store) and pay for without having any contact with the pharmacist. In theory, its dispensing by the pharmacist should be accompanied by advice on the indication for and the safe use of the product. The advice should include information on the prevention, recognition, and treatment of any possible ADRs.

BENDECTIN: A WELL-KNOWN FALSE ALERT

Bendectin is a fixed combination of three active ingredients used for the nausea and vomiting of pregnancy:

■ Doxylamine, an H_1 antihistamine that acts as an antinausea and antivomiting agent
■ Pyridoxine, vitamin B_6
■ Dicycloverine, removed from the product shortly before market withdrawal of Bendectin

This product was incorrectly suspected of causing congenital abnormalities. Several case-control studies were performed, and their results formed the basis for the exoneration of this product. It had been on the market for about 27 years and used by some 33 million pregnant women in the United States, representing 20–40% of all pregnant women. It was voluntarily withdrawn from the U.S. market and never returned even after its exoneration. It was sold under the name Debendox in other countries (Fleming, 1981;283:99; CSM/MCA, *Curr Probl Phamacovigil* 1981;6; Editors, *Lancet* 1984;2:205 and *Br Med J* 1985;271:918).

RETURN TO THE MARKET IN CANADA

A laboratory was authorized to sell a product containing doxylamine and pyridoxine under the name *Diclectin*. In order to reduce the remaining suspicions held by obstetricians, it was specified in the product labeling that the therapeutic category for which this combination was approved was "Anti-nausea agent for the nausea and vomiting of pregnancy." A group of Canadian experts published a statement on 11 August 1989 affirming that this fixed association was safe; the British authorities had also expressed the same opinion. The Canadian government has thus maintained a marketing authorization for this product for a Canadian manufacturer (CSM/MCA, *Curr Probl Pharmacovigil* 1981;6; Editors, *Lancet* 1984;2:205; Medico-Legal Committee Opinion, *J Soc Obstet Gynecol Can* 1995;17:162; Koren, *Can J Clin Pharmacol* 1995;2:38).

BENEFITS

A *therapeutic benefit* is the improvement in the state of health of the patient exposed to a treatment. The decision to use a particular treatment is based on the analysis of the *benefit/risk ratio* (sometimes also called, somewhat negatively, the *risk/benefit ratio*). It should be recalled that the therapeutic benefit should be greater than the simple pharmacologic effect achieved. The benefit should be *clinical,* not just pharmacologic. The benefit can be manifested in numerous ways: increased lifespan, improved quality of life, complications avoided, and so on.

CRITERIA FOR THE EVALUATION OF A BENEFIT IN CLINICAL TRIALS

In controlled clinical trials in clinical pharmacology, it is necessary to choose *outcome measures.* When the objective of the treatment is a prophylaxis or preventive effect, it is necessary to make the distinction between a *pharmacologic effect* (also called a *surrogate outcome* or *surrogate marker*) and a true *clinical benefit.* Pharmacologic effects can often be seen in short-term clinical trials whereas clinical benefits often require large-scale, long-duration, and costly clinical trials, which are difficult to perform and are not frequently done.

In an individual patient, a benefit is sometimes very easy to measure (e.g., pulmonary function, ankle swelling, vital capacity, disappearance of a rash or of gastric lesions on endoscopy). However, it can be very hard to measure if no objective measurements exist (e.g., quality of life outcomes, course of depression) or, if the benefit is prophylactic or preventive, it may be almost impossible to measure in an individual patient (e.g., slowing of the progression of emphysema, myocardial infarcts avoided, fractures avoided). In determining the risk/benefit ratio for a specific patient this can pose enormous challenges to the clinician.

TYPES OF TREATMENTS AND BENEFITS

After the prescriber has made a diagnosis and decided to pursue a therapy, he or she must decide on a therapeutic objective and choose among those pharmacologic agents (i.e., drugs, vaccines, biologics) that are available.

- *Corrective agents*: antidotes, antagonists
- *Diagnostic agents*: contrast agents, radioisotopes, allergens
- *Curative agents*: antibiotics, antivirals, gene therapy
- *Prophylactic agents*: hypolipidemics, antihypertensives, antiaggregants, antiarrhythmics, vaccines, anticoagulants
- *Substitution therapies*: hormones (e.g., insulin), electrolytes (e.g., potassium), metabolites (e.g., glucose), blood products, vitamins
- *Symptomatic therapies*: analgesics, antiemetics

BENOXAPROFEN: MARKET WITHDRAWAL

This product was launched in 1980 and withdrawn from the market in the United Kingdom in 1982 because of the hepatorenal syndrome. It has been stated that it could have been withdrawn sooner if more attention had been paid to the pharmacokinetics in elderly people who received "adult" doses (Editors, *Br Med J* 1982;285:519). It was withdrawn from the American market after only 2.5 months in 1982.

BENZYL ALCOHOL: NEONATAL MORTALITY FROM AN EXCIPIENT

In 1981, the Food and Drug Administration was notified of the death of newborns exposed to a preservative in saline solution that was used to rinse central vein catheters in premature babies. In one hospital, 10 cases occurred in 6 months; in another hospital 6 cases were seen in 12 months. After the FDA recommended that the use of this excipient be stopped, the "epidemic" ended. This result can be considered as a *positive collective dechallenge*. This episode clearly illustrates that deaths can be due to ADRs that are related to excipients as well as to active ingredients of a drug product (Gershanik, *Clin Res* 1981;29:895a; MMWR 1982;31:290).

BIOLOGIC PRODUCT

A medical product prepared from biologic material of human, animal, or microbiologic origin (such as blood products, vaccines, insulin, and antibiotics) in contrast to products made from chemical substances. Usually governmental regulation and surveillance of blood products (hemovigilance) and vaccines (vaccinovigilance) are given to agencies separate from those that oversee drug products. Biologics (including recombinant deoxyribonucleic acid (DNA) products) may be regulated by the same division that controls drug surveillance; or, as in the United States, a separate division may handle biologic products (Center for Biologics Evaluation and Research (CBER)).

BIOTECHNOLOGY

Development of new biologic products by genetic manipulation or techniques of cellular multiplication. In the European Union they are evaluated and approved by the European Medicinal Evaluation Agency (EMEA). In the United States they are usually evaluated by the Center for Biologics Evaluation and Research (CBER) of the Food and Drug Administration, with oversight from other health agencies.

BLOOD SAFETY SURVEILLANCE; HEMOVIGILANCE

Surveillance of the AEs associated with blood products and blood derivatives. Scandals concerning blood contaminated with hepatitis virus and human immunodeficiency virus (HIV) have occurred in Canada, Japan, and France. In France some people were convicted and imprisoned after a criminal inquiry.

BOSTON COLLABORATIVE DRUG SURVEILLANCE PROGRAM (BCDSP)

This group, associated with Boston University, was established in 1966 to conduct formal epidemiologic research to quantify adverse effects of drugs by inhospital monitoring. Resources used include the Group Health Cooperative of Puget Sound (United States) as well as the General Practice Research Database (United Kingdom).

The BCDSP was the first to do systematic pharmacoepidemiologic follow-ups of cohorts. All hospitalized patients were followed in order to measure their medication use just before and during their hospitalization. In addition, AEs that occurred during the hospitalization were noted and the relationship of these AEs to the medications administered was evaluated (Danielson, *JAMA* 1982;248:1482; Lawson, *Pediatr Clin North Am* 1972;19:117). They have published many papers; three of the more recent are those by Meier CR et al, *JAMA* 1999; 281:427, Vasilakis C et al, *Contraception.* 1999;59:79, and Sturkenboom M et al, *Arch Intern Med* 1999;159:493. See their website (www.bu.edu/bcdsp).

In spite of its high costs, this technique became the paragon of its type. It permits the determination of ADR frequency (at least in the short term) as well as helping to differentiate those factors likely to be related to the drug compared to those factors related to the patient. Newer techniques using secondary data in health insurance- and medical records-linked databases are now employed in addition, and perhaps in preference, to this technique; although exposed to more biases, they are cheaper and faster and cover larger populations.

BRITISH NATIONAL FORMULARY (BNF)

A pharmacotherapy guide published by independent experts under the authority of a Joint Formulary Committee that comprises representatives of the publishers—Royal Pharmaceutical Society and British Medical Association—and of the Department of Health. The *BNF* aims to provide doctors, pharmacists and other healthcare professionals with sound, up-to-date information about the use of medicines. Electronic versions of the *BNF*, including Internet versions, are produced in parallel with the paper version. An Internet version is being developed. The executive editor's address is at the Royal Pharmaceutical Society of Great Britain, 1 Lambeth High Street, London SE1 7JN. (e-mail: editor@bnf.rpsgb.org.uk). See their website (www.bnf.org). Number 40 appeared in September 2000.

BROMFENAC: MARKET WITHDRAWAL

On June 22, 1998 the US Food and Drug Administration withdrew this nonsteroidal antiinflammatory drug (NSAID) from the market because hepatotoxicity led to fatalities and liver transplants in several cases. The clinical trials had shown this product to produce a greater elevation of hepatic enzyme levels than other NSAIDs. This is an example of a serious signal whose confirmation changed the risk/benefit ratio to such an extent that withdrawal was warranted (*US Federal Register* 1998;63(195):54082).

BROMOCRIPTINE: WITHDRAWAL OF AN INDICATION

This agent is useful for stopping lactation in women who are not breast-feeding. However the observation of rare but severe ADRs markedly changed the risk/

benefit ratio of this product in this indication. Cerebrovascular accidents, hypertension, myocardial infarcts and death were observed with its use. Between 1980 and 1994 the Food and Drug Administration received a total of 531 cases of serious ADRs, of which 32 fatalities were seen in postpartum women who took this product to suppress lactation. The manufacturer voluntarily withdrew this indication for the product from the U.S. and Canadian markets. It is still marketed for other indications including parkinsonism and acromegaly (FDA Press Release August 17, 1994; www.fda.gov/bbs/topics/ANSWERS/ANS00594.html).

BULLETINS, ADVERSE DRUG REACTION AND PHARMACOVIGILANCE

In 1962 the first bulletin of summaries of published or litigated case reports was created under the name *Clin-Alert*. Each eight-page issue reviews ADRs that have been published or are the object of litigation in the United States. The amount of money obtained as compensation, as a result of the trial or of an outside settlement, is often available and is of interest to those in the medicolegal domain (*Clin-Alert*, Technomic Publishing, 851 New Holland Avenue, Lancaster, PA 17604; www.techpub.com). *Clin-Alert 2000* is now available in book form.

The Adverse Drug Reaction Bulletin has historic importance as the first bulletin aimed as discussing drug safety issues. It was created in 1966 by Professor D.M. Davies in the United Kingdom. Each edition contains a fully referenced analysis prepared by invitation covering the ADRs of a particular class of drugs and their effect on the risk/benefit ratio. See their website (www.lww.com).

Today the most useful international bulletin is *Reactions Weekly,* published by ADIS. It provides an accessible and up-to-date summary of case reports and regulatory information published in the major pharmacovigilance and other medical journals. It is available in print or electronically. It is indispensable to anyone working daily in the field of pharmacovigilance. See their website (www.adis.com).

BULLOUS ERUPTION

In dermatovigilance, this category of cutaneous disease includes erythema multiforme, Stevens-Johnson syndrome, and toxic epidermal necrolysis and (Lyell's syndrome).

Erythema multiforme is the least severe and is often due to a nondrug cause, whereas the other two pathologic conditions are much more dangerous and are generally of drug origin.

BUNDESINSTITUT FUR ARZNEIMITTEL UND MEDIZINPRODUKTE (BfArM)

The Bundesinstitut fur Arzneimittel und Medizinprodukte (Federal Institute for Drugs and Medical Devices) is the official national drug agency in the Federal Republic of Germany. It is the counterpart of the Food and Drug Administration in the United States, the European Medicinal Evaluation Agency (EMEA) for the European Union, and the Commitee on Safety of Medicines (CSM) in the United Kingdom. It was formerly called the Bundesgesundheitsamt (BGA). In regard to pharmacovigilance, they examine AEs and may take various measures under what is called the *Stufenplan* or graduated plan. See their English-language website (www.bfarm.de/gb_ver).

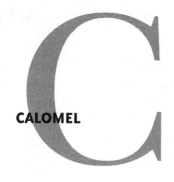

CALOMEL

A mercury-based purgative used in the past to treat yellow fever. Of historical interest because mercury intoxication was discovered by "spontaneous reporting" in the United States at the end of the 18th century, though its use continued until the end of the 19th century. In modern times, withdrawal of toxic products from the market usually occurs more quickly.

CANADIAN ADVERSE DRUG REACTION NEWSLETTER

An increasingly useful national bulletin of pharmacovigilance, produced by the Therapeutic Products Programme of Health Canada, published quarterly, inserted in the *Canadian Medical Association Journal* (the Canadian counterpart of the *Journal of the American Medical Association* (*JAMA*)). It includes the section Drugs of Current Interest. Readers are encouraged to report suspected ADRs to the Canadian ADR Monitoring Programme in Ottawa, to a regional center, or on reporting forms available on the Internet (www.hc-sc.gc.ca/hpb-dgps/therapeut/zfiles/english/forms/adverse_e.pdf).

CARDIAC ARRHYTHMIA SUPPRESSION TRIAL (CAST)

The CAST trial was a placebo-controlled clinical trial that demonstrated a fatal proarrhythmic effect of two class 1C antiarrhythmics: encainide and flecainide. This trial is noteworthy for two reasons. First, it demonstrated the detection of a *paradoxical* ADR at the pharmacologic level (proarrhythmic rather than antiarrhythmic) and at the therapeutic level (increased mortality rate rather than decreased mortality rate). Second, it also demonstrated again the usefulness of placebo controls in clinical trials even when hard data are used as end points, since this effect would not have been seen as readily without such controls (Cast, *N Engl J Med* 1989;321:406).

CAST, which was financed by the U.S. National Institute of Health, clearly showed that these new type I antiarrhythmics increased the relative risk of fatal cardiac arrest by 2.5 times whereas the attributable risk due to the drugs was estimated at 5.88 per 100 patient-years. Before this trial, signals had been observed in phase III clinical trials that led to the CAST trial. It is rare that an ADR as serious as sudden death, appearing very frequently (1/17 patients per year) and very rapidly after treatment was started, becomes the subject of a controlled clinical trial.

CASE CAUSALITY ASSESSMENT

Instead of presenting the various causality aids, such as questionnaires, algorithms, and decision tables, that have been devised over the last two decades, we present the logical basis of those questionnaires, using a simplification of the Bayesian model. The causality criteria can be considered as belonging to four classes: general prior odds, risk factors, and temporal and nontemporal event characteristics. The first two may be called *predictive* because they are present *before* the occurrence of the AE; the last two may be called *diagnostic* because they are gathered as evidence *after* the occurrence of the AE and are expressed by epidemiologists as likelihood ratios.

PREDICTIVE: GENERAL PRIOR ODDS

For the epidemiologist, the numerator is the *attributable risk* of the suspect drug in patients exposed to the suspect drug, and the denominator is the *reference* or *baseline risk* from the most likely alternative cause in comparable subjects not exposed to the drug. This ratio is based on *general evidence* (Miettinen, *Can Med Assoc J* 1998;158:215), the type or class of suspect drug, the type of ADR, and the general type of patient treated. The source of information is the medical and epidemiologic literature.

For example, the frequencies of hematemesis are determined in "typical" arthritis patients treated with a nonsteroidal antiinflammatory drug (NSAID) and in such patients not treated with an NSAID. This is done without referring to the specific patient being studied. It answers the question, *Will* this drug produce this type of AE in *groups* of patients with a given indication, to what extent, with what probability?

Here is an example where attributable risk is available.

A pharmacovigilance investigation of zimeldine done predominantly in Sweden found that the underlying baseline risk of Guillain-Barré was 20 cases per million person-years, whereas in those exposed to zimeldine it was 580 cases per million person-years. These data permitted the calculation of the following:

Relative risk: 29:1 (580:20)
Attributable risk: 560 per million person-years (580 - 20)
General prior odds (in bayesian analysis): 560/20 = 28/1

Here is an example where only relative risk is available.

If we assume that the risk of hematemesis is three times greater in those patients taking an NSAID during a 1-year period compared to similar patients not taking an NSAID during this period, then the relative risk is 3:1. This means that for every three cases of hematemesis in those taking the NSAIDs, two are attributed to NSAIDs and one is due to an underlying pathology. (For epidemiologists, relative risk minus 1 equals attributable risk in this context: $3 - 1 = 2$. Attributable risk of 2 divided by baseline risk of 1 yields prior odds of 2:1.)

PREDICTIVE: RISK FACTORS

The *specific evidence* is based on the details of an analysis of the drugs the patient has taken and his or her medical workup (history, physical exam, and lab tests). For example, we could consider a 20-year-old patient who has taken a large overdose of acetaminophen (paracetamol) in a suicide attempt. The details are confirmed by a family member who was an eyewitness on the scene and who stated that the patient took no other medications or illicit drugs and had no history of liver problems. This allows us to predict that liver toxicity is imminent. It is not necessary to determine whether liver damage has occurred to make a *specific prediction*.

It answers the question, *Will* this drug, in *this* particular patient, produce this AE? The answer is based on whether there were positive or negative prechallenges, presence or absence of risk factors such as comedication or intercurrent illnesses, excessive dosage, previous occurrences of the AE without drug exposure, and so on. Risk factors are expressed as *relative risks*. When prior odds are modified (multiplied) by risk factors, we obtain the *case prior odds as modified by history*.

LIKELIHOOD RATIOS OF EVENT CHARACTERISTICS

Let us consider a time to onset of 30 minutes for an asthmatic reaction after ingestion of a tablet of an NSAID. Let us assume that from an analysis of other series of cases of NSAID-induced attacks, the time to onset is within 30 minutes in 10% of cases. Let us ask a pharmacoepidemiologist about the probability that a non-drug asthma attack will occur during any 30-minute period in this type of patient; suppose he answers 0.1%. If you divide 10% by 0.1% you get 100. This is your likelihood ratio, 100 to 1.

TEMPORAL CHARACTERISTICS

There are several critical factors to examine when evaluating the time course between the administration of a drug and the occurrence of an AE. They may be divided into three main categories: time to onset, course (including dechallenge), and rechallenge.

> **Time to Onset (Delay in Appearance) of the Event**

This refers to the interval between the *critical dose* for this patient (e.g., first dose, last dose, incorrect dose, overdose) and the first manifestation of the event. This should be evaluated in conjunction with the kinetics of the drug and its metabolites

> **Type of Course in Relation to Dechallenge (see DURATION OF AN ADVERSE EVENT)**

The duration of the event may have different interpretations. The total duration of the event normally refers to the period of the event during treatment with the suspect drug, plus the period after dechallenge. The clinical course after the cessation or reduction in dose may give a clue to a dose-dependent effect. If the event is irreversible, then the duration per se is not meaningful, and it is thus preferable to refer to permanent sequelae (such as myocardial infarct). If the event is transient, it may appear and disappear during treatment with the suspect drug. If the event occurred only after the final dose or only after a single dose, the duration refers only to the period during which the actual event was present. The latter case is the situation that usually applies in vaccinovigilance.

> **Rechallenge**

This refers to whether the event recurred after the reintroduction of the suspect drug. The rechallenge may be fortuitous or voluntary. The clinical records should be very carefully examined to be certain that the event truly disappeared before rechallenge, for AE/ADRs that are intermittent (e.g., arrhythmias). This may be difficult to ascertain.

ABOUT PRECHALLENGES

It is also necessary to take into account, during the causality assessment, any previous exposures to the drug (*prechallenges*), whether and when they occurred, and whether the AE appeared at that time. They are generally considered part of the *case risk factors* alluded to previously.

NONTEMPORAL CHARACTERISTICS

The nonchronologic criteria can be subdivided into four categories: based on pharmacology, pathology, topography, or semiology.

> **Pharmacology**

Based on the nature of the ADR: Beta-blockers provide an example. If the AE is bradycardia and if one of the suspect drugs is a beta-blocker, then this is a pharmacologic criterion favoring the beta-blocker as the causative agent.

Based on response to an antagonist/antidote. Naloxone, for instance, is used to treat narcotic (morphine, codeine, etc.) overdoses. It may prove useful if a patient arrives in the emergency room in a coma or with a respiratory depression that responds very rapidly to an injection of naloxone. The rapid correction of the problem argues in favor of a narcotic cause of the problem.

▶ Pathology (Pathognomonic)

Some rather rare adverse reactions are always due to medications. One example of this is a *fixed drug eruption.* Others are virtually specific to a product such as the corneal microdeposits seen in the majority of patients taking amiodarone over a long period. Also known as *pathognomonic.*

▶ Topograpy: In Situ Reactions

Reactions seen at the application (administration) site, a transit site, or a site of high concentration should be considered as nontemporal factors favoring the causality of the suspect drug. Examples include injection site pain or scarring, transit site esophageal obstruction by a sticky drug, and nephrolithiasis from a drug metabolite concentrated and crystallized in urine.

▶ Semiology: Altered Clinical Presentation

Certain diseases (or AEs) manifest themselves differently when they are due to drugs than when they occur "on their own." Although this is quite rare, when it does occur, it is very useful to the clinician in determining the cause of the disease.

Drug-induced *lupus* erythematosus has been known for more than 40 years and differs from idiopathic lupus erythematosus as it presents with an incomplete clinical picture: fever, malaise, and polyarthalgia are frequent whereas pleuritis and pericarditis are less likely and renal complications quite rare. In drug-induced lupus erythematosus, the clinical signs and symptoms generally disappear more rapidly than the laboratory abnormalities, after dechallenge.

Torsades de pointe are a particular form of ventricular tachycardia often of drug-induced origin. Prolongation of the QT (or QTc) interval on the electrocardiogram (ECG) is typically seen. Clinically, it is characterized by syncope, which may lead to ventricular fibrillation and cardiac arrest. What distinguishes torsades from other ventricular tachycardias is an oscillation on the ECG due to cyclical variations of the duration and amplitude of the QRS waves. The nonsedating H_1 antihistamine terfenadine was withdrawn from the market because of this adverse reaction. It was noted in 2000 that cisapride can also produce this reaction; certain restrictions were added to its labeling and it was removed from the U.S. market in July 2000. This is a serious AE/ADR that health authorities are now paying great attention to.

CASE REPORT

In pharmacovigilance, the summary of one or more undesirable or AEs suspected of being due to a medication observed in a patient, ideally accompanied by a discussion of the evidence for and against a drug-related cause. This summary can be sent to the pharmaceutical company or the health authority (*a notified case report*) or submitted in a journal (*published case report*).

CASE SERIES; SERIES OF CASES

In pharmacovigilance the word *case* applies to a patient who has suffered one or more AEs. However, the term *case series* is used in three different ways (Strom 1995).

SPONTANEOUS ADVERSE DRUG REACTION REPORTS

When a series of case reports presents a strong signal, one of the first steps undertaken if a pharmacovigilance investigation is justified, consists in examining spontaneous report databases to discern as quickly as possible the dose, time to appearance, risk factors, outcomes, treatment durations, time to disappearance after dechallenge, response to various treatments, clinical course and laboratory tests that help to distinguish a drug-related cause from other causes (if any) of the adverse effect.

The use of spontaneous reports of AEs permits the development of the safety profile of a new drug more rapidly than the use of structured clinical studies. The results of the examination of the first series of cases are usefully presented in various national pharmacovigilance bulletins such as *Current Problems* in the United Kingdom, *ADRAC Bulletin* in Australia, and the U.S. Food and Drug Administration website, or published as articles in medical journals.

CASES IN AN EXPOSED COHORT

Prospectively observed cases in a series of patients exposed to the suspect product. The cohort can be small and chosen for convenience (*convenience cohort*) if the study is limited to one or two hospitals but the cohort could be rather large when health authorities require the manufacturer to undertake surveillance on the first 1000 or more patients exposed to the drug. Alternatively a Prescription Event Monitoring (see PRESCRIPTION EVENT MONITORING) program, as done in the United Kingdom, could be set up.

REGISTRY OF CASES

A listing and tracking of cases that have occurred in a hospital, a region, or a country. The frequency of prior exposure to the suspect drug is measured in the cases in the registry; when a group that did not suffer from the AE in question is constituted to resemble as closely as possible the registry group, it becomes a control group. A registry can be used to verify whether the launch of a new drug is associated with an increased frequency of a particular AE/ADR and, conversely, when a drug is withdrawn from the market to verify whether the frequency of the AE/ADR decreases.

CAUSALITY: THREE TYPES

It is useful to consider three different types of causality:

■ Medical (or case) causality
■ Epidemiologic (statistical) causality
■ Legal causality (liability): civil or criminal

MEDICAL (CASE)

The probability (measured on any scale) that an AE is due to a drug refers to individual *cases* and the assessment of what a clinician would call the *clinical likelihood* that the event was due to the drug. It is usually not possible to make a rigorously precise quantitative assessment. Rather, ordinal (ranking) terms such as *definitely, probably, possibly,* and *unlikely* related to the drug are used in the same way that a clinician makes medical judgments without being absolutely sure in his or her daily practice when treating individual patients. In the case of drugs, the determination of causality is based on predictive criteria (general and specific to the case from epidemiologic and medical knowledge) and on diagnostic criteria (temporal and nontemporal) linked to the adverse effect.

EPIDEMIOLOGIC (STATISTICAL)

Case-control studies, cohort studies, and comparative therapeutic clinical trials can produce results in which a statistically significant difference is seen between patient *groups.* These statistical associations may be considered causal associations inasmuch as the sources of bias have been, at least in theory, eliminated. This type of causality judgment may be applied to groups of patients; it is also used to determine the general prior odds in case causality assessment. For example, if an antihypertensive agent causes cough in 1% of patients exposed, it does not mean that in a particular patient's case the AE "cough" has a 1% chance of being due to the drug; after examining the case risk factors (case prior odds) and the temporal (time to onset, etc.) and nontemporal characteristics (productive vs. dry cough, etc.) of the AE, it could turn out that the confidence in drug cause is less than 1% or more than 95% in this patient's case.

LEGAL

▶ In a Criminal Trial

In general (legal systems obviously differ from country to country), when an accusation of criminal negligence involving a serious or fatal adverse drug event is made, three conditions must be present:

- *Harm* (tort in legal jargon) must have been done.
- An *offense* must have been committed (either by negligence or with criminal intent).
- There must be a *causal link* between the harm and the offense.

In criminal cases the law generally requires a very strong causality link (e.g., nearly 100%, or "beyond any reasonable doubt") before a guilty verdict can be handed down.

▶ In a Civil Trial

The party that has been harmed in a civil suit demands financial compensation from the party alleged to be responsible for the damage. In these situations it is not necessary to have proof "beyond a reasonable doubt"; but rather, "in the weighing of probabilities, the balance of proof must weigh in favor of the drug etiology." This implies that the case causality need only be superior to 50%, a much lower threshold than in criminal cases.

The two views of threshold levels of legal causality (either above 50% or nearly 100%) are markedly different from the approach taken in medical causality in which causality can be "calculated" at any level between 1% and 100% on an infinite scale and where, moreover, confidence intervals may be calculated and sensitivity analyses may be done (at least in Bayesian analyses). Explaining this distinction to judges is difficult; explaining it to juries is nearly impossible.

An interesting article looking at this issue is that by Angell (*N Engl J Med* 1996;334:1513–1518). For a review on the (unique) American legal situation regarding AEs, see the review by Ruger and Willig (Strom 2000).

CAUSALITY SCALE

In case causality assessment, most scales are of the ordinal, ranking type. Six levels are sufficient to summarize the majority of publications on the subject, if we include the class *unknown, unassessable*. For convenience a number may be attached to equivalents in words. The results may be obtained by a questionnaire, algorithm, decision table, bayesian analysis, or clinical intuition of experts:

Level 4	Definite, very probable, certain
Level 3	Probable
Level 2	Possible
Level 1	Improbable, unlikely
Level 0	Unassessable, unassessed, unknown
Level - 1	Excluded, ruled out

In a standard textbook, 36 methods have been counted (Stephens 1999:308).

CENTER FOR BIOLOGICS EVALUATION AND RESEARCH (CBER)

A section of the Food and Drug Administration that evaluates biologic products (as opposed to drug or device products). It is involved in safety issues in pharmacovigilance. It has some 29 offices and divisions including a division of Biostatistics and Epidemiology. It is located in Rockville, Maryland (http://www.fda.gov/cber/index.html).

CENTER FOR DRUG EVALUATION AND RESEARCH (CDER)

A section of the Food and Drug Administration that evaluates drug products (as opposed to biologics or devices). It has an Office of Post-Marketing Drug Risk Assessment (OPDRA), which is further divided into two Divisions of Risk Evaluation. It is located in Rockville, Maryland (http://www.fda.gov/cder).

It has an extensive section on Drug Information at the website (www.fda.gov/cder/drug/default.htm), which includes New Drug Approvals, Consumer Information, Adverse Event Reporting System (AERS) (www.fda.gov/cder/aers/index.htm), the Annual Adverse Drug Experience Report with its summary of FDA's year of pharmacovigilance, Warning Letters, Dear Doctor Letters, and updates on some of the new and controversial drugs recently approved. There is an automatic e-mail notification service of important new drug information; see the website (http://www.fda.gov/cder/cdernew/listserv.html). In addition there is now a CD-ROM subscription service available with quarterly updates of the AERS raw data (www.ntis.gov/fcpc/cpn8762.htm). This information represents a treasure trove of information that anyone working in the field of pharmacovigilance must be familiar with.

CHALLENGE

In pharmacotherapy the word *challenge*, used as a noun or a verb, refers to the exposure of a patient to a particular medication, usually as a valid therapeutic treatment, to determine whether a particular reaction (either positive, producing beneficial effects, or negative producing an ADR) occurs ("We gave the patient with ulcerative colitis a steroid challenge").

Another use of the term *challenge* occurs when the dose of a drug that is suspected of producing a type A (dose-related) adverse reaction is increased ("We've raised the dose of the nonsteroidal anti-inflammatory drug (NSAID) because of his arthritis pain; I hope this challenge doesn't produce any gastric problems").

In pharmacovigilance this term is limited to the exposure preceding the adverse effect being analyzed for drug causality. When the AE has occurred on numerous exposures to the suspect drug, the exposure called the *challenge* will be the one that offers the most complete and valid account (such as the AE being recorded during a hospital stay). The prior exposures are called *prechallenges*. ("He had three prechallenges with steroids last year before the problem arose this year").

This term is also used in contrast to *rechallenge*, which refers to a re-exposure to the drug after an AE has appeared and disappeared. The rechallenge may be done in an attempt to clarify the risk/benefit ratio. Alternatively, the rechallenge may be done knowing that the drug will produce an effect (e.g., thrombocytopenia seen with certain oncologic drugs) but whose benefit outweighs the toxicity. Obviously, in both of these situations the patient's benefit must be the prime reason for the rechallenge and the patient must be very carefully monitored.

Note that allergists often use the term *challenge* or *challenge test* when reintroducing a medication as a diagnostic test, though in fact this constitutes a rechallenge to find out whether the same AE is reproduced. They often use a less dangerous route of administration, such as a skin test.

CHLORAMPHENICOL

This antibiotic is capable of producing aplastic anemia. The signal that this was a possibility first occurred after initial marketing in the 1950s at a time when the formal pharmacovigilance system that exists today was not even "on the radar screen." This observation is of important historical interest because it led the Council on Pharmacy and Chemistry of the American Medical Association (AMA) to create the Committee on Blood Dyscrasias in 1954 to produce a registry of such problems. This registry took over the duty of monitoring all adverse effects in 1961 (Erslev, *JAMA* 1962;181:1140). However, the Food and Drug Administration took over the duty of pharmacovigilance in the United States in 1961 and effectively ended the AMA's role several years later.

The mechanism of the aplastic anemia is probably partly allergic and partly toxic. The confirmation of the signal was done primarily by the registry and then by a case-control trial. Chloramphenicol remains on the market in some countries and is still useful since the risk/benefit ratio is still thought to be positive, as the ADR in question, though serious and sometimes fatal, is quite rare, whereas the drug's efficacy remains good (Wallerstein, *JAMA* 1969;208:2045).

CHRONIC INTERSTITIAL CYSTITIS AS AN UNSUSPECTED ADVERSE DRUG REACTION

Nonsteroidal anti-inflammatory drugs (NSAIDs) such as tiaprofenic acid can rarely produce a drug-induced chronic cystitis that can easily be confused with biopsy-proven aseptic interstitial cystitis. This misdiagnosis can lead to inappropriate and ineffective pharmacologic treatment followed by major urologic surgery (e.g., cystoplasty). The literature reports several cases of unnecessary and sometimes risky surgery. The ADR is not limited to this drug and may occur with other NSAIDs. We mention this ADR because it is a perfect example of *diagnostic interference* when the adverse effect resembles the natural form of the disease (interstitial cystitis) and drugs are not suspected because the ADR is very rare and urologists may not be sufficiently aware of it.

CIOMS I WORKING GROUP

The Council for International Organizations of Medical Sciences (CIOMS) I Working Group, made up of representatives from industry and government created the Expedited Report Form (also known as the *CIOMS I form*) that manufacturers and sponsors must use when submitting ADRs to governmental health authorities. This form is usually used for *15 day reports* or *alert reports* which sponsors must submit for serious and unexpected (*unlabeled* or *unlisted*) adverse effects from foreign countries (see ALERT REPORTS). It is important to note that this form does not include any judgment regarding causality, as is consistent with the precepts enunciated in ICH E2A-CIOMS (see ICH E2A). Another key document with which all those working in pharmacovigilance should be familiar; to order copies see the CIOMS website (http://www.who.int/dsa/cat98/zcioms8.htm).

CIOMS II WORKING GROUP

The Council for International Organizations of Medical Sciences (CIOMS) Working Group proposed the standardization of the format and contents of the periodic reports (see ICH E2C PERIODIC SAFETY UPDATE REPORTS) regarding the safety of marketed drugs that sponsors must submit to the governmental health authorities. It largely corresponds to the E2C document (Periodic Safety Update Reports for Marketed Drugs) published by the International Conference on Harmonization (ICH). (See Final Report of CIOMS Working Group II. International reporting of periodic drug-safety update summaries. Geneva: CIOMS, 1992. 21 pages.) A key document that all those working in pharmacovigilance should be familiar with.

See their website for ordering (http://www.who.int/dsa/cat98/zcioms8.htm).

CIOMS III WORKING GROUP

This Council for International Organizations of Medical Sciences (CIOMS) Working Group proposed the standardization of the pharmacovigilance data that should appear in the Core Safety Data Sheet that contains the basic safety information on a marketed drug. This group also tried to attack the problem of what is the necessary and sufficient amount of data needed to make additions to the Core Safety Data Sheet after marketing. The knotty issue here is that before marketing, the core safety data are (usually) based on controlled clinical trials ("the gold standard"), whereas postmarketing safety data usually consist of uncontrolled spontaneous adverse effect reports with all the inherent problems (confounders, comedications, lack of controls, causality difficult to establish, etc.) therein. It is hard to separate the wheat from the chaff; this report was the first attempt to do so in a formal manner. This document has been superseded by the CIOMS V Working Group Report (Report of CIOMS Working Group III. Guidelines for preparing core clinical-safety information on drugs. Geneva: CIOMS, 1995). See their website for ordering (http://www.who.int/dsa/cat98/zcioms8.htm).

CIOMS IV WORKING GROUP

This Council for International Organizations of Medical Sciences (CIOMS) Working Group took on the difficult task of defining what a pharmacovigilance investigation (inquiry) and signal evaluation should consist of. This evaluation can lead to significant changes in the marketing of a drug (e.g., market withdrawal, loss of an indication, additional adverse effects or warnings in product labeling) if the result of the investigation concludes that the risk/benefit ratio has changed. The report (Benefit-risk balance for marketed drugs: evaluating safety signals. Geneva: CIOMS, 1988, 1998) can be ordered from the CIOMS website (http://www.who.int/dsa/cat98/zcioms8.htm). A key document that all those working in pharmacovigilance should be familiar with, it includes seven case studies of drugs that produced important signals and describes the evaluation and workup that occurred:

- Quinine: allergic hematologic events
- Felbamate: blood dyscrasias
- Dipyrone: agranulocytosis
- Temafloxacin: renal impairment and hypoglycemia in the elderly
- Remoxipride: blood dyscrasias
- Clozapine: agranulocytosis
- Sparfloxacin: phototoxicity

CIOMS V WORKING GROUP

This Council for International Organizations of Medical Sciences (CIOMS) Working Group issued its report covering the minimal drug safety information that should be communicated by manufacturers to physicians and other prescribers in 1999. It describes the Company Core Safety Information document intended for marketed drugs and the Development Core Safety Information as a discrete safety section for Investigator's Brochures. This document supersedes the CIOMS III report and is a key document that everyone in the field of pharmacovigilance should be familiar with (Guidelines for preparing core clinical-safety information on drugs. Geneva: CIOMS, 1999). For information on ordering see the CIOMS website (www.who.int/dsa/cat98/zcioms8.htm).

CLAIMS DATABASE

A health insurance database (either public or private) that includes bills (claims) linked to specific medical, diagonostic, hospital, or pharmaceutical services provided. These databases can be used for pharmacoepidemiologic studies, including: pharmacovigilance, pharmacoeconomic, and drug utilization review. Examples of such databases are Medicaid (U.S., public), Kaiser (U.S., private), and Health Insurance of Quebec & Saskatchewan (Canadian, public). Claims databases may or may not contain actual medical records. If they do not, they can be linked electronically to medical databases containing these patients' medical information. However, the medical data, whether in the claims database or in a linked database, may be of varying completeness (e.g., only inpatient information, no information on over the counter medications, no source documents available).

A claims database should not be confused with a database of medical records such as the General Practice Research Database (GPRD) in Great Britain (see GENERAL PRACTICE RESEARCH DATABASE).

The results obtained from a study done in a database must be interpreted carefully, taking into account the purpose of the database and the way the information was gathered.

CLINICAL EPIDEMIOLOGY

An applied science that examines the determinants and impacts of medical decisions made regarding diagnostic, prognostic, preventative, curative, and palliative procedures. Professor M. Jenicek has proposed calling it simply *clinical science*.

CLINICAL PHARMACOLOGY

Medical science applied to interactions between drugs and the human organism. This interface between pharmacology and human physiology is mainly based on controlled clinical trials in humans done during phases I, II, and III of a drug's development. This term is also used to indicate clinical trials done in humans as opposed to those done in animals (*preclinical trials, animal pharmacology and toxicology*).

CLINICAL RESEARCH ORGANIZATION; CONTRACT RESEARCH ORGANIZATION (CRO)

A private company that does clinical research and handles the methodologic, technical, logistic, analytic, regulatory, and other details of research. The CRO may be contracted by the investigational new drug (IND) holder (see INVESTIGATIONAL NEW DRUG APPLICATION) to plan, perform, prepare and present to the health authorities the complete dossier of the preclinical and clinical trials as well as other data required for the approval of the NDA or marketing application (see MARKETING AUTHORIZATION). Some pharmaceutical companies hire CROs to perform only a part of the process (e.g., setting up sites and monitoring) and others hire CROs to perform all other duties. This is often done (it is believed) to save time and/or money in the development of a new drug without having to hire and train new personnel.

Some CROs are now specializing in various aspects of the drug development process such as handling only pharmacovigilance or only regulatory affairs. There is now a market consolidation of CROs as many small "mom and pop" companies are bought or merged into the fewer and larger remaining ones.

Some pharmaceutical companies are now considering the delegation or "outsourcing" of the pharmacovigilance of a product to a CRO. This practice may be useful for some pharmaceutical companies, particularly small ones with little staff and few resources, but can be risky. In any case, it does not eliminate the legal responsibility and liability of the pharmaceutical company.

CLINICAL TRIAL DRUG SAFETY

The study of AEs/ADRs that occur in the course of clinical research trials or structured studies of a drug in accordance with drug development and/or postmarketing laws and regulations.

CLIOQUINOL: MARKET WITHDRAWAL

This oxyquinoleone-derived amebicide caused a veritable epidemic of subacute myelo-optic neuropathy and produced one of the great dramas of modern pharmacovigilance. In spite of an active pharmacovigilance investigation, there was a long delay until market withdrawal. It was only after major toxicity occurred in Japan in the form of subacute myelo-optic neuropathy that the product was taken off the market. Up to 15% of people with this adverse reaction ended up in wheelchairs and as many as 30% had their vision affected. It was nearly 45 years between the first publication of this adverse reaction in Argentina in 1935 and its market removal in Japan in 1979. It has been estimated that 11,000 people were victims of this adverse reaction in Japan between 1955 and 1970. Such a long delay between the initial reports and market removal is very disquieting. It is hoped that improvements in our pharmacovigilance system since that time will forestall any similar delay.

DISCOVERY OF THE SYNDROME

This compound was first synthesized in Germany at the beginning of the 20th century and was initially sold as a cutaneous disinfectant. It was later used as an intestinal antiseptic for the treatment of diarrhea, including travelers' diarrhea (*turista*). In 1930, this product was first proposed as an intestinal amebicide. It was commercialized in Japan in 1934. In December 1935, two articles written in Spanish were published by the Argentine physicians Grawitz and Barros reporting neurologic complications that followed excessive doses of clioquinol. These two articles were not seen or acted upon by the scientific community. The first reports in animals indicating that convulsions and neurologic disorders can occur in the cat appeared in 1939. In 1944, neurotoxicity was demonstrated in three other species, but these observations were not published. In 1952, Dr. Kiyono in Yomagata described the syndrome of encephalopathy, a peripheral sensory-motor neuropathy, and optic nerve problems.

In 1955, the use of clioquinol began increasing, as did the observation of this neurologic syndrome. This clinical signal began to appear in Japan beginning in 1956. The term subacute myelo-optic neuropathy (SMON) was given to this syndrome during a meeting of Japanese internists held in 1964. The Japanese epidemic was now undeniable.

NEW OBSERVATIONS

In 1965, new reports of animal toxicity appeared. Veterinarians reported convulsions and behavioral changes in dogs and cats taking therapeutic doses of clioquinol. In 1966, an English article reported optic atrophy leading to blindness. In 1967, 1452 additional cases were reported; in the worst cases paralysis or permanent blindness developed. In 1968, 1653 cases and in 1969 another 1240 cases were reported.

REGULATORY ACTIONS

A pharmacovigilance investigation began in 1968. On August 7, 1970, the Japanese report concluded that clioquinol was the cause of this syndrome—15 years after the beginning of the "epidemic." One month later, the Japanese health authorities removed the product from the market along with 186 other halogenated hydroxy-quinolones. The impact on public health was swift and dramatic: only 18 cases were seen in the 3 years after withdrawal. This was truly a "collective positive dechallenge." Similar drops in the syndrome occurred in other countries as the products were withdrawn from the market.

WHY JAPAN?

This epidemic was almost entirely limited to Japan. Only 200 cases were reported outside Japan through 1980. Japanese people who immigrated to South America were spared. Other countries in South East Asia were similarly spared even though they were large users of clioquinol. Several hypotheses have been advanced but none has been proved. The existence of some sort of predisposition is postulated, and, because the mean dose of clioquinol in Japan was higher than in other countries, it is possible that this combination produced the great number of cases. It was known that the most severe of the AEs were dose-related. Others have hypothesized that the Japanese are more susceptible to ADRs in general because their average body weight is less than that in other countries. Others have proposed environmental interactions or a viral cause.

EPILOGUE

In 1982, the sponsor announced its intention to decrease the sale of the product outside Japan gradually. Yet, as late as 1989 clioquinol was still sold in the third world by generic laboratories (Kono R, in Soda T, Editor. Drug induced suffering. Princeton, NJ: Excerpta Medica, 1980:11; Grawitz, *Semana Med* 1935;42:525, in Spanish; Barros, *Semana Med* 1935;42:907, in Spanish; Dukes MNG and Swartz B. Responsibility for drug-induced injury. Amsterdam: Elsevier, 1988:77–79; Claeson, *Br Med J* 1989;299:527; Mann R, Drug-induced disorders of the central nervous system in iatrogenic disease, 3rd edition, D'Arcy P and Griffin J, Editors. London: Oxford, 1986). An examination of the animal data can be found at the website of the Research Defence Society (www.rds-online.org.uk/ethics/clioquin.html).

COCHRANE COLLABORATION AND LIBRARY

The Cochrane Collaboration is an international group of centers dedicated to evidence-based medicine. It developed in response to Dr. Archie Cochrane's call for systematic, up-to-date reviews of all relevant randomized controlled trials in health care. The Cochrane group suggested that the methods used to prepare and maintain reviews of controlled trials in pregnancy and childbirth should be applied more widely (Chalmers, *Br Med J* 1992;305:786; Editorial, *Lancet* 1992;340:1131).

The organization aims to help people make well informed decisions about health care by preparing, maintaining, and ensuring the accessibility of systematic reviews of the effects of health care interventions. The collaboration is built on nine principles:

- Collaborating
- Building on the enthusiasm of individuals
- Preventing duplication
- Minimizing bias
- Keeping up to date
- Ensuring relevance
- Ensuring access
- Improving the quality of its work continually
- Ensuring continuity

The collaboration maintains a computerized collection of data that includes four databases useful in medical decision making by using the principles of *Evidence Based Medicine*:

- A collection of review articles on the effects of health care *(Cochrane Database of Systematic Reviews)*
- A registry of clinical trials, both published and unpublished; references; and summaries *(Cochrane Controlled Trials Register)*
- A collection of critical analyses and structured reviews of the best review articles available worldwide on the efficacy of health care interventions *(York Database of Abstracts of Reviews of Effectiveness)*
- A bibliography on meta-analysis methods *(Cochrane Review Methodology Database)*

This unique electronic library is of great importance in the practice of evidence-based medicine and in health care decision analysis. It also allows pharmacoepidemiologists to obtain information on the AEs seen in the course of clinical trials. It is updated quarterly and is available on CD-ROM or diskette. It is available at multiple websites around the world (http://www.update-software.com/ccweb/cochrane/crgs.htm#CENTRES; in Canada, http://hiru.mcmaster.ca/cochrane/default.html; in the United States, http://www.cochrane.org/: in Australia: http://som.flinders.edu.au/fusa/cochrane/acc/accbroch.htm; in the United Kingdom, http://www.update-software.com/ccweb/default.html).

CODING SYMBOLS FOR THESAURUS OF ADVERSE REACTION TERMS (COSTART)

Used in the past by the U.S. Food and Drug Administration , this is a standardized classification of terms and synonyms used for the coding of AEs. It is available in printed and electronic versions. The FDA has stopped using *COSTART* and is now using *MedDRA* (see *MedDRA*) in pharmacovigilance.

COHORT STUDIES

Observational (i.e., nonexperimental, noninterventional) clinical studies and trials that are structured, analytic, and prospective. They are done in three steps:

- Selection of a group of patients exposed to the suspect drug and the selection of another group (*reference group*) of patients who were not exposed to the suspect drug but who are otherwise reasonably comparable to the exposed group
- Follow-up over time to determine the occurrence of the particular AE under study in each group
- Comparison of the rate of the AE in question by calculating the relative risk and attributable risk in each group

The method of the cohort study can be applied to data that are already in existence and computerized. Medical and pharmacologic data can be cross-linked and analyzed. However, the statistical analysis of such data, originally collected for financial or bureaucratic purposes for medical or pharmacologic studies, should be done with great care and prudence.

It is also possible to do *single cohort* studies composed of only a single group of patients exposed to the suspect drug. This type of "study" cannot really be called an analytic or comparative study since there is no comparison group.

COLLABORATING CENTRE FOR DRUG STATISTICS METHODOLOGY (CCDSM)

This center, located in Oslo, Norway, is responsible for the determination of "defined daily doses" (see DEFINED DAILY DOSE). See the website (http://www.medfarm.unito.it/pharmaco/events/eurodurg.html).

COMMITTEE FOR PROPRIETARY MEDICINAL PRODUCTS (CPMP)

The principal scientific body of the European Medicines Evaluation Agency (EMEA), this committee, made up of representatives from each of the European Union member states and associated states (Norway, Liechtenstein, and Iceland currently), is responsible for the evaluation of new drugs and their Marketing Authorization as well as for pharmacovigilance. It works closely with the national health agencies of its member and associated states. See the EMEA website (http://www.eudra.org/en_home.htm).

COMMITTEE FOR THE SAFETY OF MEDICINES (CSM)

The British governmental department responsible for pharmacovigilance inside the Medicines Control Agency (MCA). "The committee's responsibilities include advising the UK Licensing Authority to ensure that medicines meet the standards of quality, efficacy and safety the public and health professions would expect." See their website (http://www.open.gov.uk/mca/csmhome.htm).

COMPANY CORE DATA SHEET (CCDS)

This document, prepared by the Marketing Authorization holder, is a summary of the key characteristics of the product. It is updated as necessary and accompanies the Periodic Safety Update Reports (PSURs), as described in the ICH E2C proposals. It includes, in addition to pharmacovigilance data, information on indications, dose, pharmacology, and other characteristics. This document (as well as the PSURs) is not always made public though many companies compile a product monograph (see LABELING) that is quite similar and contains much if not all of the information in the CCDS. It includes information (particularly in regard to indications) that is not necessarily applicable in all countries where the product is sold (see CIOMS V).

COMPANY CORE SAFETY INFORMATION (CCSI)

This document contains the entirety of or a summary of the pharmacovigilance section of the Company Core Data Sheet (CCDS). It is intended to be the minimal safety information appearing in the labeling of this product in all the countries of the world where the drug is marketed. The exclusion in one particular country's local labeling of safety information in the CCSI must be justified either by medical or regulatory considerations. For example, a drug interaction could be left out in one country if the drug being interfered with is not marketed there. Alternatively, some national health authorities might not feel the weight of evidence merits the inclusion of a particular AE and thus officially refuse the company's request to list this AE in the local labeling. The CCSI is usually an internal company document maintained by the Marketing Authorization holder and used to aid in the preparation of local national labeling and the Summary of Product Characteristics (see LABELING). It is not always available to the public.

According to the recommendations of ICH E2C this document is used as a reference in preparing the Periodic Safety Update Reports (PSURs) and for determining whether a particular AE is *labeled* or *unlabeled* (*expected* or *unexpected*) for regulatory safety reporting (see CIOMS V).

COMPENDIUM OF PHARMACEUTICALS AND SPECIALITIES (CPS), 35TH EDITION

This large compendium includes all the products available to Canadian prescribers and constitutes a national formulary. Most of the book summarizes or extracts sections of the Company Core Data Sheets (CCDS) or product monograph that the sponsor voluntary submits (Ottawa, Canada: Canadian Pharmaceutical Association, 2001). A CD-ROM version is available; see the website (http://www.cdnpharm.ca/).

COMPLETENESS OF CASE REPORT

The case report of a patient suffering from an AE/ADR may sometimes require a wide range of information if causality is difficult to establish. Some short reports are sufficient in simple cases. The following list of possibly useful data can be checked when a report seems to be a serious signal occurring in complex medical circumstances. Consulting the reporting forms of several manufacturers and of several national schemes locates additional elements that are useful in applied pharmacovigilance (see APPLIED PHARMACOVIGILANCE).

▶ Reporter

Name (printed), signature (if a written form is used), profession, medical specialty, medical license number, address, telephone, fax, e-mail address; all may be useful.

Comment: The identification of the reporter is not a part of the case information but a part of the validation of the case. The medical license number supports the report's validity by eliminating jokesters, charlatans, and malicious reporters; in addition, if the physician has multiple offices this section indicates the office where the patient's records would usually be found. Because of privacy laws, this information may be withheld in some cases.

▶ Report

Date of report, initial or follow-up, who else has been notified (i.e., health authority, manufacturer), case-control number, or identification number assigned by health authority, company, and other information are included.

Comment: These data help to prevent duplicate reporting and allow follow-up reports to be tied to the initial report.

Will the patient (and reporter if other than the patient) allow the authorities to transmit the information elsewhere?

▶ Patient

Identification and demographic characteristics, to include sex, age, birth date, initials, and country.

Comment: This demographic element is important in the comparison of drug use and reporting rates of an AE, among countries. It is also useful in the search for alternative causes of an AE, in which geography may play a role (e.g., the rate of heat prostration with dehydration would be lower in the differential diagnosis of syncope in a case in Norway than in one in a tropical climate). It is also a very important fact to know in examining concomitant medications used,s as these medications are often reported by brand name rather than by generic name. It is thus necessary to search in the compendium from the appropriate country to find out what the product is.

This demographic information is necessary in every AE/ADR report, whether expedited or periodic. It may indicate the country where the AE/ADR occurred and the country where the product was obtained, which may differ. Particular attention should be paid to the country in which the suspect product(s) were obtained as identical trade names may be used for products with different ingredients (both active and excipients). The ICH E2B document notes two special situations:

■ The AE/ADR occurred in a foreign country during the course of a trip that the patient was making, but the medication was obtained in the home country of the patient. The report may originate in the home country or in the country being visited.

■ The suspect product was obtained abroad. It may be necessary in such cases to search out the manufacturer in order to identify the product.

Country Differences in Reporting Rates: An Example

Suprofen was associated with a specific form of "lumbago." It is not clear why a particular syndrome (flank pain syndrome) characterized by lumbar pain and a type of renal colic seen with this new oral nonsteroidal anti-inflammatory drug (NSAID) was rapidly reported in the United States but passed unnoticed in Europe. The reason may be that a large number of samples were given to U.S. physicians, who used the samples themselves rather than giving them to their patients. It is worth noting also that when the AE/ADR is experienced by the physicians themselves, they are rapid and exemplary reporters of AEs! The oral forms of the product were voluntarily withdrawn from the U.S. market in May 1987 (Rossi, JAMA 1988;259:1203).

Comments About Age

For adults, the age in years at the *beginning* of the AE should be noted. The Food and Drug Administration suggests the following units for infants:

Age	Units
< 3 years old	Months
< 1 year old	Months, weeks, days
< 1 month old	Days
Newborns	Hours

The birth date is useful for ruling out duplicate reports and for validating the age at reaction onset. The age and sex may be risk factors for or against a drug-related cause.

▶ Case or chart number

Case or chart number (office/hospital), weight, height, race, occupation, parity, date of last menstrual period (to calculate the beginning of the pregnancy) are listed.

Comment: The case number is necessary to record follow-up information correctly when it is requested and received from the clinician and when the course or outcome of the event necessitates additional testing or visits to the physician. Weight is mainly useful at the "extremes of life" (babies and the elderly), when the pharmacokinetics and dose are risk factors for an ADR. Height in adults is useful only if the calculation of the degree of obesity/cachexia is done and is a risk factor; in babies, height is useful to follow the growth of the child. Race and ethnicity may be useful in relation to alternate causes that might produce a problem of increased susceptibility (e.g., thalassemia). Occupation may be useful if workplace exposure to toxins or allergens is an issue. Parity and date of last menstrual period are useful in teratovigilance and in the context of assisted pregnancy.

▶ Prior ADR History

Previous use of the suspect product followed by the AE/ADR in question? If yes, this is a positive prechallenge and the details of this occurrence should be included.

Previous use of the suspect product without reaction? If this is the case, this is a negative prechallenge.

Same reaction with a different suspect product? If yes, this can be a case of a cross reaction or "cross intolerance."

Same AE without exposure to a drug product? If yes, this represents an argument in favor of an alternate cause of the current AE.

▶ **Chronology of the AE/ADR**

Time to onset

Time from the first dose or from the last dose (as applicable)

Time from a single, unique dose (if applicable)

Dates of the critical doses (first/last/unique) (see CRITICAL DOSE)

Dechallenge

Cessation or reduction of the suspect product? No, unknown, yes

If yes, date of cessation or reduction; improvement of the reaction: yes (positive dechallenge), no (negative dechallenge); if yes, date of the beginning of the improvement, date of complete disappearance, calculation of the time to improvement and time to disappearance

Rechallenge

Reintroduction of the suspect product? If yes, date of restarting and dose used in reintroduction

Reappearance of the reaction? Yes (positive rechallenge) or no (negative rechallenge); if yes, date of reappearance and calculation of the time to reappearance and time to disappearance if drug is stopped again

▶ **Medical Condition and Past Medical History**
Weight, functional status of the key organ systems (renal, hepatic, immunologic, cardiovascular, respiratory, cerebral, etc.), as well as genetic and enzyme abnormalities, alcohol and tobacco use, exercise, sun exposure, hydration, nutritional status, and other factors

Concomitant medical problems: acute, chronic, recurrent, subclinical, in remission, other

▶ **Search for Alternative Etiologies (Hypotheses)**
Current illness (i.e., the indication for the use of the suspect product), new illness, underlying, subclinical, intercurrent, concurrent, latent

Concomitant medications: indication, name, dose, start and stop dates, including prescription drugs, over the counter (OTC) products, "natural products," medicinal herbs, homeopathic products, and illicit drugs (the indication for each concomitant product aids in understanding of the global medical condition of the patient; the medical reviewer may decide to consider a concomitant medication as a suspect medication or as a part of a drug-drug interaction)

Concomitant interventions: surgery, anesthesia, dialysis, others

▶ **Examination of Risk Factors in Favor of a Drug Cause, related to the use of the suspect product**

Excessive dose (if the pharmacologic effect is dose-related)

Excessive duration of treatment

Administration too rapid

Incorrect administration (Blood level of the suspect product, if taken may be useful to confirm excessive dosage.)

▶ **Examination of Risk Factors in Favor of a Drug Cause, related to the underlying status of the patient**

Organ dysfunction: renal or hepatic insufficiency, other

Genetic predisposition (enzyme deficiency, etc.)

Nutritional issues (alcohol, dehydration, obesity)

Physiologic state: pregnant, nursing mother, newborn

Drug-drug interaction

Allergies: previous history, testing

Medical device issues (hemodialysis, etc.)

SUSPECT PRODUCT

The following information is useful: Trade name, generic name, manufacturer, formulation (capsule, gel cap, suspension, solution etc.), route of administration, single-dose unit, daily dose, prn dose, compliance with prescribed and labeled instructions, total cumulative dose taken, total duration of treatment, blood level in case of autopsy, massive overdose, and/or narrow therapeutic index (window) lot number.

ADVERSE EVENT

The event and its course (including dechallenges and rechallenges) are detailed:

Medical term or syndrome or major manifestations, medical coding (*MedDRA*, *WHO-ART*, or *COSTART*), start date, date of beginning of improvement or date of ending of the AE, calculation of total duration of the reaction, and, if applicable, details of treatment given for the AE

Pertinent laboratory test results: date, units, type of test, result, normal values

Details of lab tests done for repeated analyses

Before the first dose (reference value)

First abnormal result (to calculate the time to appearance)

Most abnormal result (to evaluate the severity)

Last abnormal result (to calculate the duration of the reaction)

First improved result (to calculate the time to disappearance)

First normal results

OUTCOME

Classification as serious or nonserious according to the regulatory criteria in force

Outcome of the reaction in the case report: recovered, not recovered, unknown

Details of the disability, hospitalization, death (in the case of death: circumstances, autopsy results, reported causes of death, date of death)

For hospitalization: copy of the discharge summary

Description of the treatment required to prevent disability, hospitalization, or death.

COMPLIANCE

IN PHARMACOTHERAPY

The degree of compliance of the patient in taking his or her prescribed medication; that is, the degree to which the patient followed the prescriber's instructions regarding dose, scheduling, use with or without food, and so on. Compliance is a function of many factors, one of which is ADRs. An ADR, even if mild and of no significant medical consequence (such as a dry cough), can be ruinous for compliance. In general, compliance is not rigidly accounted for in normal clinical outpatient practice. The patient is usually quizzed qualitatively about his or her compliance. Rarely does the physician or pharmacist ask that the bottles of medications be returned so that the contents can be counted at each visit. On the other hand, inpatients and those in clinical trials usually are subject to rigid compliance checks.

The level of discontinuation of a prescribed drug can be used as an index of the lack of satisfaction with the product, although the following example concerning cessation of treatment for hyperlipidemias indicates lack of satisfaction may be only partly due to ADRs.

> A study using linked databases by two American health insurance companies identified 2369 patients taking medications for hyperlipidemia. The likelihood of stopping treatment during the first year was examined. The probabilities for stopping were 46% for niacin, 41% for cholestyramine, 37% for gemfibrozil, and 15% for lovastatin. In 56% of the cases, ADRs were considered as risk factors for abandonment of treatment and in 18% as the primary reason for stopping. (Andrade, *N Engl J Med* 1995;332:1125)

IN CLINICAL PHARMACOLOGY AND CLINICAL TRIALS

The same definition applies, except that the patient is receiving experimental pharmacotherapy. In clinical trials, there is rigid control; all drugs dispensed are counted and compliance percentages calculated. Unused drugs must be returned. During such trials, compliance measures must be made and taken into account during the statistical analyses and interpretation of the results—both statistically and pragmatically. Drug blood and urine levels, measured to study pharmacokinetics, are also used to estimate compliance.

Note that *protocol compliance* refers to other requirements of the study in addition to just the medication.

Levels of compliance can also be used as surrogate markers for subjective ADRs. That is, the less the compliance, the more likely that the subjective ADRs were troubling to the patients.

> During clinical trials of antihypertensors, compliance can be used as a surrogate marker for symptomatic ADRs. It is generally felt that good compliance reflects the absence of any significant unfavorable effects on quality of life. (Boissel, *J Hypertens* 1995;13:1059)

CONCENTRATION SITE REACTION

This type of reaction is rare. They may have very long latency periods. They are characterized by an ADR at the site or in the organ where the drug is concentrated, metabolized, or excreted. Here are four body sites as examples of such concentration.

IN THE THYROID

Radioactive iodine administered for hyperthyroid disease may cause hypothyroidism many years later after the iodine is concentrated in the thyroid.

IN THE KIDNEYS

The diuretic triamterene can be concentrated in the kidney and produce a nephropathy. Indinavir can produce crystalluria and calculi leading to renal colic, renal insufficiency, and renal failure.

IN THE BRAIN

Concentrations of silver in the brain and plasma at levels over 100 times normal produced coma in a patient with end-stage kidney disease after 2 weeks of treatment with silver sulfadiazine for second degree burns. At autopsy, profoundly elevated levels of silver were found in brain tissue (Iwasaki, *Am J Kidney Dis* 1997;30:287).

IN THE GALL BLADDER

Ceftriaxone can precipitate in the gall bladder as a calcium salt and produce calculi (*pseudolithiasis*), which can be detected on echography. The latency period can be very short.

Dipyrimadole can be found as gallstones after prolonged usage (mean 10 years). An 85-year-old female was hospitalized, and a biliary calculus that contained 70% dipyrimadole was noted. She had been taking this product for 15 years (Moesch, *Lancet* 1992;340:1352; Editors, *Prescrire Int* 1999;8(39):20).

CONCOMITANT INTERVENTIONS

In the context of an ADR case report, the investigation of the event must include all medical interventions that might be possible alternative causes of the event. These concomitant possibilities are of two types:

> *Pharmacologic:* concomitant medications particularly polymedication, over the counter (OTC) products, "natural" products, nutritional supplements, medicinal plants, use of illicit drugs, and others

> *Nonpharmacologic:* food, alcohol, hydration, surgery, hospitalization, bed rest, posture, stress, exercise, sun exposure, hemodialysis, plasmaphersis, transfusion, and others

CONCOMITANT MEDICATION

In the context of an ADR case report, any pharmaceutical product that is not suspected of having caused the event but was taken (shortly) *before* the event occurred is considered to be a concomitant medication. How much time is "shortly before"? That depends on the kinetics of the drug and the boundaries of the temporal window between the consumption of the drug and the appearance of the AE. Concomitant medications must be distinguished from *suspect medications* as well as antidotes or other drugs given to treat the AE. These three types of medications must be noted on the ADR case reporting form (e.g., CIOMS I form) to amass the optimal information to evaluate the event.

CONSUMER ADVOCACY GROUPS

Associations of consumers may put pressure on the health authorities or pharmaceutical companies to make the use of drugs safer. Their philosophy is that one is best served by oneself, and their views of companies and health agencies may vary from "trust but verify" to "trust nobody."

Public Citizen/Health Research Group, a well-known group in the United States (Dr. Sidney Wolfe) that publishes *Worst Pills–Best Pills* for the general public (www.citizen.org)

Health Action International, which publishes the bulletin *Problem Drugs* (www.haiweb.org)

Consumers' Association, a British association (www.which.net)

DES-Action, a mutual aid association for women exposed to DES in utero and their descendents (www.desaction.org)

Social Audit, a British group headed by Charles Medawar, an investigative journalist and author (www.socialaudit.org.uk/)

Medical Lobby for Appropriate Marketing (MALAM), a consumer organization whose aim is to induce manufacturers to produce better balanced advertising and drug monographs that clearly inform the user of risks, warnings, and problems seen with the product (www.camtech.net.au/malam/)

CONTINUING MEDICAL EDUCATION

The lack of initial and continuing pharmacovigilance education is a major shortcoming in the medical education systems in a majority of countries. A brief introduction should constitute an essential element in the initial undergraduate curriculum, and continuing training should be provided to medical professionals who deal with pharmacotherapy, such as prescribers, dispensers, diagnosticians, and therapists of adverse effects, medical educators, hospital administrators, and drug insurance scheme consultants. Pharmacovigilance should be part of any graduate course in pharmacoepidemiology.

CONTROVERSY

In pharmacovigilance, a signal may produce major controversy when one or more of the following occurs:

- The signal is difficult to confirm or disprove.
- A very early signal (e.g., one based on epidemiologic data of questionable quality) gets significant play and publicity in the lay or medical press before the proper pharmacovigilance investigation can be performed.
- Confirmation of the signal may produce an addition to the label of a new AE, a new warning, or a new precaution, leading to decreasing sales or even market withdrawal.
- Unconfirmed signals or "accusations" circulate in the media or on the Internet.

The controversies may be scientific (conflicting or contradictory evidence or interpretations of the evidence), administrative (regulations differing from one country to another), legal (lawsuits pursued by individuals or groups), and media-associated.

CORRECTIVE MEASURES; TREATMENT OF THE ADVERSE EVENT/ADVERSE DRUG REACTION

A clinician who observes an AE in a patient who is being treated with medication and suspects that one of the drugs may be causally associated with the problem can take corrective measures in the best interests of the patient:

Definitive cessation of the suspect product

Dosage reduction

Change in the route of administration

Cessation of the suspect product

Substitution of

Another product with a similar mode of action from the same drug class

Another product with the same active ingredient

Another product from a different class of drugs

Cessation of the product followed by intentional rechallenge, to confirm the diagnosis of a drug-induced AE, if appropriate

Continuation of the treatment when it is deemed unacceptable to stop it (i.e., the risk/benefit ratio is still in favor of treatment)

Continuation of the treatment without stopping even briefly because it is deemed unacceptable to stop it (i.e., the risk/benefit ratio is still in favor of treatment)

Addition of a drug (treatment) to correct the AE/ADR (e.g., a specific or nonspecific antagonist)

Cessation of the product and addition of a corrective treatment of the AE/ADR

COUNCIL FOR INTERNATIONAL ORGANIZATIONS OF MEDICAL SCIENCES (CIOMS)

An international nongovernmental committee formed in 1949 under the auspices of the World Health Organization (WHO) and (UNESCO). Working groups that dealt with AEs have been designated CIOMS I, II, III, IV, and V. Several documents on the conclusions of these working groups have been published. In particular the documents covering CIOMS I, II, IV, and V should be familiar to anyone working in the field of pharmacovigilance. CIOMS can be contacted at its headquarters, CIOMS, WHO, avenue Appia, CH-1211 Geneva 27, Switzerland (www.who.int/dsa/cat98/zcioms8.htm).

COURSE

This term can refer to the pharmacologic treatment, to the AE/reaction and to the outcome of the AE/ADR:

PHARMACOLOGIC TREATMENT
The *treatment course* here refers to the duration of the treatment or cycle for an individual patient.

EVENT

The course of the event is a temporal characteristic; its duration in relation to the suspect drug administration (challenge, dechallenge) is an important criterion for causality determination.

OUTCOME IN A BROAD SENSE

The *course* (or *hospital course* if the patient is hospitalized) here refers to what happens to the particular patient after the event has occurred. It includes subsequent procedures, secondary events, treatments of the AE, lab tests required to assess the AE, and other factors, as well as other aspects of the outcome: recovered, not recovered, unknown, hospitalized, died. This information helps to determine the severity of the AE.

CREUTZFELDT-JACOB SYNDROME

A fatal spongiform encephalopathy presumably due to a prion and characterized by a long (8 to 15 years) latency period resulting from pharmacotherapy with growth hormone derived from human cadavers before the development and use of synthetic somatotrophin around 1988. A closely related syndrome was described in Great Britain and Europe during the epidemic of Mad Cow Disease starting in the late 1990s, a matter of growing concern in Europe.

CRISIS IN DRUG SAFETY

A pharmaceutical company can face a crisis when a series of unexpected AEs/reactions occurs in a short period whose seriousness, if confirmed, would throw into question the risk/benefit ratio. The crisis is usually provoked by a signal from spontaneously reported AEs. This is most likely to occur after a new drug is launched in a country that has a strong and well-developed system of pharmacovigilance. The company must move into "crisis management" mode. It must begin an immediate pharmacovigilance investigation to confirm or disprove the signal. Simultaneously the company must negotiate with the health authorities (often in multiple countries), prepare responses to questions from journalists and the public, prepare for possible legal action, and prepare for the implementation of regulatory measures that may be required to maintain the safe use of the product.

The term *crisis* also has a broader meaning, as exemplified by a recent DIA workshop on this topic, in which the following situations were given as possible examples: "new animal studies showing additional toxicity, changes in risk/benefit ratio, government call for additional data or unannounced inspection, media reports, tampering or extortion, consumer group allegation."

CRITICAL DOSE

The dose used to calculate the interval from drug exposure to the appearance of the ADR (see TIME TO ONSET).

CURRENT CONTENTS

This bulletin is a collection of the tables of contents of scientific and medical journals, published by the Institute for Scientific Information. Consultation of *Current Contents* is essential to any systematic and complete collection of AEs on an ongoing basis. *Current Contents* is also useful for examining letters to the editor, which are found in the tables of contents, but are often not found in other automated databases of the published literature (www.isinet.com/isi/products/cc/ccconnect).

CURRENT PROBLEMS IN PHARMACOVIGILANCE

The respected British national bulletin of pharmacovigilance. The four to six page periodical is published three or four times a year by the Committee for Safety of Medicines (CSM) and the Medicines Control Agency (MCA). For information, contact Editor, Current Problems in Pharmacovigilance, Medicines Control Agency, Market Towers, 1, Nine Elms Lane, London SW8 5NQ, UK. It is now available on the Internet (www.open.gov.uk/mca/cuprblms.htm).

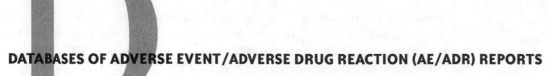

DATABASES OF ADVERSE EVENT/ADVERSE DRUG REACTION (AE/ADR) REPORTS

Also called *pharmacovigilance databases*. All pharmacovigilance units—be they academic, governmental, or industrial—must maintain a computerized database for spontaneous reports from health care professionals (and, in some countries, consumers) who have made case reports of AEs that they suspect may be of drug related origin. Reference to these databases is required in pharmacovigilance investigations that all pharmacovigilance units are obliged to do on various occasions. The largest database in the world is that of the World Health Organization's Uppsala Monitoring Centre, which is a depository of listings of information from the national databases of participating countries. For each individual branded product the largest database is that of the manufacturer. Most units are also obliged to maintain computerized databases of clinical trial AEs for regulatory reporting purposes.

Each country that maintains a governmental pharmacovigilance structure, whether centralized as in the United States or regional as in France, has a *national database*. One issue is the lack of transparency of data. Most of the databases, whether governmental or industrial, are confidential. Most databases maintained by pharmaceutical companies are considered to be proprietary and thus secret. Many governmental databases are also considered secret and allow minimal or no access at all to the general public. Two significant exceptions exist. The first is the U.S. Food and Drug Administration database, which makes spontaneous AE data available to the public either directly from the U.S. government (from whom one can obtain line listings and individual MedWatch forms for a nominal cost) or at its website, where line listings are available as (enormously large) files that must be downloaded to be used, or on CD-ROMs that are updated regularly. The second is the WHO database in Uppsala, Sweden. Line listings are available from this database either as hard copy or directly on-line for a nominal cost. However, these data are less complete as only line listings are available (CIOMS I or MedWatch forms are not available); furthermore, some participating governments do not allow their data to be made public.

DATA CUT-OFF POINT; DATA LOCK-POINT

A regulatory term used regarding Periodic Safety Update Reports (as defined in ICH E2C) or, in the United States, IND annual and NDA periodic reports. It refers to the last day in the period covered by the report. The duration of the period is usually 3 months, 6 months, 1 year, or 5 years, usually depending on the original approval date (*birth date*). The report is usually due in the health authority 30, 60, or 90 days after the data lock-point. The health authority, however, has the right to alter the duration and the preparation time as they see fit.

DATA SHEET

The British term for the official product monograph, Summary of Product Characteristics (SPC or SmPC), labeling; the ADRs mentioned in these documents are considered *labeled*.

DATA SHEET COMPENDIUM

The British national compendium of drugs, produced by the Association of the British Pharmaceutical Industry (ABPI).

DEAR DOCTOR LETTER (DEAR PHARMACIST LETTER, DEAR HEALTH CARE PROFESSIONAL LETTER)

A letter mailed to some or all of the target audience with the aim of rapidly and immediately informing the readers of a safety concern about a product. Two objectives are possible.

A CALL FOR THE REPORTING OF A SPECIFIC ADVERSE EVENT/ADR

This type of active pharmacovigilance (*prompted reporting*) is aimed at an important signal that must be confirmed, supported, or rejected. Health care professionals are requested to notify the authorities of all observations of the particular AE/ADR in question. This request is part of a safety signal evaluation.

A SAFETY WARNING MESSAGE

This type of letter is written far more often and takes the form of a warning to prescribers. It informs health professionals of an important safety problem that was recently discovered or confirmed. The letter usually describes the reaction and proposes the means to prevent it, to detect it, and/or to treat it. The letter may be written by health authorities or by a pharmaceutical company. The letter may also limit the usage in certain groups at risk or may remove or limit an indication. Such a letter might be one of the measures taken after a pharmacovigilance investigation. In many countries the format, color, font size, and other features of the letter are specifically regulated. Often the letter must be approved by the health authority before its release. In addition to the mailing of the letter to health professionals, many authorities are now posting the letters on their own websites or on pharmacovigilance websites.

▶ **Some American Examples**

In July 2000, a letter to health professionals was sent out to note an update to the Warnings section of a brand of divalproex sodium delayed-release tablets indicating that cases of life-threatening pancreatitis have been seen in adults and children taking valproate (www.fda.gov/medwatch/safety/2000/depako.pdf). Also in July 2000, health professionals were notified of severe hypersensitivity reactions that followed reintroduction with abacavir sulfate (www.fda.gov/medwatch/safety/2000/ziagen1.htm). In January 2000, a letter was sent to health care professionals regarding cisapride, noting changes to the Boxed Warning, Drug Interactions, and Dosage and Administration. The changes included the recommendation that a 12-lead electrocardiogram (ECG) should be obtained before administration, that cisapride should not be initiated if the QTc value exceeds 450 milliseconds, that it is contraindicated in patients with electrolyte disorders, and that levels of serum electrolytes should be assessed in diuretic-treated patients before initiating cisapride and periodically thereafter (www.fda.gov/medwatch/safety/2000/propul.htm).

These letters are available on the FDA website, and a free notification e-mail service is also available (www.fda.gov).

▶ **A Few British Examples**

In 1986 the CSM required the mailing of a letter to discourage pediatricians from using aspirin because of risk of Reye's syndrome and to remind allergists of the danger of anaphylaxis from allergy desensitizers. In 1990 a letter was posted to announce the withdrawal of L-tryptophan from the market and in 1991 a letter was sent to warn of the cardiotoxicity of terodiline. In 1993 a letter went out noting the cases of colonic stenosis in infants with mucoviscidosis after the use of pancreatin combinations high in lipase and reminding prescribers of the risk factors for thromboemboli in women using combination birth control pills (Waller, PEDS 1996;5;363).

UK information is available on the British Committee Safety of Medicines website (www.open.gov.uk/mca/csmhome.htm). Safety alerts from the French agency are also available on their website (http://agmed.sante.gouv.fr/).

DEATH, RELATED

This expression designates the consequences and outcome of an AE/ADR. It implies three notions:

- An outcome: death
- A suspicion of causality between the AE/ADR and the death
- A suspicion of causality between the product in question and the AE (i.e., it is an ADR, not only an AE)

There is a double causality judgment here and the strength of the judgment of causality can differ in second and third points. For example, a death would probably be unrelated if the person died of a ruptured cerebral aneurysm while reading the newspaper a week after receiving a flu vaccine even if an ADR (e.g., fever) that was due to the vaccine occurred immediately after vaccination. The following example shows the thread inexorably linking death to a simple constipation induced by narcotics:

> A coroner's inquest in Toronto, Canada, done after the death of a 31-year-old female, attributed her death to a septicemia that followed peritonitis due to the rupture of her sigmoid colon from severe constipation due to prolonged usage of several constipating narcotic analgesics (Ontario Medical Association, *Drug Rep* 1994;49). In this report, the primary ADR is constipation. The death is the outcome. The likelihood of a drug-related cause of the constipation is very high. The contribution of the narcotics in the death was tempered by several risk factors.

FREQUENCY OF DEATH RELATED TO MEDICATION USE IN THE POPULATION

The true level of death due to medication in the general population is not known for several reasons:

> The level of underreporting of drug-related fatalities is high and variable, sometimes attaining 100%. Oncologists, for example, usually do not notify the manufacturers or health authorities of drug-related deaths though it is clear that a significant number of their patients die of the effects of chemotherapy.

> The level of medication use in the general population is not known and is poorly estimated at best.

> It is also not clear how to calculate risk in a way that is meaningful to the clinician. A patient who takes a few doses a year of a drug (e.g., an antihistamine for seasonal allergic rhinitis) cannot be counted with the same weight as someone who takes it daily (e.g., for perennial rhinitis). To try to get around

this, statisticians convert the data, where available, into episodes of "AEs per patient-days of exposure." This method allows relative comparisons of drugs but does not always aid the clinician in deciding a specific patient's risk.

The level of drug-related deaths in the hospital is higher than in the outpatient population because of the severity of the diseases for which these patients are being treated and because of the "polypharmacy" they undergo. There may also be more reporting of hospital-based AEs and deaths than of outpatient AEs and deaths.

FREQUENCY OF DEATH IN PHARMACOVIGILANCE DATABASES

In various publications, the level of fatalities in spontaneously reported AEs hovers around 2%:

In Ontario, Canada, 1% (Gowdey, *Can Med Assoc J* 1985;132:19)

In the United States, 2% (Faich, *JAMA* 1989;257:2068)

In Quebec, Canada, 2% (Biron, *Thérapie* 1996;51:578, English abstract)

In France, 2% (Moore, *Thérapie* 1995;50:557, English abstract)

In Canada, 2.3% (Mittmann, *PEDS* 1997;6:157)

Data of these kinds cannot be used as a substitute for the true level of drug related mortality in a population, which can only be obtained from observational studies (which are very difficult to perform). The rare studies that are done to look at drug-related deaths are usually limited to inpatient studies.

DECHALLENGE, COURSE UPON

This concept has two components. The first is qualitative and refers to severity of the event and whether it improves or worsens. The second is quantitative and refers to the duration or persistence of the AE/ADR after the suspect drug was last taken (and then stopped) or after the dosage of the suspect drug was lowered (for those ADRs that are dose dependent). A very close synonym is *outcome*, which is more rigorously defined by the Council for International Organizations of Medical Sciences (see CIOMS).

The AE/ADR can have the following courses:

- Worsening
- Persisting
- Abating (improving)
- Disappearing (resolving)

The correct interpretation of the evolution of the dechallenge can be a true diagnostic challenge and requires the clinician to be familiar not only with the medical assessment of the patient but also with the disease or event in question and with the profile of *the suspect drug* or drugs. It is worth reading the Yale questionnaire (Kramer, *JAMA* 1979;242:623).

DECHALLENGE, DISCONTINUATION

In case causality assessment, the cessation (stopping) of the administration of the product in question. Dechallenge may sometimes be used to designate a simple reduction in the dose of the suspect product without completely stopping it. This may occur if the ADR is dose-dependent and regresses or stops after this dosage change. The term *discontinuation,* however, is not used to indicate a decrease in dosage.

If the ADR disappears after a dechallenge or discontinuation it is said to be a *positive dechallenge* and if it does not disappear it is a *negative dechallenge.*

DECHALLENGE, INCONCLUSIVE

This is a medical judgment. A dechallenge is said to be inconclusive if

The patient improves but the improvement is felt to be "spontaneous" (e.g., a headache improves spontaneously a few hours after taking a suspect drug and without any treatment).

The problem persists but is "pathophysiologically" irreversible (e.g., the patient has a stroke and the neurologic damage does not improve significantly).

The event disappears coincident with treatment given for it (e.g., a patient develops anginal chest pain for which nitroglycerin is given, producing relief of pain).

The adverse event/reaction is a "one time only" occurrence that cannot abate (e.g., a myocardial infarct whose symptoms may abate though the infarct, itself, remains).

It is mistakenly made without allowing sufficient time for the drug to be cleared or for the AE/ADR to abate (e.g., digoxin toxicity persists longer than expected if its long half-life is forgotten).

Follow-up is inadequate or is not possible.

There is no clear way to measure, quantitate, or track the AE.

DECHALLENGE, NEGATIVE

This determination is a medical judgment that is made when a (theoretically) reversible adverse reaction persists in spite of discontinuation of the suspect drug. In making this decision it is necessary to take into account the natural course of the event and the pharmacokinetics of the suspect drug.

A negative dechallenge is said to occur if the event worsens or persists, presuming that the pathophysiologic characteristics of the event and the pharmacokinetics of the drug allow improvement. That is, if the event were irreversible (e.g., a myocardial infarction) or the kinetics indicate persistence of the drug (e.g., digoxin or a depot preparation of a drug), then a negative dechallenge may be harder to define.

A negative dechallenge may argue against a drug causality of the adverse effect.

DECHALLENGE, POSITIVE

This is a medical judgment that is made when a (theoretically) reversible adverse reaction regresses or disappears after the suspect drug is stopped. A positive dechallenge is usually an argument in favor of a causality due to the suspect drug. It is necessary to be careful not to ascribe too much weight to positive dechallenges when factors other than the suspect drug may be acting, such as the following:

The event is naturally transient (e.g., a headache).

The event may have been due to other medications that were stopped at the same time.

Treatments that were administered may have caused the abatement of the event.

The kinetics of the suspect drug are such that the abatement of the event is unlikely to be a true positive dechallenge (e.g., the rapid disappearance of an arrhythmia presumed to be due to a digoxin overdose)

DECHALLENGE, COLLECTIVE (OR POPULATIONAL)

By analogy to the stopping of a drug in an individual patient, a *collective dechallenge* refers to the withdrawal of a product from the market that forces all patients taking the drug to stop. A positive collective dechallenge has occurred if the event in question disappears from the population after withdrawal, as demonstrated by public health statistics, registry information, a case-control study, or a secular trend. A positive collective dechallenge argues in favor of a drug cause of the event.

- The withdrawal of thalidomide from the market was followed by a return to the baseline incidence of phocomelia.
- Clear cell cancer of the vagina became a rare event after the cessation of the use of DES in pregnant women (see DIETHYLSTILBESTROL).
- Cases of pulmonary hypertension dropped markedly in Switzerland after the market withdrawal of Aminorex.
- The withdrawal of clioquinol ended the epidemic of SMON in Japan (see CLIOQUINOL).

DEFINED DAILY DOSE (DDD)

The daily maintenance dose recommended in the adult for the primary indication of the drug. The dose represents one day of treatment for one person in the population. The World Health Organization (WHO), uses the DDD per 1000 inhabitants as an international unit for comparing the consumption from country to country. Because the reality is sometimes different and the concept of the *mean daily dose* has been developed. The determination of the DDD is done by the WHO Collaborating Centre for Drug Statistics Methodology in Oslo, Norway.

DEFINITIONS BY CONSENSUS

Following an earlier French model, the Council for International Organizations of Medical Sciences (CIOMS), the World Health Organization (WHO) and several pharmaceutical companies began holding international conferences with the aim of preparing consensus definitions of various AEs. They attempted to define them both qualitatively (nature of the event) and quantitatively (severity of the event) by using three criteria: risk of misinterpretation, importance, and frequency of appearance in databases. The selection was done by using high-level critical terms from WHO and preferred terms in the *WHO-ART* dictionary (Bénichou, *Drug Inf J* 1989;23:71 and 1991;25:251). The following are a few published articles:

- Digestion: hemorrhagic colitis, ulcers, pancreatitis (*PEDS* 1992;1:133)
- Circulation: anaphylactic shock, arrhythmias, cardiac failure, hypertension, thrombosis, embolus (*PEDS* 1992;1:39); cardiovascular disease terms (*PEDS* 1993;2:591)
- Liver: (*J Hepatol* 1990;11:272 and *Int J Clin Pharmacol Ther Toxicol* 1990;28:317)
- Skin: Photosensitivity: principal skin toxicities (CIOMS, *PEDS* 1997;6:115)
- Lungs: principal problems (CIOMS, *PEDS* 1997;6:115)

- Urinary system: principal problems (CIOMS, *PEDS* 1997;6:203)
- Blood: medullary aplasia and hypoplasia, coagulation problems, agranulocytosis, thrombophlebitis (CIOMS. *PEDS* 1992;1:191); cytopenias (Bénichou, *Int J Clin Pharmacol Ther Toxicol* 1991;29:75)
- Nervous system: dyskinesias, depression, myopathy, neuropathy, paralysis, convulsions (CIOMS, *PEDS* 1993;2:149)
- Eyes: visual disturbances, keratitis, cataracts, retinopathies (CIOMS, *PEDS* 1993;2:189)

Here are a few examples of ADR definitions by consensus:

DYSPNEA
Awareness by the patient of difficulty in breathing. It can be the result of a medication that produces bronchoconstriction, laryngeal edema, cardiac failure, or psychiatric symptoms.

INTERSTITIAL LUNG DISEASE
The presence of inflammatory cells or other abnormal substances in the interstitium of the lung. It is usually diagnosed radiologically. It can be produced, for example, by bleomycin, gold salts, amiodarone, or sulfonamide antibiotics (CIOMS, *PEDS* 1997;6:115).

PNEUMONITIS
Noninfectious pulmonary inflammation producing a diffuse alveolitis or a slowly progressive fibrosis (CIOMS, *PEDS* 1997;6:115). As an example, a thiazide diuretic can be rarely associated with an acute pneumonitis that presents as pulmonary edema (Biron, *Can Med Assoc J* 1991;145:28).

PSEUDOMEMBRANOUS COLITIS
This iatrogenic disease (which has a characteristic colonoscopic appearance) associated with the prior use of antibiotics should not be confused with a simple diarrhea. Pseudomembranous colitis has been defined by the following three criteria:

The *severity* of the diarrhea and

The presence in the stool of the cytotoxin of *Clostridium difficile* or

The presence of pseudomembranes on sigmoidoscopy

AGRANULOCYTOSIS
A frequently used term in hematovigilance, it designates a cytopenia that affects the white blood cell granulocyte line. The criteria for diagnosis have been defined as follows:

An acute, severe, and isolated neutropenia defined as a polymorphonuclear neutrophil count less than 500,00/l (0.5 x 10^9/l)

Without anemia (hemoglobinemia greater than 100g/l)

Without thrombocytopenia (platelet count greater than 100 million/l) (CIOMS, *PEDS* 1992;1:1911; Bénichou, *Int J Clin Pharmacol Ther Toxicol* 1991;29:75)

APNEA AND RESPIRATORY ARREST
Apnea is defined as temporary cessation of ventilation that lasts at least 10 seconds as determined by the lack of airflow in the nose or mouth. It can be pro-

duced by opioids or other drugs. The cessation of airflow for a longer period and with medical intervention would constitute a respiratory arrest (CIOMS, *PEDS* 1997;6:115).

ACUTE PANCREATITIS

A clear definition of this AE is necessary in pharmacovigilance because of its gravity. Delcenserie (*Gastroentérol Clin Biol* 1992;16:761, English abstract) has suggested limiting usage of this term in AE reporting to those patients exposed to a drug who have the following three characteristics (definition by consensus):

- A clinical presentation suggestive of pancreatic pain and
- An elevation of pancreatic enzyme concentration (amylase, lipase levels) in the blood and urine, and
- A positive pancreatic echogram finding (a negative abdominal echography result requires that the serum enzyme level be at least four times normal to support the diagnosis)

If these criteria were adhered to, the following case report, which could be called an "orphan ADR," would not be acceptable under this definition.

Pancreatitis occurred in a female after taking a single dose of an nonsteroidal anti-inflammatory drug (NSAID) for dysmenorrhea. She presented with acute abdominal pain radiating to the back. A dechallenge was positive after several days. Elevation of the levels of serum lipase and of the pancreatic isoenzyme of amylase was found. Using Delcenserie's definition, the diagnosis has not been fully established, thus casting doubt on whether this was truly drug-induced acute pancreatitis. Even though a drug etiology is unclear, it is doubtful that anyone would rechallenge this woman with an NSAID (Du Ville, *Am J Gastroenterol* 1993;88:464).

PHOTOSENSITIVITY

An exaggerated cutaneous response to ultraviolet radiation. It is familiarly described as an exaggerated "sunburn" whether induced by a drug or not. There are two clinical and pathophysiologic forms: phototoxicity and photoallergy (CIOMS, *PEDS* 1997;6:115). This dermatovigilance ADR provides an example of an interaction with a physical factor (ultraviolet radiation) as a risk factor.

DELAY IN DISCOVERY

Some ADRs were not recognized for many years or even decades. Although this point is mainly of historic interest, it does cause one to pause and reflect. Let us consider several examples:

Analgesic nephropathy: chronic nephrotoxicity associated with long-term exposure to analgesics. The products in question were usually phenacetin-based with fixed doses of nonsteroidal anti-inflammatory drugs (NSAIDs), aspirin, antipyrine, acetaminophen, caffeine, and/or codeine. The kidney lesions seen were papillary necrosis and interstitial nephritis. This iatrogenic syndrome was described in Switzerland in 1950. Phenacetin remained on the market for 80 years in the United Kingdom and 83 years in the United States.

Aspirin: digestive hemorrhage: 39 years to be recognized and 59 years to alert the medical community.

Aspirin: Reye's syndrome: 83 years between the time aspirin was first introduced in 1899 and the removal in the United States of the indication of fever in the infant. However, the syndrome was not recognized until 1963.

Amidopyrine: aplastic anemia: recognized 47 years after the first signs were described.

Chloramphenicol: blood dyscrasias: the information was made widely known more than 20 years after the first detection of the risk in the 1950s.

Chloroform: cardiac problems: first used as an anesthetic in 1831; cardiac arrests were noted 46 years later in 1877.

Cincophen: icterus: Described 15 years after first use, and a public alert after 26 years.

Clioquinol: subacute myelo-optic neuropathy (SMON): 35 years passed between the first publications in Argentina in 1935 and the removal from the market in Japan in 1970. A signal that takes a very long time to be recognized can obviously cause a delay in regulatory actions and market withdrawal. In December 1935 two articles in Spanish appeared (Grawitz, *Semana Med* 1935;42:525; Barros, *Semana Med* 1935;42:907) reporting neurologic complications after excessive doses of clioquinol. These two index cases were not acted upon; it was only 21 years later in Japan that the syndrome was widely recognized (see CLIOQUINOL: MARKET WITHDRAWAL).

Neuroleptics: malignant hyperthermia syndrome: 8 years between the index case first reported in 1960 and the full recognition of the syndrome by the same team in 1968 (Delay, *Ann Med Psychol* 1960;118:145).

Warfarin: thrombosis: Cutaneous necrosis produced by oral antivitamin K anticoagulants can result from the thrombosis in peripheral venules and capillaries after a rapid fall in the level of the coagulation inhibitor protein C. Warfarin has been implicated in more than 300 published cases over the last 40 years. The loss of a limb, a penis, one or both breasts, and other organs testifies to the serious ADRs this drug may produce. The suspicion of a drug effect was not the immediate reaction after the first publication by Flood (*NY State J Med* 1943;43:1121) since the second report did not occur until eleven years later (Verhagen, *Acta Med Scand* 1954;148:453). These ADRs were not fully recognized until two other cases were described 18 years after the first publication by Kipen (*N Engl J Med* 1961;265:638).

DERMATOVIGILANCE

ADR surveillance of the skin and mucosal membranes. The reactions can be systemic or topical. The principal systemic manifestations are acne, alopecia, eczema, erythema, exanthema, exfoliative dermatitis, fixed drug eruption, pigmented erythema, lichenoid eruptions, lupus, photosensitivity, pigmentation, porphyria, pruritus, purpura, vesicular-bullous toxiderma (Stevens-Johnson syndrome and toxic epidermal necrolysis (TEN)), urticaria, angioedema, stretch marks, and vasculitis. The major local reactions are contact dermatitis (eczema), irritations, and photostimulation.

A WEBSITE ON THE CUTANEOUS DRUG REACTIONS

Dartmouth University maintains a website that has restricted access (gopher://gopher.dartmouth.edu/11/research/biosci/cdrd). To aid in causality assessment, questionnaires have been proposed. Some general principles are presented in Shear (*Arch Dermatol* 1990;126:94). The Free University of Amsterdam publishes a periodically updated guide that contains a listing of cutaneous ADRs associated with drug products (Bruinsma W. *A guide to drug eruptions, the European file of side-effects in dermatology*. DeZwaluw: Oosthuisen, Netherlands 1996).

DES ACTION

A consumer protection movement that includes women exposed in utero to diethylstilbestrol and their descendants (see DIETHYLSTILBESTROL).

DES ACTION INTERNATIONAL

This organization is represented in several countries including Australia, Belgium, Canada, England, France, Ireland, the Netherlands, and New Zealand. Its aims include the tracking down of women exposed in utero, the creation of a group that can take collective action, and the dissemination of medical information on this subject to the health profession and to the women exposed. This movement has shown the important role that consumer groups can play in the follow-up of populations exposed to pharmaceuticals. It has also shown how critical it is to follow these women for their entire lives and for the entire lives of their daughters—the third generation.

DES ACTION USA

Created in 1977, it is located at DES Action USA, 610 16th Street, Oakland, CA 94612 (hotline, 1-800-DES-9288; phone, 510-465-4011; fax, 510-465-4815; website http://www.desaction.org; e-mail desact@well.com).

They publish a quarterly bulletin, *DES Action VOICE, A Focus on Diethylstilbestrol.* There are regional (state) sections in the United States. The problem is important since up to 5 million American women may have been exposed to DES between 1941 and 1971 (*DES Action VOICE*, Summer 2000).

DES ACTION CANADA

Founded in 1982, DES Action Canada aims to inform the public and professionals of the health consequences of this synthetic estrogen on the estimated 200,000 to 400,000 Canadian women exposed to this drug at the beginning of their pregnancies between 1941 and 1971. This nonprofit organization, subsidized by Health Canada, publishes a bulletin and a list of gynecologists and urologists across Canada. Their mailing address is POB 233, Snowdon Station, Montreal, QC, Canada H4A 1G2.

DETECTION OF NEW ADVERSE REACTIONS

The fourth edition of *Detection of New Adverse Reactions* (London: McMillan References, 1999), abbreviated as Stephens 1999 in this book, was edited by MDB Stephens, JCC Talbot, and PA Routledge. This superb classic textbook on pharmacovigilance is recommended to anyone involved in the field. It contains 15 chapters, 6 appendices, abbreviations, websites, a bibliography, and an index, all in 546 pages.

DIETARY SUPPLEMENT

Dietary supplements can be considered as drugs in some cases but for historical or political reasons are not treated or regulated as drugs. They can produce adverse effects. Pharmacists sometimes refer to them as *nutriments* or *nutriceutics.* Consider three examples: iron, tryptophan, and vitamin A

PARENTERAL IRON

This mineral can produce significant and unexpected AEs. For example, there is a report of loss of taste in an 80-year-old woman that lasted for 3 days after each intramuscular injection of an iron–sorbitol–citric acid complex. Fatal anaphylaxis has also been reported, though fortunately it is exceptional. Iron taken by mouth can also cause discoloration of teeth (ADRAC, *Med J Aust* 1979;2:204; *Aust ADR Bull* 1992;11(4):14).

L-TRYPTOPHAN

Eosinophilia-myalgia syndrome is an unusual syndrome that attracted the attention of the Center for Disease Control (CDC) in Atlanta. The first 154 reports of this syndrome were published in a report in *Morbidity and Mortality Weekly Report* dated 17 November 1989. The eosinophilia was significant, with levels above $10^9/l$ and accompanied by myalgia, fever, and rash. A veritable "epidemic" of this syndrome was described and by May 1990 the Food and Drug Administration had already been informed of 1500 cases, of which 23 were fatal.

Contamination of the product was suspected, and this hypothesis was supported by the finding of an abnormal chromatography peak, which was found to be a dimer of L-tryptophan. However, since not all of the cases could be explained by this contamination hypothesis, the FDA ordered a market withdrawal of all products containing the active moiety. Great Britain and Germany followed suit.

VITAMIN A

Taking excessive amounts of vitamin A can produce hepatotoxicity, which manifests itself as cirrhosis, hepatic failure, and ascites. In one reported case of a 51-year-old Australian female with ascites, her medical history revealed that she had been taking large amounts of vitamin A daily for 6 months (ADRAC, *Case Studies* 1981:21).

DIETHYLSTILBESTEROL (DES): MARKET WITHDRAWAL

INTRODUCTION

Diethylstilbesterol is an estrogen first synthesized in 1938. It presents a good example of modern pharmacovigilance on a grand scale in terms of the number of persons exposed to the drug (the pregnant women) and persons reported to be affected by the adverse reaction (the female offspring). In 1941 DES was approved for human use by the FDA. In 1947 the agency approved the use during pregnancy for the treatment/prevention of spontaneous abortion (i.e. miscarriage) based largely on the work of Harvard researchers, George and Olive Smith.

The suspicion of a problem arose in 1970, when clinicians observed a rare vaginal cancer occurring in women 14–22 years old. This cancer, clear cell adenocarcinoma (CCA), was usually only seen in women in their 70s. No explanation seemed apparent until the mother of one of the young cancer patients mentioned that she had taken DES to prevent a miscarriage. Questioning of the other mothers revealed that they too had taken DES and Dr. Arthur Herbst confirmed the association between DES and CCA in a case control study in 1971.

DELAYED ONSET OF MALIGNANCY (LONG LATENCY)

The delay in the appearance of the ADR after the last dose (latency period) is among the longest ever seen. The delay in detection has several explanations:

■ The adverse event did not occur in the women who took DES but in their female offspring exposed during the critical window of vaginogenesis
■ The adverse event was not visible in the female offspring at birth

- The adverse event was not evident until after puberty during a gynecologic examination
- The obstetric problems appeared only when a pregnancy occurred

The spontaneous reporting consisted of a publication of the first series of cases and a case-control study.

The reported risk of developing CCA in DES-exposed women is approximately 1 in 1,000 from birth to 34 years of age. The risk increases rapidly from the onset of puberty until the late teens and early 20s. Subsequently, the risk drops dramatically, although a few cases have been reported in women in their 40s. Other less serious but more frequent obstetric and gynecologic problems in the DES-exposed progeny have also been commented on in the medical literature:

- Vaginal adenosis, cervical ectropion (normal, albeit misplaced columnar epithelium)
- Structural anomalies such as cervical hoods, hypoplastic and T-shaped uterus
- Functional problems such as decreased fertility, ectopic pregnancy, spontaneous abortions (RR = 92:1) and pre-term births (RR = 5:1)
- Possible abnormalities in children of daughters whose mothers received DES (i.e., third generation)
- Benign malformations, such as small testicles and epididymal cysts in males exposed in utero

ACTIONS TAKEN

In 1971, the FDA banned the use of DES in pregnant women (FDA Drug Bulletin 1971). In the same year, a Registry was established with Dr. Arthur Herbst as the Chairperson and in 1978 the DESAD Project was developed to promptly study DES-exposed women with adenosis. In 1973 the National Institutes of Health (NIH) notified medical schools and gynecologic oncologists about increased cancer risk. In 1977 France withdrew the obstetric indication. A movement known as DES Action (see DES ACTION) was created in the United States in 1977, in Canada in 1982, in France in 1987 and in the U.K. in 1989.

In the U.S. in 1999 Congress directed the National Cancer Institute to fund a three-year DES National Educational Campaign housed at the Centers for Disease Control and Prevention (CDC)(Herbst; *N Engl J Med* 1971;284;878-881; Wilcox *N Engl J Med* 1995; 332:1411; Giusti, *Ann Intern Med* 1995; 122:778; *DES Action VOICE*, Summer 2000).

DIGITAL SIGNATURE (see ELECTRONIC SIGNATURE)

DIGITALIS INTOXICATION

Historically one of the first ADRs correctly and spontaneously described by Dr. Withering in 1785.

DINITROPHENOL

A product of historical interest since it was the first to be associated with drug-induced cataracts in 1935. This product, 2,4-dinitrophenal, was tried for obesity after a chance observation of a possible weight loss effect. The cessation of its use was as rapid as its introduction. Good sense prevailed as the risk of cataracts was too great compared to the benefit of a transient loss of a few pounds.

DIPHENOXYLATE: APNEA

It was originally thought that this antidiarrheal could only produce apnea in the infant after an overdose. However, thanks to pharmacovigilance, this adverse reaction was detected after the administration of normal pediatric doses. After the receipt of 45 cases (one is described here) the Australian pharmacovigilance authorities decided to revoke the Marketing Authorization of this product.

> A baby boy of 2 years of age was found blue and apneic in his bed and required 14 hours of resuscitation. Diphenoxylate was found in the gastric contents (ADRAC, *Med J Aust* 1980;2:292).

DIRECT (PRIMARY) EFFECT

This term is used to describe an adverse effect produced by the suspect product in question. This is in contradistinction to a secondary or indirect effect, which is not produced by the drug product but results from a cascade of indirect effects that occur after an earlier direct effect. For instance, a diuretic may directly cause a hypokalemia through its action on the renal tubule, leading to an arrhythmia in a patient on digitalis.

DISCONTINUATION

In regulatory matters, this is a more neutral term than *suspension* or *withdrawal* of a product from the market. It may be permanent or temporary. In pharmacotherapy matters, this term is equivalent to the cessation or interruption of the suspect product. It should not be confused with stopping treatment in patients, a term used in the clinical setting. It is often abbreviated *D/C* (as a verb) in medical records (e.g., "D/C morphine on June 16" or "Morphine was D/Ced on June 16").

DOCUMENTED, WELL

REACTION

The expression *well documented ADR*, refers to a previously confirmed ADR with the suspect product in other patients. It concerns an adverse reaction that is clearly accepted to be due to the suspect medication. In this work we avoid this meaning, in favor of *expected* ADR or *labeled* ADR to prevent confusion between expectedness and the other two meanings presented next.

REPORT

The phrase *well documented report* is synonymous with a *valid report* in the broadest sense of the word, meaning a report whose validity includes completeness, factual correctness, and plausibility. We do not use this term and prefer the use of *valid report*.

Some authors use *documented report* as a synonym for *causally related report*, which confuses validity and causality. We avoid this use and prefer to use a rank on a causality scale ranging from *excluded* to *definite*.

DOPING

The use of substances, often prescription medications, with the aim of improving sports performance. The objective is neither medical nor therapeutic since the subjects are in good health and are not "patients." The substance is obtained illicitly or with the complicity of a medical professional who writes a prescription that is filled through normal channels. The prescriber who truly has the best interests of the patient in mind should not prescribe such substances. A prescriber who provides it with the attitude that the athlete will obtain the substance anyway and that medical surveillance is better than illicit use with no surveillance should redouble his or her vigilance regarding the prevention, detection, and correction of adverse reactions—some of which may be severe, have long latency periods, or even be fatal.

DOSSIER, CLINICAL (FOR DRUG APPROVAL, FOR THE NEW DRUG APPROVAL)

Documents presented to the authorities to obtain the Marketing Authorization (NDA in the United States) for a new product or formulation in at least one indication. It contains the results of the phase I, II, and III studies. In the case of a product already on the market, new data containing additional studies for a new indication or formulation must be submitted. The dossier is confidential under the terms of *industrial secrets* or *proprietary information*. This unfortunately prevents the medical and pharmacoepidemiology world from obtaining full knowledge of all the ADRs observed in the course of the clinical trials (see PHARMACOTRANSPARENCY: DECLARATION OF ERICE).

DRUG INFORMATION CENTER

An entity whose goal is to aid practitioners in their use of *pharmacotherapy*, in particular in the surveillance of patients taking new products with which the clinicians are not yet fully familiar. These centers may be national, regional, hospital-based, or private companies. They must have complete access to the latest information on the products at the national level and even at the international level. They must have data on indications, dosing, contraindications, AEs, overdose data and treatments, warnings, and pregnancy/lactation information to help the clinician prevent, detect, and treat ADRs.

DRUG; DRUG PRODUCT; MEDICINE (IN THE UNITED KINGDOM); MEDICATION

A chemical substance used to modify the functioning of a biologic organism for medical reasons and administered in the form of a pharmaceutical product. For the World Health Organization (WHO), a drug is "any substance administered to man for the prevention, diagnosis or treatment of a disease or for the modification of a physiologic function."

A medication is prepared as a *commercial product* whose galenic form includes the active ingredient (moiety) and excipients. The regulatory definition of a *drug* versus a *device* can differ from country to country, so that the same product is considered a device in one country and a drug in another, producing peculiar and even paradoxic reporting situations. Note that in some pharmacovigilance regulatory situations, the term *drug* may also include biologics. A *molecule* can be used for other purposes, however, as illustrated in the following situations:

CONSUMER-INITIATED

▶ **Illicit Drugs (Street Drugs, "Drugs"):**
Usage of the products here is not "approved" and is "recreational." The drugs may be commercial products created by the pharmaceutical industry (either unchanged or adulterated on the street) or may be products of questionable origin, content, and quality. The word *drugs* thus has two senses in English: those that are used for medical purposes to treat disease, and drugs that are used for recreational ends and often become addictive.

▶ **Sports Drugs (Doping)**
The use of illicit or commercial drugs with the aim of improving athletic performance. Drugs used include anabolic steroids, erythropoietin, and amphet-

amines. Their use is almost always outside approved indications (for legal drugs) and is forbidden by the International Olympic Committee and several other professional and organized amateur sports.

▶ Food Supplement

This expression refers to substances that are used for nutritional reasons (vitamins, minerals, etc.). However, in some countries the definition is rather broad; in the United States, this includes such products as melatonin. Food supplements are not regulated by the Food and Drug Administration in the United States. *They may produce significant adverse reactions.*

MEDICALLY INITIATED

▶ Diagnostic Agent

The clinician can administer a pharmaceutical product whose goal is purely diagnostic (radiocontrast agents, histamine test, etc.) with no expectation of a direct therapeutic benefit.

▶ Pharmacologic Agent

This term refers to the use of products for biologic testing (e.g., in receptor research).

Let us consider two substances.

> *Iodine*: iodine given to populations at risk for goiter is considered to be a nutritional supplement (e.g., in table salt). It has also been used as a preventative when given to people living near nuclear reactors from which radioactive iodine accidentally escaped. The iodine serves as a competitor to the radioactive iodine accumulating in the thyroid, thus decreasing the risk of thyroid problems.

> *Melatonin*: for physiologists, melatonin is a hormone secreted by the pineal gland. For others, it is a natural product and a food supplement not governed by the drug laws of the country and readily available in "health food" stores and supermarkets. To researchers in the pharmaceutical industry, it is the starting point for the development of analogues as medical drugs with fewer ADRs and better targeted efficacy for the treatment of jet lag or other problems. Whether a molecule is a drug or a food supplement depends on the point of view of the scientist, the health professional, the regulator, the producer, and the consumer.

DRUG IN A SPONTANEOUS REPORT

As proposed by ICH E2B, a drug or drugs may be categorized by the reporter, the manufacturer or the health authority in one of three ways in a spontaneous report of an AE/ADR:

> *Suspect drug*: The drug is suspected of having contributed to the AE/ADR

> *Concomitant drug*: The drug is not suspected of having contributed to the AE/ADR but was taken by the patient

> *Suspected of interaction*: Two drugs are suspected of interacting together to produce the AE/ADR.

DRUGDEX

A drug dictionary, covering the products sold in the United States, is available on CD-ROM and electronically from the company Micromedex. A large section is devoted to ADRs and is well referenced and annotated. It is available in many libraries and is a useful reference tool (http://www.micromedex.com/products/pd-main.htm).

DRUG INFORMATION ASSOCIATION (DIA)

This organization created in 1964 in the United States describes itself as follows: The DIA is "a non-profit, multi-disciplinary, member-driven scientific association with a membership of over 22,000. These members are primarily from the regulatory agencies, academia, contract service organizations, pharmaceutical, biological and device industry, and from other health care organizations." Members are entitled to receive the following:

The *Drug Information Journal*, published quarterly

DIA Newsletter, which keeps members posted on services, seminars, activities, membership, and other information

DIA Membership Directory, with over 22,000 members' names, affiliations, and addresses

Pharmaceutical/Biotech Contract Support Organization Register, a listing of companies offering various services

Calendar of Events, announcements of more than 100 educational activites over the course of the year including workshops, seminars, courses, and symposia.

The cost of membership is quite modest, and whether one is in the pharmaceutical industry, academe, or government it is well worthwhile. Conferences, courses, and meetings are held on both sides of the Atlantic. Topics covered include the following drug safety (pharmacovigilance) issues: *MedDRA*, good clinical practices, the role of poison control centers, ADR labeling, pediatric surveillance, safety and drug promotion, CIOMS IV, risk/benefit ratio, safety of biotechnology products, electronic submission of safety data, safety in hormone substitution therapy, the periodic report, ADRs during clinical trials, and information technology issues (website: www.diahome.org. U.S. address, 501 Office Center Drive, Suite 450, Fort Washington, PA 19034-3211; fax, (215) 641-1229; e-mail, dia@diahome.org; European address, Postfach, 4012, Basel, Switzerland; e-mail, dia@diaeurope.org).

DRUG INFORMATION JOURNAL

The official journal of the Drug Information Association (DIA) is peer-reviewed and publishes articles concerning the pharmaceutical industry and pharmaceutical medicine involving the production, processing, and use of information in all of the phases of drug development including safety surveillance (www.diahome.org/English/dhp5a.htm). This quarterly journal has articles (and occasionally complete issues) devoted to pharmacovigilance. Recommended to anyone in the field to keep abreast of new developments in regulations, methodology, safety investigations, Internet uses, databases, other topics.

DRUG MONITOR

Also known as the *Local Safety Officer*, the person responsible for pharmacovigilance, either during clinical trials or after marketing, in the pharmaceutical industry.

DRUG MONITORING

In pharmacoepidemiology, the term is synonymous with *pharmacovigilance, drug surveillance,* and *drug safety surveillance;* it comprises the duties of collection, processing, analysis, and communication of AEs and ADRs.

In pharmacotherapy, the term refers to the very tight and scrupulous surveillance of the patient who is undergoing drug therapy, with the goal of maximizing the benefits (efficacy) and minimizing the ADRs (risk). Also referred to as *therapeutic drug monitoring,* it often includes the measurement of plasma drug levels (e.g., lithium) or of a marker of drug action (e.g., glycemia for insulin).

DRUG SAFETY

This expression has two different meanings, according to context:

Synonymous with harmlessness: the lack of danger that a particular medication presents ("safety of a drug") in a given patient, as in "Drug safety in Mr. Jones is of primary importance since he is 96 years old, is in moderate renal failure, and is taking four different medications."

Synonymous with pharmacovigilance: drug safety surveillance, as in "Every pharmaceutical company must, by law, have a department of Drug Safety."

DRUG SAFETY

A monthly publication from Adis International, it publishes "comprehensive reviews of adverse drug experience and risk benefit evaluations in disease management." Articles on the methodology of pharmacovigilance are also published. This journal is recommended to anyone in the field (http://www.adis.com; U.S./Canada office, Suite F-10, 940 Town Center Drive, Langhorne, PA 19047, U.S.A.; in the United Kingdom, Chowley Oak Lane, Tattenhall, CH3 9GA).

DRUGS AND THERAPEUTIC BULLETIN

Founded in 1963 in Britain with the support of the Consumers' Association, this journal developed the original notion of putting the letter *S* next to those references that are symposia financed by pharmaceutical laboratories since these references are not always given the same rigorous peer review that other articles in journals normally receive. The circulation surpassed 100,000 in 1997. Member of the International Society of Drug Bulletins (ISDB).

DRUGS UNDER SURVEILLANCE

In pharmacovigilance bulletins, this refers to a list of products that are the subject of intensified reporting of adverse effects (either a specific AE or all AEs seen with the product). This may be done for different reasons.

The product is very new on the market.

It belongs to a family of drugs for which there is a specific risk.

A signal regarding this drug has already been reported and a call for intensified scrutiny and reporting of AEs is required.

The placing of a drug on the intensified scrutiny list is done for scientific reasons to gain further information in order to be able to decide whether a signal is confirmed or rejected and, in some circumstances, in order to find out whether signals are generated.

The *Australian ADRs Bulletin* lists the products under surveillance in the section *Drugs of Current Interest*. Most of these products are new and powerful medications, some of which have already been the subject of important signals (http://www.health.gov.au/tga/docs/html/aadrbltn/aadrbidx.htm).

The national pharmacovigilance bulletin published by the Therapeutic Products Programme in Canada now has a Drugs of Current Interest section.

DRUG UTILIZATION RESEARCH GROUP (DURG)

This European group performs drug utilization reviews in order to follow prescribing habits. There are affiliated groups in many European countries. It works in collaboration with the World Health Organization (WHO) Collaborating Centre in Uppsala, Sweden (www.eurodurg.org).

DRUG UTILIZATION REVIEW (DUR)

Research on quantitative and qualitative aspects of drug use and therapy, the determinants of drug use and the effects on patients, specifically on the population in general (Stockholm DURG Meeting 1994) (www.eurodurg.org/presentation.htm).

These studies examine the use of particular drugs by particular physicians for particular indications. Comparisons from one geographic area to another are then done. These studies are done for three major reasons:

- Cost control by insurance companies, health maintenance organizations (HMOs), hospitals, and others
- Marketing tools by the pharmaceutical companies to clarify who is prescribing which drugs
- Academic motives of enhancing the understanding of actual pharmaceutic prescribing practice compared to ideal (theoretic) pharmacologic prescribing

DUPLICATE CASE

The second notification of the same adverse effect case report in the product database or the second publication of the same AE in the literature: "Same patient, same reaction, same product, same date." The reporter is not necessarily the same. It is the most misleading in pharmacovigilance when the reaction is very serious or critical (e.g., aplastic anemia, Stevens-Johnson syndrome, torsades de pointes) and it cannot be ascertained whether there are two reports or only one.

Duplicate reports come about in an interesting way. Sometimes duplication is malevolent as the same report is published in slightly different contexts in different journals. More innocently it might be published alone and later published as one of a series of similar events but with insufficient detail to ensure that it is a true duplicate. In other cases, an event might be reported to a national agency that then reports it to the World Health Organization (WHO) Collaborating Centre where it is not always clear that it is a duplicate report because of coding differences. Similarly, a spontaneously reported AE sent to the national agency may also be reported to the manufacturer and/or other national agencies (e.g., a report originating in Canada is reported by the company to the HPB but also to the U.S. Food and Drug Administration, and others). Transcription errors, recoding into different drug dictionaries, and incomplete data may all produce duplicate reports.

A more subtle problem arises when there is a single AE in question, but the information in the two reports is complementary. For example, a pharmacist reports a case that does not contain exactly the same demographic or medical details as the report of the prescribing physician. Another problem occurs when the telephone report to the manufacturer does not contain the same information as the written or electronic version sent to the authorities.

Finally, a new problem is arising with the tightening of privacy (data protection) laws around the world. In many cases the identity of the patient must be anonymized as any identifiers such as birth date, age, initials, sex, or even country of origin are removed. In these situations, it is often hard to know whether similar reports represent one or two different instances of the reaction.

The benefit of duplicate reporting that contains complementary data is that combining the information from both reports allows a more complete report to be obtained. For example, the notification made by the treating physician may contain clinical details of the AE, whereas the report from the pharmacist may contain the details of the suspect drug dosage, route of administration, and other points. Perhaps a better term for this is *complementary reports*, as long as the authorities and manufacturer are aware of the situation.

In vaccinovigilance, it is recommended that two reports be made if one reaction is a local site reaction and the other a systemic reaction since the causalities of the two reactions may be entirely different.

In pregnancy surveillance, ICH E2B recommends the filling out of two separate forms if the mother and fetus/infant both have a suspected ADR.

DURATION OF AN ADVERSE EVENT

In case causality assessment, the course of the event over time is one of the temporal charcteristics of the event and is of great diagnostic value. We would propose to divide this period into two segments: the *dechallenge dependent* segment and the *dechallenge independent* segment.

THE DECHALLENGE-DEPENDENT SEGMENT (COURSE AFTER DECHALLENGE)

The interval between the last dose of the product and disappearance of the reaction. Two courses can then occur:

> *The event disappears and the disappearance can be interpreted as being in favor of a causal link between the medication and the event (positive dechallenge)*: If the dechallenge is positive (i.e., the event ceases), then the time between the last dose and the beginning of the disappearance (*time to improvement*) or the time between the last dose and the complete disappearance (*time to resolution*) should be noted. This value should then be interpreted in light of the half-life and clearance of the drug. That is, if the drug takes many days to be eliminated, but the event disappears quickly after the last dose, this fact may argue against a drug cause. The time to disappearance is often a critical element in the causality assessment and is likely to be more validly observed than the time to onset, when the dechallenge is performed with the purpose of assessing drug causality. Clearly this concept is meaningful only if the AE began before and ended after the last dose of the suspect drug.

> *The event persists or worsens:* This can be interpreted as an argument against the event's being related to the drug in question. However, there are *first dose phe-*

nomena (see FIRST DOSE PHENOMENON) that only occur after the first dose; also, some ADRs are self-limited in duration.

THE DECHALLENGE INDEPENDENT SEGMENT

There are circumstances in which dechallenge-independent segments may be observed during the course of an adverse effect/ADR depending whether the event began before or after the last dose of the drug in question. Two situations are possible:

If the event began before the last dose, two possiblities exist:

- The event lasts as long as the treatment with the suspect drug. When the event persists during the entire treatment period the interpretation requires clinical acumen. For example, a diarrhea lasting the full 10 days of treament with an antibiotic in a child would argue in favor of drug causality if the child suffers from an uncomplicated viral upper respiratory tract infection, in which diarrhea is usually short-lived.

- The event disappears before stopping of the suspect drug. This occurs when the drug treatment is not stopped even though there is an AE. The occurrence of this type of situation might suggest an intercurrent non-drug-related cause of the event but clinical skills are needed since some AE/ADRs are self-limited.

If the event began after the last dose, although it occurred "outside the treatment window," a causal relationship to the drug is still possible, though it must not be confused with a rebound or withdrawal effect. Keep in mind that for "single-use" drugs (injections, etc.) and vaccines this is always the case: that is, the first dose is the same as the last dose.

ELECTRONIC SIGNATURE (DIGITAL SIGNATURE)

Signature refers to the verification of authenticity of an electronically transmitted file. It is the counterpart of the written signature on a paper document. Legislation in this area is pending or has been passed in many countries. The relevance here is that adverse effect reports will soon be sent electronically (see ICH E2B) and the assurance that a signature currently gives on paper documents will be required for the electronic transmissions. Two definitions of an electronic signature have been proposed:

- "An electronic sound, symbol or process attached to or logically associated with a record and executed or adopted by a person with the intent to sign the record."
- "Information in electronic form that a person has created or adopted in order to sign a document and that is in, attached to or associated with that document."

EPIDEMIOLOGIC STUDIES: WHY THEY ARE NOT SUFFICIENT

One of the great advantages of the spontaneous reporting system (SRS) is that its sensitivity is high and exceeds that of other types of systems or studies known to date. The SRS, unlike an observational study, captures information on all suspect products, all body systems, and all categories of patients exposed to the products. Very rare ADRs can be picked up in the SRS, whereas they may be missed in cohort studies even those that have 10,000 or more patients. Similarly, promotional studies do not seem to pick up significant safety signals. Prescription event monitoring systems (surveillance of adverse effects after prescription of a drug) are better but do not seem to be as sensitive as the SRS for signal detection.

Studies done in cross-linked databases with hundreds of thousands (or more) of prescriptions also have certain limitations and can miss an ADR if there is no adequate and clear coding term for it, if the drug is not on formulary, if over the counter (OTC) medications are not recorded, and for other reasons.

When *H2 antihistamines* came on the market for use in the treatment of peptic ulcers, the Food and Drug Administration required a cohort study, although they had retrospectively demonstrated the lack of usefulness of prospective phase IV trials compared to a well organized spontaneous reporting system for AEs (Rossi, *JAMA* 1984;252:1030). The end point measured here to compare each approach was the addition of new ADRs in the product labeling. The largest proportion of such new ADRs was obtained from the spontaneous reporting rather than from the alternative and very costly follow-up trials on thousands of patients.

A retrospective study suggested that patients with arthritis were less frequently exposed to *beta-blockers* than control patients without arthritis (Waller P, *Br Med J* 1985;291:1684). However, a British publication noted 18 cases of arthritis associated with one beta-blocker (Savola, *Br Med J* 1983;287:1256) and the FDA published five other case reports (*JAMA* 1986;255:198) with two positive rechallenges. Which is correct? It is clear that this case-control study did not have the sensitivity needed to detect what is possibly a very rare ADR.

EUROPEAN MEDICINES EVALUATION AGENCY (EMEA)

The EMEA (also called the European Agency for the Evaluation of Medicinal Products) is a European Union (EU) agency for the authorization of medicinal products. It was created by the European Council in 1993 and came into being in 1995. In addition to evaluating and approving new medications for the entire European Union (and certain affiliated nations, Iceland, Liechtenstein, and Norway currently), the EMEA also has as its mission to control the safety of medicines through a pharmacovigilance network. The agency has an executive director, a management board, a technical and administrative secretariat and a scientific committee (the Committee for Propriety Medicinal Products (CPMP)) responsible for formulating the agency's opinion on human medicines. There is a similar committee for veterinary products (CVMP).

The EMEA is based in the United Kingdom at 7 Westferry Circus, Canary Wharf, London E14 4HB, UK. They have a very extensive website with thousands of documents available (www.emea.eu.int).

EUROPEAN PUBLIC ASSESSMENT REPORT (EPAR)

Since 1995 the European Medicinals Evaluation Agency and its Committee for Propriety Medicinal Products publish in writing and on the Internet (www.eudra.org/humandocs/humans/epar.htm) summaries of their evaluations of products approved by the "centralized" procedure (see APPROVAL PROCEDURES – EUROPE). Many are now published in modular format, easing access to specific parts of the document, as detailed on the website.

These reports are somewhat similar to the Summary Basis of Approval (SBOA) reports that the U.S. Food and Drug Administration issues. Two important problems regarding these EPARs were noted by the International Society of Drug Bulletins during a 1997 conference held in London on transparency and data access. First, these data are available only for products approved by the centralized procedure and not for those approved by the national authorities in the EU. Second, these summaries are too succinct because they exclude the following:

■ The details of the clinical trials including the adverse reactions
■ The expert opinions (expert reports) submitted to the committee
■ The minutes of the discussions held by the committee
■ The reasons for the lack of approval of a new product or indication

EUROPEAN SINGLE CASE PHARMACOVIGILANCE EXCHANGE (EUROSCAPE)

A system of electronic transmission of spontaneous ADRs in individual patients. It was tested from 1994 to 1996 in France, the U.K., Spain, and Germany. The harmonization of the format and contents of such reports was the object of the E2B group of the International Conference on Harmonization (ICH). The M2 Working Group of ICH has developed standards for the electronic transmission of information.

EUROPEAN UNION DRUG REGULATORY AUTHORITY NETWORK (EUDRANET)

A network of computerized databases in Europe. Its goal is to link the databases of the European Medicinal Evaluation Agency (EMEA) and the 15 member states to permit electronic transmission of pharmacovigilance data. Its goal is to add industry to the network for electronic transmission after the national health authorities and the EMEA have been successfully linked. A website carries the latest news on EUDRANET's status (www.eudraportal.eudra.org); another website provides additional details (http://www.ispo.cec.be/ida/text/english/dissemination/PartTwo/IDA3IIp20.html).

Read also Maistrello (*PEDS* 1998;7:183).

EVOLUTION

A term used in two ways:

Duration and course (worsening, stabilization, improvement, death, reappearance, unknown) of an AE; also referred to as the *clinical course*

Outcome, as in the expressions *favorable evolution, fatal evolution*, and *unknown evolution*

EXCIPIENT; INACTIVE INGREDIENT

In the broad sense of the word, a biologically inactive component added to the galenic formulation of a pharmaceutical product. This category includes diluants, fillers, binders, lubricants, disintegrators, colorings, flavors, solvents, and preservatives. It is not unusual to find a dozen or more in each galenic formulation. For a compilation of excipients used in medications, foods, and cosmetics see N. Weiner and I. L. Bernstein (Editors. *ADR to Drug Formulation Agents: A Handbook of Excipients*. Marcel Dekker, 1989) and S. C. Smolinske (*Handbook of Food, Drug and Cosmetic Excipients*. Boca Raton, FL: CRC Press, 1992). On the Internet see the website created by the International Pharmaceutical Excipients Council (IPEC) (www.ipec.org).

Dr. Edward Napke has been instrumental in convincing the international community of the importance of excipients in the production of ADRs and of the usefulness of the term *suspect product* rather than limiting the evaluation to the *suspect active ingredient.* He has also played a critical role in convincing the World Health Organization (WHO) to begin a surveillance program to this effect (Napke, *Can Med Assoc J* 1984;131:1449 and 1994;151:529).

A classification of *intrinsic* (type A or B, linked to the active ingredient) versus *extrinsic* (linked to a defect associated with the production, and not due to a problem in labeling) ADRs has been proposed. Thus ADRs related to harmful excipients would be a type of extrinsic ADRs (Drew and Myers, *Med J Aust* 1997;166:538).

BENZYL ALCOHOL: NEONATAL MORTALITY

The FDA was notified in 1981 of the death of newborns exposed to a preservative in saline solution used to rinse central venous catheters in premature infants weighing less than 2.5 kg: 10 cases occurred in 6 months in one institution and 6 were seen in another institution over a 16-month period. After the FDA recommended the cessation of the use of benzyl alcohol in this clinical setting, the "epidemic" ended. This could be considered a "positive population dechallenge" (Gershanik, *Clin Res* 1981;29:895a; MMWR 1982;31:290).

ANTINEOPLASTICS AND ALCOHOL: INTOXICATION

About 2 hours after the beginning of a rapid high-dose infusion of an antineoplastic agent, a woman who had breast cancer and pleural metastases and was also receiving opiates developed neuropsychiatric symptoms (ataxia, dysarthria, agitation), which lasted several hours in spite of naloxone given as an antagonist to the opiates. During a reported positive rechallenge a serum alcohol level of 0.98 g/l due to the presence of 50 ml of the excipient ethanol in one of the infusions was noted (Wilson, *Ann Pharmacother* 1997;31:873).

ANTIEPILEPTIC AND CALCIUM SULFATE: ABNORMAL BIOAVAILABILITY

Shortly after a change in the galenic formulation of an antiepileptic by its Australian manufacturer, 51 previously stable epileptics had very serious ADRs including coma. It was discovered that the substitution of calcium sulfate for lactose produced a marked increase in absorption that led to toxic levels of the active ingredient (Tyrer, *Br Med J* 1970;4:271).

SULFANILAMIDE AND DIETHYLENE GLYCOL

It is of historical importance that an elixir of sulfanilamide killed 50 adults and a similar number of children at the beginning of the twentieth century. It was discovered that the cause was the excipient diethylene glycol (Leech, *JAMA* 1937;109:1724; Calvery, *South Med J* 1939;32:1105).

EXPECTED (LABELED)

This term is used in three different contexts: the *regulatory* usage, the *pharmacological* usage and the *toxicology* usage.

REGULATORY USAGE (LABELED)

An AE is considered *expected* if it appears in the Summary of Product Characteristics (SPC or SmPC) (i.e., the official labeling). It is equivalent to "level 4 = expected, fully labeled" in terms of documentation. It answers the question, Can it cause this ADR? Is it accepted to be capable of causing this event?

The term *listed* has recently been added to the pharmacovigilance vocabulary to refer to an AE that appears in a Company Core Safety Information (CCSI) document for a drug but which may or may not appear in the SPC.

The FDA also uses the term *expected* to mean any event that appears in the officially approved package insert (labeling). An important nuance of this, however, applies to AEs that are part of class labeling. An AE that is listed only as class labeling in a particular drug's package insert is not considered expected for FDA reporting purposes. The EU health authorities hold similar views on this subject.

PHARMACOLOGY USAGE (PREDICTABLE)

A *pharmacologically expected or predictable* event is one that would be predicted on the basis of the pharmacologic properties and mechanism of action of the active ingredient. The ICH E2A document recommends that the pharmacologic definition (*anticipated from the pharmacological properties of a medicinal product*) *not* be used in pharmacovigilance.

An event can be *predictable* (i.e., expected in this usage) if it acts in an exaggerated manner on a targeted receptor, or in an exaggerated or normal manner on an untargeted receptor. Events of this nature are known as *type A* and are generally dose-dependent and less severe and less frequent than *type B* events.

TOXICOLOGY USAGE

In toxicology usage an event is *predictable* from *background knowledge* or *prior documentation*. It is the theoretical possibility that an ADR might occur with a particular drug but has not yet been observed. The possibility that the ADR may occur with continued use may be based on the following:

> Preclinical animal toxicity—particularly chronic toxicity studies
>
> Phase II and III trials that have shown a subclinical form of the AE (e.g., minor liver enzyme level elevations may predict a more severe hepatotoxicity that would occur in the postmarketing situation)

EXPECTEDNESS

This term usually is used to express the documented capability of the drug in question to produce an ADR. It answers the question, Can it? (see EXPECTED). That is, in regulatory terms, is the ADR included in the product labeling?

MEASUREMENT SCALE

Ordinal scales have been proposed. The official French scale used for *extrinsic imputability* or expectedness, has four levels (B-0 to B-3). The following scale is a modification of the French scale that differs by the inclusion of a fifth level (Moore, *Lancet* 1985;2:1058; Biron, *PEDS* 1993;2:579).

Level 4: expected, fully labeled

Level 3: recognized, not fully labeled

Level 2: anecdotal or predictable

Level 1: unpublished, unpredictable

Level 0: unknown worldwide

EXPEDITED REPORT (ALERT REPORT, 15-DAY REPORT)

Regulatory term designating a case report of a serious AE that is sent to a health authority in an urgent manner (usually 7 or 15 calendar days).

EXPEDITED REPORTING

The regulations regarding domestic and foreign reports of serious and/or unexpected AEs are usually based on the definitions and proposals of the Council for International Organizations of Medical Sciences (CIOMS) I Working Group.

THE ALERT (EXPEDITED, PRIORITY) REPORT

A document containing the report of a serious AE/ADR to be submitted to the health authorities on a CIOMS I form (or local equivalent such as the MedWatch 3500A form in the United States) in a very rapid time frame. The time allowed for submission depends on whatever local regulations, which may vary from country to country, apply and whether the event is from a clinical trial of a new product or from a spontaneous case report of a marketed product. For a serious ADR from a phase I–III clinical trial the time allowed for submission may be as short as *immediately* to 7 calendar days for a life-threatening unexpected ADR to as long as 15 calendar days for a serious event associated with a marketed product. Other time frames (e.g., 3, 5, 7, or 10 days) may still be found in some countries. There is, however, a tendency to move to the standardized 7- or 15-calendar-day proposals of the International Conference on Harmonization (ICH) for clinical trial reports. For marketed drugs, the ICH proposals for 15-calendar-day expedited reporting have largely been adopted.

EXPEDITED REPORTING FORM (ALERT REPORTING FORM)

A "universal" form developed by the CIOMS I group for expedited case reports that must be sent by manufacturers to health authorities within 15 calendar days of first notification when the adverse effect is serious and unexpected (unlabeled). This form may be used for reports that are domestic, foreign, or both, depending on the country. Some countries will require a local form, usually in the language of the country, for all domestic alert reports or, in some cases, all domestic serious reports. For other serious cases (i.e., foreign cases), the CIOMS I form in English is often accepted. The original form was created in English and has been translated into other languages.

EXTRINSIC EFFECT

This expression is used to designate those ADRs that are not due to the active ingredient but rather to such diverse causes as a reaction to an excipient; contamination; defective material; manufacturing, packaging, labeling, or storage problems; or inadequate preparation (Drew and Myers, *Med J Aust* 1997;166:538).

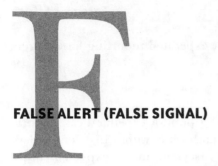

FALSE ALERT (FALSE SIGNAL)

Any signal that is not confirmed is theoretically a false signal or alert. However, in pharmacovigilance, the term *false alert* is usually meant to be a signal of a serious and unacceptable AE that, since it was not confirmed or perhaps even clearly disproved, nevertheless is followed by negative consequences for the manufacturer and even for public health.

The most dreaded consequence to the manufacturer is a sudden and dramatic "free fall" of the use of a product. This can be due to one or more causes: negative publicity, severe regulatory measures restricting its use, market withdrawal ordered by the authorities (or done in a voluntary or "semivoluntary" manner by the manufacturer), multiple lawsuits (e.g., Bendectin which was falsely suspected of producing congenital malformations). It raises the interesting philosophical question, At what point should a signal and its investigation be made public? It is no longer possible to restrict information to the medical press as the media and the Internet rapidly pick up and propagate such information as soon as it is made public, for example, from the Food and Drug Administration website and some other national pharmacovigilance bulletins/websites. (see BENDECTIN; RESERPINE)

FACTUAL RELIABILITY (IN AN ADVERSE DRUG REACTION CASE REPORT)

This term refers to the conformity of the reported "facts" to the reality of what occurred. A synonym is *authenticity*. The determination of factual reliability is one of the elements of *validation* or *quality control*. The facts that need to be verified include those discussed in the following sections.

THE ADVERSE EVENT

The event itself must be confirmed, or *medically substantiated*. The medical confirmation of the event is one of the primary duties of the manufacturer upon receipt of a report of a spontaneous AE. The confirmation of the data may be one of the criteria in the determination of whether the event meets the reporting requirements for a 15-calendar-day alert report (for serious and unexpected—unlabeled—events) or for inclusion in the next periodic report.

For example, one must not confuse the following:

A drug fever with a fever due to an infection

Syncope due to a drug effect, followed by convulsions, with an epileptic seizure followed by loss of consciousness

A febrile convulsion with a nonfebrile convulsion in an infant

Angina pectoris of cardiac origin with chest pain due to a gastrointestinal (GI) problem (e.g., esophagitis, recurrent ulcer)

A report of what appears to be the first episode of an adverse effect that, upon careful patient follow-up, turns out to be a recurrent but intermittent problem (for example, an episode of atrial fibrillation that at first appears to be new and due to the drug but that a careful history reveals occurred in the past before the drug was given)

In the analysis of an undesirable event, particularly that of an abnormal laboratory exam result, the examiner must be sure that the abnormality was correctly reported by the patient or health care professional and that the laboratory test was performed and interpreted correctly in comparison with the normal values of the test in that laboratory. If there is doubt about the validity of the result, it is useful to repeat the test (e.g., liver enzymes levels, potassium) before incriminating the drug.

In vaccine surveillance (vaccinovigilance) serious incidents that occur after vaccination should be confirmed by a physician, especially if they are of the following types: cellulitis, anaphylactic shock, convulsions, encephalopathy, meningitis, encephalitis, paresthesias, paralysis, Guillain-Barré syndrome, thrombocytopenia.

THE SUSPECT PRODUCT

The identity of the product (brand name or generic), the dose taken, the times and duration of the product taken, the route of administration (or misadministration), and whether the drug was taken by the person to whom it was prescribed must be verified. Sometimes it is useful to obtain the lot or batch number as well.

THE MEDICAL HISTORY AND WORKUP

The presence of other alternative causes that may have caused the AE must be verified, excluded, or confirmed as well as risk factors favoring a drug cause, and those favoring other possible nondrug factors as a cause of the AE.

THE REPORTER

The identification and authentication of the reporter are rarely difficult to verify if the reporter is a medical professional. The identity of the (medical) reporter must be confirmed to evaluate the reliability of the report and the differential diagnosis. This can be done by a phone call or fax to the reporter for follow-up information and by confirmation in medical directories or websites (e.g., www.ama-assn.org) of licensed physicians, pharmacists, etc., when necessary. Reports from consumers or nonmedical professionals should always be validated by contact with the treating physician or medical professional, though some health authorities require nonvalidated consumer complaints to be reported as if they were validated medical reports (e.g., in the United States and Canada).

The introduction of electronic mail has raised the question of how the sender can be verified. Various proposals have been made by governments to produce "electronic signatures" (see ELECTRONIC SIGNATURE) of validity equal to that in a written and signed letter. It is necessary to guard against pranks or, worse, malicious reports of AEs intended to "punish" a manufacturer. Any governmental agency or company that accepts spontaneous e-mail reports of AEs must have the means to follow up and validate such reports by regular mail ("snail mail"), fax, or telephone.

Validation by e-mail poses privacy issues and should be avoided, though, if there is only an e-mail return address, there may be no choice—at least for the first communication back to the sender. Most manufacturers prefer to use more classic means of communication with guarantee of receipt (certified mail with return receipt requested, use of overnight or 2-day couriers with receipt trackable on the Internet, etc.) (Cobert B, *Drug Saf* 1999;20(2):95).

THE CASE REPORT

Several issues arise in the evaluation of individual case reports.

Duplicate reports must be detected before they are entered into the database in order to prevent a false increase in the reporting frequency and number of cases in NDA periodic reports and PSURs.

An initial report must be clearly distinguished from a follow-up report in order to prevent false increases in frequency and to ensure that the complementary follow-up information is entered into the database. In fact, the Council for International Organizations of Medical Sciences (CIOMS 1) form requires that a box be filled in indicating whether the report is an initial or a follow-up report. In the daily flow of paper entering a pharmaceutical company or health agency this distinction may be hard to make if a specific case number is not assigned to a case and used on all documents.

False duplicate cases must also be carefully prevented. This term refers to duplicate but complementary reports on the same AE from different sources. For example, a physician might make a report containing the clinical details of the event whereas the report made by the pharmacist (often unbeknown to the physician) may contain important dosing information on the suspect product. Combining the information makes the case more complete and better able to be analyzed.

FARMACOTHERAPEUTISCH KOMPAS

A respected Dutch-language guide to pharmacotherapy. It is independent of industry both in its editorial content and in its financing. It uses a specific logo to identify new chemical entities during their first 2 years of commercialization to remind the prescriber to use caution in their use and to report serious and unexpected (i.e., unlabeled) AEs. It is edited by the Centrale Medisch Pharmaceutisch Commissie, a commission of the Ziekenfondsraad.

FETAL DEATH

If a drug is suspected of having contributed to fetal death or to a spontaneous abortion, the recommendation of ICH E2B is to routinely file a report on the mother. The report is known as a *parent-fetus report*.

FIRST DOSE PHENOMENON

An ADR of type A that is seen almost exclusively after the first dose of the drug in most of the patients who experience this reaction. It can be due to an exaggerated pharmacologic effect (easily prevented if the drug is given in smaller and/or divided doses) or a paradoxical effect. Some examples follow:

■ Neuropsychiatric reactions have been reported after the first dose of a nonsedating H_1 antihistamine, subsequently removed from the market for another reason (rare but unacceptable arrhythmias) (Napke, Lancet 1989;2:615).
■ A drug of a subclass of calcium antagonists has been shown rarely to produce angina after the first dose in some patients, possibly as a result of an exaggerated reflex tachycardia or coronary steal (Schanzenbacher, Am J Cardiol 1984 Jan 15;53(2):345–346; Radice, Clin Cardiol 1992;15:98).

FIXED DRUG ERUPTION

In dermatovigilance, this is probably the only cutaneous ADR whose cause is clearly associated with a drug or xenobiotic taken systemically. The time to appearance, each time in the same spot, varies from 30 minutes to 8 hours or more, although it is rare after 16 hours. Rechallenge by the same route of administration at a lower dose under medical supervision and with the consent of the patient is a very sensitive method to verify the causality of the suspect product. The sensitivity of cutaneous allergy testing is low but a positive result is useful (Knowles, *Can J Clin Pharmacol* 1994;1:145).

FOLLOW-UP LETTER

A letter, e-mail, of fax from a pharmacovigilance center (e.g., a pharmaceutical company, or a health authority) asking the addressee for additional medical information about a particular ADR report. The addressee either has not responded to the first letter sent out or has not sent sufficient detail on the case. The addressee may be the patient, the primary physician, a consulting physician, nurse, pharmacist, emergency room, ambulance squad, or other. All pharmacovigilance centers should have formal policies requiring such follow-up; in many countries follow-up is required by law for certain types or categories of AEs. The follow-up is imperative when the case or signal is serious and/or unexpected and the public health consequences may be important. On the other hand, excessive zeal in tracking down the details of a penicillin rash, for example, would be a waste of valuable and limited resources.

FOOD AND DRUG ADMINISTRATION (FDA, "THE AGENCY") (see ORGANIZATION OF PHARMACOVIGILANCE: UNITED STATES AND THE FDA)

FREEDOM OF INFORMATION (FOI)

Government information in the United States, unless classified, is available to the public. The Freedom of Information Act (FOIA) was passed by Congress in 1966 and amended in 1974. Based on the premise argued by Madison and Hamilton in the eighteenth century that openness in government will assist citizens in making the informed choices necessary to a democracy, FOIA creates procedures whereby any member of the public may obtain the records of the agencies of the federal government. The 1996 amendments to the act mandate publicly accessible "electronic reading rooms" with agency FOIA response materials and other information routinely available to the public, with electronic search and indexing features. See the American Civil Liberties website (www.aclu.org/library/foia.html) for an excellent overview of the concept as well as the U.S. Department of Justice site (www.usdoj.gov/04foia/index.html). FOI information is available on the FDA website (www.fda.gov/foi/foia2.htm).

FREQUENCY OF AN ADVERSE EVENT/REACTION: DEFINITIONS

This is a very tricky and difficult area in pharmacovigilance. First, it is necessary to distinguish between the *reported frequency* of an adverse event and *actual frequency*. The *reporting or reported frequency* of an AE refers to the reports received by manufacturers and/or health authorities divided by a usage figure (discussed later). The *actual or true incidence* of an event includes those events (both reported and unreported) divided by the true usage of the drug.

The true incidence is usually not known. Nonetheless, it is sometimes useful and often required that an attempt be made to calculate the reported frequency of various AEs in periodic reports sent to health agencies on marketed drugs. The numerator is the reported cases of an AE, and the denominator is patient exposure for an average course of treatment or for a specified course of treatment (e.g., days, months, years). The expression of frequency as commonly specified (e.g., in Periodic Safety Update Reports) is the number of reported cases divided by the number of tablets sold (e.g., 3 cases per million tablets sold). This requires the reader to make a conversion into a clinically useful figure (e.g., 5 cases per million patient-days of treatment) by calculating the mean duration of treatment or the mean daily dosage. The need to harmonize this expression was noted in the literature in the 1970s (Hollister, *Clin Pharmacol Ther* 1973;3:309). Spontaneous AE data cannot be used to produce data similar to that from clinical trials. One cannot say from spontaneous AE data that 1% of patients taking drug X develop headaches.

The E2C ICH document on Periodic Safety Update Reports recognizes the frailty of these data and requests "where possible an estimation of accurate patient exposure." The methodology used in determining the number must be provided but may be chosen by the preparer of the report. If it is "impossible to estimate or is a meaningless metric," then other measures can be used such as patient-days, number of prescriptions, or number of dosage units. If even these amounts are unavailable, then bulk tonnage may be used.

An additional problem arises with the loose usage of terms *frequent, common, rare.* The Council for International Organizations of Medical Sciences (CIOMS) has proposed a standardization of the terms as noted in the table. Given the difficulties in determining frequencies for AEs/ADRs with marketed drugs these terms are useful only for data obtained in clinical trials.

Very frequent or common	>10%	>1 in 10
Frequent or common	1%–10%	between 1 in 10 and 1 in 100
Infrequent or uncommon	0.1%–1%	between 1 in 100 and 1 in 1000
Rare	0.01%–0.1%	between 1 in 1000 and 1 in 10,000
Very rare	0.001%–0.01%	between 1 in 10,000 and 1 in 100,000
Exceedingly rare	<0.001%	<1 in 1,000,000

It must be remembered that the acceptability of an ADR (risk/benefit ratio) lies not only in the frequency of the ADR but also in its severity, duration, and importance, as well as in the importance, duration, and frequency of the benefit of the drug when analyzed against alternative treatments available and the disease being treated (see also RULE OF THREES).

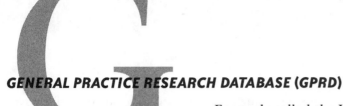

GENERAL PRACTICE RESEARCH DATABASE (GPRD)

Formerly called the Value Added Medicinal Products (VAMP) database, this contains the medical records of a large number of British general practitioners. A limited amount of information is recorded by the physician in the records collected by the database. The quality of the data is a function of the assiduousness of the participating physicians. This database allows for linked database studies on both medical practices and prescribing profiles (Jick, *PEDS* 1992;1:347). See the website of the Boston University Boston Collaborative Drug Surveillance Program (http://www.bu.edu/bcdsp/gprd.htm).

GUAR GUM: WITHDRAWAL FROM MARKET

This hydrophilic residue, which was sold as a weight loss product, began to produce some problems in the United States starting in 1985 when a new brand was introduced. In August 1989, a 39-year-old male entered the emergency room complaining of being unable to swallow his saliva several hours after swallowing three tablets. Rigid esophagoscopy was required. However, the esophagus was torn during the procedure and surgical repair was required. Several days later the patient had a fatal pulmonary embolus: a striking example of an indirect, secondary effect. The pharmacovigilance investigation done in the Food and Drug Administration database revealed 17 additional cases of esophageal retention; though none was equally serious, one patient required hospitalization and endoscopy. Guar gum was removed from the market and stocks that were already in the distribution channels were recalled, a preventive measure that is rarely performed. This ADR is in the category of transit site reactions. See two documents on the FDA website (www.fda.gov/bbs/topics/ANSWERS/ANS00386.html and www.fda.gov/medwatch/report/desk/casestud.htm).

GRANDFATHER DRUG

A term proposed by the Food and Drug Administration to designate older medications (e.g., aspirin) that entered the market before the current regulations came into force. Periodic safety reports are not required for these drugs because of their longtime use without any apparent risk. The issue of possible drug interactions between an old drug and new products, however, is not addressed.

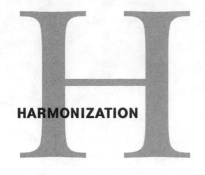

HARMONIZATION

The attempt to reach agreement in the pharmaceutical world (sometimes narrowly defined as the United States, the European Union, and Japan) on common procedures and requirements in drug development and surveillance. This took the form of a series of international meetings and working groups starting in 1990 and continuing today, the International Conference on Harmonization. See their website for full details (http://www.ifpma.org/ich1.html). In the pharmacovigilance world, similar harmonization has been done by the Council for International Organizations of Medical Sciences (CIOMS). See their website (http://www.who.int/dsa/cat98/zcioms8.htm).

The international harmonization of coding terms (*MedDRA*), of definitions (E2A), of forms (CIOMS I form), of procedures for periodic reporting of AEs and reactions (E2C), and of good pharmacovigilance practices are the objectives and results of several groups, most particularly CIOMS and the International Conference on Harmonization (see CIOMS and the INTERNATIONAL CONFERENCE ON HARMONIZATION).

HEALTH ACTION INTERNATIONAL (HAI)

An international group for the defense of consumers based in the Netherlands, who publish *Problem Drugs* (HAI-Europe, Jacob van Lennegekade 334T, 1053 NJ Amsterdam, the Netherlands, fax 31.20.685.50.02; www.haiweb.org).

HEMATOVIGILANCE

Pharmacosurveillance of AEs/ADRs affecting the blood (red and white cells, platelets) and blood forming organs. Distinct from hemovigilance, sometimes used to designate the surveillance of ADRs associated with the adminsitration of blood products.

HEMATOX AND HEPATOX

A database of the number of cases published in the literature associated with hematotoxic medications and hepatotoxic medications. It contains references indexed for each medication and for the various types of hematologic problems. This database is kept in Paris at the Regional Center for Pharmacovigilance Paris-Saint-Antoine and is updated periodically. Antineoplastic and immunosuppressant medications, well known for their hematotoxicity, are not included in the database in keeping with the classic separation of oncovigilance and hematovigilance. A frequency table is produced twice a year. For example, the January 1999 edition of Hematox counted 10,254 bibliographic references from 1983 to date covering 846 medications arranged by hematologic problem. Similar databases are maintained for two other target organs: Nephrotox (renal ADRs) and Pancreatox (pancreatic ADRs) (Dr. M. Biour, CRPV Paris-Saint-Antoine, Hôpital Saint-Antoine, 184, Rue du Faubourg St-Antoine, F-75571 Paris Cedex 12, France).

HEMOVIGILANCE

A term sometimes used to designate the surveillance of ADRs associated with the administration of blood products.

HIGH-LEVEL TERM (HLT)

In a coding dictionary such as *MedDRA* or *WHO-ART*, *high-level terms* (HLTs) are medical terms that are more general and inclusive than preferred terms (PTs) but more specific and less inclusive than system organ class (SOC) terms. Thus the hierarchy is SOC < HLT < PT < LLT (included term). For example, LLT: headache, PT: headache not otherwise specified, HLT: headache not elsewhere classified, SOC: nervous system disorder.

HISTORY, PAST ADVERSE DRUG REACTION

When a clinician questions a patient about his or her past medical history during the causality assessment of a suspected ADR, it is necessary to inquire about all past ADRs as well as the one in question.

It is necessary to distinguish between past history of ADRs in general and the specific history of prior occurrence of the ADR under suspicion. This distinction is necessary because the simple fact of having already experienced one or more ADRs constitutes in and of itself a nonnegligible risk factor for experiencing further ADRs even if the past ADRs are somewhat different from the current one in question and even if the drugs that produced the past ADRs are different from the current suspect drug. Relative risks ranging from 1.5 to 3.6 have been reported, confirming the clinical intuition that some patients do not tolerate drugs very well (Levy, *Eur J Clin Pharmacol* 1980;17:25; Hurwitz, *Br Med J* 1969;1:536).

The specific *history of the ADR in question* is obtained by determining which of four possibilities regarding the patient's previous exposure to the suspect drug (*prechallenge*) has occurred and whether the ADR in question has ever occurred without drug exposure. All ADR reports should contain this information or indicate that it is unavailable. There are four possible results:

- A positive prechallenge: The ADR in question occurred when the patient was exposed to the suspect drug in the past.
- A negative prechallenge: The ADR in question did not occur when the patient was exposed to the suspect drug in the past.
- The ADR in question occurred without a prior exposure to the drug. In this case then, the ADR was actually an AE.
- The ADR in question did not occur in the past, and the patient has never been exposed to the suspect drug.

I

ICH E2A DEFINITIONS AND STANDARDS FOR EXPEDITED REPORTING

An International Conference on Harmonization (ICH) working group that defined and normalized the criteria and definitions for expedited (alert) reporting of AEs. Their work was significantly influenced by that of the Council for International Organizations of Medical Sciences (CIOMS) I group. These proposals have been largely adopted in North America, Europe, Japan, and elsewhere (www.ifpma.org/pdfifpma/e2a.pdf).

ICH E2B DATA ELEMENTS FOR TRANSMISSION OF ADVERSE DRUG REACTION REPORTS

An International Conference on Harmonization (ICH) working group that defined and normalized the format and contents of expedited (alert) reports that are transmitted electronically. Their objectives were similar to those of the Council for International Organizations of Medical Sciences (CIOMS) Ia Working Group. These proposals have been modified and, for the moment, are final. They have been or are in the process of being adopted by many of the major health agencies in the world that are working on electronic transmission of safety data (www.ifpma.org/pdfifpma/e2b.pdf).

ICH E2C PERIODIC SAFETY UPDATE REPORTS (PSURs)

An International Conference on Harmonization (ICH) working group that defined and normalized the format and contents of periodic safety update reports that are sent to health authorities for marketed drugs. Their objectives were similar to those of the Council for International Organizations of Medical Sciences (CIOMS) II Working Group. E2C has been adopted by the European Union, Canada and Japan. The United States had not adopted E2C as of early 2001 (www.ifpma.org/pdfifpma/e2c.pdf), though a draft guidance (March 2001) by FDA indicates that the PSUR format may be used upon request.

ICH M1 STANDARDIZATION OF MEDICAL TERMINOLOGY FOR REGULATORY PURPOSES

An International Conference on Harmonization (ICH) working group that worked on the harmonization of the medical terminology for use in regulatory reporting. The *MedDRA* dictionary was ultimately chosen (see *MedDRA*) (www.ifpma.org/ich5m.html#Terminology).

ICH M2 ELECTRONIC STANDARDS FOR THE TRANSFER OF REGULATORY INFORMATION (ESTRI)

This International Conference on Harmonization (ICH) Expert Working Group, called *ESTRI*, defined the standards for the electronic transmission of normalized information for regulatory reporting (www.ifpma.org/ich5.html#ESTRI and www.ifpma.org/m2-main.html).

INCIDENCE RATE (see also FREQUENCY OF AN ADVERSE EVENT/DRUG REACTION)

In *epidemiology*, the numerator is formed by the number of new cases (i.e., patients with a disease or AE/ADR) that appear during a specified period; the denominator is formed by the total number of subjects (the population) who could develop (are susceptible to) the disease or AE/ADR in question during the same period.

In *postmarketing spontaneous reporting (pharmacovigilance)*, the true incidence rate is generally unknowable. What is calculated and reported is the *reporting rate*. This is calculated as follows: The numerator is the number of new cases of an AE/ADR during a specified time; the denominator is the number of comparable subjects exposed to the medication during the same time. The duration or time of exposure is either specified (months, years of treatment, etc.) or estimated assuming a mean duration of treatment (e.g., 10 days of drug use). The rate of the AE in those not exposed to the drug is known as the *baseline rate* or *reference rate* and is the number of new cases over a period. It too may be very difficult to calculate (see FREQUENCY OF ADVERSE EVENT/REACTION and RULE OF THREES).

INCLUDED TERM

In a coding dictionary such as *MedDRA* or *WHO-ART* (see *MedDRA, WHO-ART*), medical or nonmedical words describing an AE/ADR. They are synonymous with *lower-level terms* (LLT) and are a hierarchic step below *preferred terms* (PT) and more specific than preferred terms. They vary from dictionary to dictionary and language to language.

INCORRECT ROUTE OF MEDICATION

This type of error can be committed by the dispenser (e.g., anesthesiologist, nurse, pharmacist) or patient. The reaction may occur locally if the mistake involves the site of administration.

> *Methylphenidate: do not chew*: An 11-year-old hyperactive boy was responding well to methylphenidate by mouth. Upon return from summer vacation he developed intermittent but daily symptoms after each dose: headache, dizziness, palpitations, and syncope after strong exercise. With careful questioning he revealed that after the summer he developed the habit of chewing his medication rather than swallowing it. This produced buccal absorption rather than absorption lower down in the gastrointestineal tract (Rosse, *Am J Psychiatry* 1995;152:811).

A CASE SERIES FROM THE CORONER OF BIRMINGHAM, ENGLAND

A total of 3277 inquests were opened during the period 1986–1991 (Ferner, *J R Soc Med* 1994;87:145). Ten of the deaths were identified as due to errors of prescribing or giving drugs. During the same period, 36 deaths were caused by ADRs. This series of cases illustrates remarkably well the diversity of possible errors and the way that drug-related deaths ofter result from indirect, secondary effects.

- A premature newborn received 2.5 mg/kg/day rather than 2.5 mmol/kg/day of potassium chloride.
- A manic-depressive patient off lithium for 6 months believed her daily dose had been 1.2 g/day. This dose in fact had been a dose given only in an emergency. Her usual daily dose was 600 mg/day, that is, three times her normal dose.
- A woman with severe lumbar pain on propoxyphene received during the course of 1 day: delayed release dihydrocodeine, intramuscular meperidine (pethidine) in the early evening, and morphine 4 hours later.

- A patient with bronchitis received 4.5 l/min of oxygen by nasal cannula rather than 1 ml/min. She died of respiratory depression. This adverse effect would qualify as a *medical device problem.*
- An Englishman who required emergency anticoagulation while abroad was given one 2.5 mg of warfarin tablet per day. Upon returning to his own physician in Britain he was given one warfarin 3.0-mg tablet per day (the formulation available in the United Kingdom). This increase in warfarin of 20% may have led to his fatal hemorrhage.
- A man in atrial fibrillation took the nonsteroidal anti-inflammatory drug (NSAID) azapropazone and the anticoagulant warfarin together. This combination is contraindicated. A fatal cerebral hemorrhage occurred.
- A psychotic patient overdosed on propoxyphene, diclofenac, and dihydrocodeine and required peritoneal dialysis. Bouts of agitation required repeated doses of chlorpromazine both orally and intramuscularly, which produced fatal respiratory arrest.
- The last case is an example of drug withdrawal. A schizophrenic was well controlled for 10 years on 5 mg of haloperidol three times a day. A computerized prescription by his general practitioner for a markedly lower dose led to fatal catatonia and pneumonia.

INCREASED FREQUENCY

This term is used in pharmacovigilance to denote an increase in the number of spontaneous reports of a particular ADR or ADRs associated with a product in a specific geographic zone over a specific period. The Food and Drug Administration gave a regulatory definition as a 100% increase in the number of cases, adjusted for volume over the preceding period for a serious ADR, whether labeled or not. However, effective 25 July 1997, the FDA withdrew the requirement that increased frequency data be sent as expedited reports. They noted that these reports have not contributed to the timely identification of safety problems. In general, an increase in frequency can serve as a signal and lead to a pharmacovigilance investigation.

INDEX CASES

The first one or two observations of a new important ADR. When a new, serious, unexpected adverse effect/ADR first appears, is valid, and has a very strong causal association with the suspect drug, it is a signal and should be communicated: submitted to a medical journal, reported to the local health authority, and/or to the manufacturer. Also called *signal cases.*

INFORMED CONSENT

The informed consent (also called the *written informed consent* or *signed informed consent*) is a document that is required before a patient may enter almost any clinical trial or research project even if no medical intervention occurs. Although the rules differ from country to country, the broad outlines are the same: The informed consent must be written in understandable language and should be in the language of the patient even if it differs from the national language. It must give information on the drug under study, the potential benefits to the patient (if any), the potential risks, the procedures that the patient will undergo in the trial, whom to contact at any hour of the day, and other information. It must be given without coercion and refusal to sign must not compromise medical care otherwise given. The patient must also have the right to withdraw at any time after the study starts for any or no reason.

In the postmarketing setting, a written informed consent may be required in the relatively uncommon situation that after a pharmacovigilance investigation has shown a problematic risk/benefit ratio, it has been determined that the drug may remain on the market only if certain exceptional measures are taken. In these cases the prescriber may obtain a written informed consent from the patient indicating that he or she understands and accepts the risks in taking this drug. Examples could include thalidomide and isotretinoin, both in the field of teratovigilance (potentially pregnant women).

INJECTION SITE REACTION

An injection site reaction is one that occurs at the place on the skin where a parenteral drug has been given, or in the blood vessel, muscle, or any other structure in the immediate vicinity of the injection site.

What is most interesting about these reactions is that the cause in almost all cases is clearly the drug in question, and thus causality can be classified as *very probable* or even *certain*. There are very few other AEs that have such clear causality.

This type of reaction can be of type A or type B. It can be due to the active product or to an excipient. It may also be due to an error of administration that may or may not be evident such as intravenous injections that are in fact given subcutaneously or intraarterially

INJURY COMPENSATION

A fund created by governments or manufacturers to provide a lump sum, no fault payment in order to compensate for damage due to a product, lower legal costs and prevent unnecessary lawsuits, promote social justice, and prevent the bankruptcy of manufacturers (e.g., for vaccine injuries). This type of fund exists in the United Kingdom for some ADRs that occur in the course of clinical research.

INTENSIFIED SURVEILLANCE (ENHANCED MONITORING, PROMPTED REPORTING, INTENSIVE MONITORING)

These terms represent a call for reporting by health care practitioners of one or more adverse effects with the aim of increasing the reports of these AEs. This is done either in the case of a pharmacovigilance investigation because the product is new on the market and is a member of a pharmacologic family of drugs that may produce significant risk ("reporting focused on a product to see if there is a signal") or in follow-up to a known signal ("reporting focused on an AE/ADR"). Other terms have been used including: *enhanced, requested, facilitated, reinforced, encouraged, incited, active,* and *stimulated* reporting. It must be emphasized that this is a *scientific measure* taken to confirm, clarify, or refute a hypothesis raised by a signal.

GLOBAL OR UNIVERSAL SURVEILLANCE

Intensified reporting of all suspected ADRs for all products. This can be directed, usually by a health agency, to the clinicians in an entire country, region, hospital, and so on. If reporting is to be effective it is necessary to ensure that sufficient budget, logistics, and competent and motivated personnel are available and the reasons are adequately explained to the reporting clinicians. This may occur when a country introduces pharmacovigilance at the national level for the first time or revamps its older drug surveillance system.

FOCUSED ON A PRODUCT

The specific product is added to the table of medications under formal surveillance in the national bulletin of pharmacovigilance; the adverse event may correspond to a *Designated Medical Event*. The readership of these bulletins is limited to governmental agencies and manufacturers and to regional pharmacovigilance centers in those countries with such centers, though the information is now more widely available when posted on a health authority website (www.fda.gov/cder/aers/slides/tsld015.htm and www.fda.gov/cder/aers). In Australia and Canada, such bulletins are known as *Drugs of Current Interest*.

In Great Britain, such surveillance can last 2 years and a list of products under intensive monitoring is published in the national bulletin. Such a medication is identified in the labeling by a black triangle (www.fda.gov/cder/aers/slides/tsld015.htm and www.fda.gov/cder/aers).

AIMED AT AN ADR

In the course of a pharmacovigilance investigation that results from a signal it is possible to ask for intensified monitoring of a particular ADR thought to be potentially due to the drug (or more than one drug). An example of this might be a specific ADR such as torsades de pointes or a suspected new drug interaction that has only become suspect since the marketing of the product. The first step consists of placing the drug on the list of *products under surveillance* in the national bulletin of pharmacovigilance. However, if the situation is very serious, additional measures such as a request for cases can be addressed to health care professionals by use of a "Dear Health Care Professional" letter through all the modern means of communication (mail, e-mail, the Internet, announcements in professional journals) as well as a call to the public through mass media (e.g., television and radio) as appropriate from either the health authority or the manufacturer or both.

> *Blindness due to practolol:* Practolol is a beta-blocker introduced in Great Britain and later withdrawn from the market because of an oculomucosalcutaneous syndrome that was quite difficult to diagnose. Blindness was recognized only after the exposure of about 100,000 hypertensive patients as a result of the clinical acuity of an ophthalmologist, Dr. Peter Wright (*BMV*, 1975;I:595). The first three publications served as a signal to the medical community and elicited reports of 200 additional spontaneous cases.

INTERNATIONAL BIRTH DATE (IBD)

The date of the first marketing authorization in any country in the world (ICH E2C). It is used to calculate the "commercial age" of a product and to define the dates when Periodic Safety Update Reports (PSURs) (see PERIODIC SAFETY UPDATE REPORT) must be submitted to health authorities. In pharmacovigilance it would be more logical to use the day of the first launch of the product anywhere in the world since patient exposure does not begin until the launch date. Surprisingly, there is sometimes a long delay between the approval of the Marketing Authorization and the launch date.

In practice the IBD has proved difficult to harmonize and agree upon for older products not approved through common centralized procedures (especially in the European Union). That is, the drug may have been first approved in one major market long before approval in another major market, or the approval of a new indication for an old drug may occur in one country many years earlier than in another country. In these cases certain regulatory authorities are quite uncomfortable waiting 5 years between PSURs for newly approved products (which were approved more than 5 years ago elsewhere) or for old products that gain new indications over the course of years (e.g., oncology drugs).

INTERNATIONAL COMMITTEE ON HARMONIZATION OF TECHNICAL REQUIREMENTS FOR REGISTRATION OF PHARMACEUTICALS FOR HUMAN USE (ICH)

This committee includes representatives from the pharmaceutical industry and from governments of three major regions: the European Union, the United States, and Japan. In addition, observers from the World Health Organization (WHO), Canada, the European Free Trade Area countries, and individual countries have sent representatives. Technical and secretarial assistance has been provided by the International Federation of Pharmaceutical Manufacturers Association (IFPMA). See the website (www.ifpma.org/ich1.html).

After more than a year of preparation, the first meeting was held in Brussels in 1991. An aggressive agenda was proposed and working groups were formed to explore many areas of the registration process of pharmaceuticals. Broadly speaking, three major areas of focus were chosen and three groups were created:

Safety: topics relating to in vitro and in vivo preclinical studies, for example, S1 Carcinogenicity Testing and S2 Genotoxicity Testing

Efficacy: topics relating to clinical studies in human subjects, for example: E4 Dose Response Studies, Carcinogenicity Testing, and E6 Good Clinical Practices

Quality: topics relating to chemical and pharmaceutical quality assurance, for example, Q1 Stability Testing and Q3 Impurity Testing

Since Brussels 1991, additional meetings have been held; ICH 5 was held in San Diego in November 2000. Further information, including the documents produced, is available on the website.

In the area of pharmacovigilance, many consensus documents (E2A, E2B, E2C, M1, M2, and others) were published, some of which drew upon the work of the Council for International Organizations of Medical Sciences (CIOMS). Note that by bureaucratic fluke the pharmacovigilance safety documents have been produced in the Efficacy Group, not the Safety Group (this later group worked on preclinical safety). Many of these documents have been officially adopted in the European Union, Japan, the United States, Canada, and elsewhere. This has produced much greater harmonization of definitions, reporting forms, procedures for reporting expedited AEs and periodic reports and electronic transmission of data than anyone might have expected in 1990. One consequence of this harmonization has been the grudging unofficial adoption of English as the world language of pharmacovigilance. Most non-English-speaking countries now routinely accept reporting of nondomestic safety information in English and some even accept English language reports for domestic events also.

The goal of this harmonization has been the hope of all parties that the unnecessary and repetitive exposure of patients to testing as well as the costs and time needed for drug development and registration will be reduced significantly. It is the belief of all concerned that this is happening. It has, however, been hard to measure this objectively since many other factors that have occurred have influenced cost and caused delays, including the Food and Drug Administration Modernization Act, the creation of the European Medicinal Evaluation Agency

(EMEA), and reforms in the health authorities in many other countries (ICH Secretariat, c/o IFPMA, 30 rue de St Jean, POB 9, 1211 Geneva 18, Switzerland; www.ifpma.org/ich1.html).

INTERNATIONAL NONPROPRIETARY NAME (INN)

A summary list of proposed and recommended designations for pharmaceutical substances that is maintained by the World Health Organization (WHO). These names are usually the same from country to country, but in rare instances the names differ. For example, *acetaminophen* is the designation in the United States *the United States Adopted Name* (*USAN*) while *paracetamol* is the designation in France. Another example is *cephalexin* which is the designation in the United States (USAN), Great Britain (British Approved Name (BAN)) and Canada whereas the French designation (Dénomination commune française (DCF)) is *cefalexinum* and the INN is *cefalexine*.

INTERNATIONAL NORMALIZED PROTHROMBIN TIME RATIO (INR)

In pharmacotherapy: A laboratory test that is used to monitor the pharmacologic action of oral anticoagulants. The results are used to adjust the dosage to stay within the narrow therapeutic window.

In hematovigilance: This test is used to discover new drug interactions between an oral anticoagulant and recently marketed drugs.

INTERNATIONAL SOCIETY OF PHARMACOVIGILANCE (ISOP)

A group made up primarily of clinicians in academia, industry, and government dedicated to advancing the study of pharmacovigilance. Formerly called the European Society of Pharmacovigilance, they hold annual meetings usually in Europe. Membership has been primarily European but is open to others who are interested. Their address is 10-11 The Stableyard, Broomgrove Road, London, SW9 9TL, UK.

INTRINSIC EFFECT

A term used to designate an ADR due to the active ingredient in the product as opposed to a reaction (an extrinsic effect) due to a nonactive component (excipient) or to a problem with defective material. (See also EXTRINSIC EFFECT.)

INVESTIGATIONAL NEW DRUG (IND) APPLICATION

The dossier or application submitted to a health authority (drug agency) after completion of sufficient preclinical research and development of a product to move into human clinical trials. Its approval by the agency is required before starting the clinical evaluation. The contents of the dossier vary from country to country but usually include results of the preclinical work done to date, the formulation and manufacturing data, and a protocol for a proposed clinical trial. The longer-term carcinogenicity and toxicology studies are usually done simultaneously with the clinical trials on a risk basis. For drugs that are already on the market, an IND may have to be opened for clinical trials of a new indication or formulation. The contents of the IND are usually proprietary and confidential.

INVESTIGATOR (OR INVESTIGATOR'S) BROCHURE (IB)

The IB is a summary of the characteristics of a product under development (i.e., in clinical trials). It contains a detailed summary of the characteristics of the product, including pharmacology, toxicology, clinical research, and postmarketing data. It is a "living" document that is updated as new data are produced. In some countries it must be updated and submitted to the health authorities at least once yearly. It is used for the study of drugs that have not yet been approved as well as for drugs that have been approved for one indication but are being studied for other (unapproved) indications. The sponsor (manu-facturer) has a legal, scientific, and ethical obligation to supply this document to clinical investigators doing phase I, II, III, and IV studies. Ethics committees and institutional review boards (IRBs) must also have access to this document before approving a clinical trial—particularly those trials with substantial risks to patients. In pharmacovigilance, it is used (for unapproved products) as labeling to determine whether a particular AE/ADR is labeled or not and thus required for submission as an expedited report or in a periodic report (e.g., a Periodic Safety Update Report (PSUR), or New Drug Applicaton (NDA) periodic re-port). After marketing approval, the product labeling replaces the IB for deter-mination of labeling.

JKL

LABELED

This term is used to indicate that an AE/ADR is contained in the official drug labeling or monograph. For regulatory purposes it is equivalent to the word *expected*. In general, an event or reaction is not considered labeled if it is not clearly specified in the label. A term that is more specific or more severe is generally considered not labeled. Thus if *hepatitis* is labeled and the patient has *hepatitis A* or *fatal hepatitis,* for regulatory purposes, the events are *not* considered labeled. If *chest pain* is labeled, *angina pectoris* or *costochondritis* is *not* considered labeled.

In general for regulatory reporting purposes, the event or reaction is *not* considered labeled if it appears only in the class labeling. For example, if a steroid is labeled only in the *class labeling* section for cataracts and not in the AE/reaction section that is specific to the product, then it is considered unlabeled (unexpected) (see EXPECTED).

There is a continued and as yet unresolved debate in the pharmacovigilance world in regard to secondary, indirect events (events that are a consequence, a *cascade* resulting from primary, direct ADRs). For example, if a drug produces anemia and this reaction is clearly and fully labeled, should angina pectoris, coronary insufficiency, and acute myocardial infarct be labeled if they are clearly a result of the anemia? Some say that it should be labeled as it is a potential medical emergency, and others say that a prescriber should know that anemia can produce cardiac events. They also believe that secondary events will clutter the label and reduce the impact of the message to be conveyed.

One other debate, however, does seem to be resolved. The use of syndromes and eponyms in labeling is now generally avoided unless the name is widely known or understood (e.g., *Raynaud's phenomenon* or *flu-like syndrome).* Obscure names are now avoided.

LABELED, FULLY

This expression is equivalent to *labeled in its full expression or sense* and used to designate an expectedness at level 4 (expected ADR as documented in the official product labeling/monograph in force at the moment the prescription is written). Ideally the labeling of an ADR should cover four elements if our priority is the communication of the drug's background knowledge "to those who need to know" (e.g., the prescribers): its specific description, severity or gravity, risk factors if appropriate, and relative and absolute frequency (when they can be evaluated in a meaningful way: very rarely).

SPECIFIC DESCRIPTION

A reaction should always be described in a specific enough manner so as to be meaningful and useful to the prescriber and user. In rare instances chronologic or historical details can be included to assist in the detection and causality assessment of the reaction:

> *Interstitial nephritis* is more specific than *acute renal insufficiency*

> *Cerebral thrombosis* is more precise than *cerebrovascular accident*

It is clear that the progressive adoption of *MedDRA* as a replacement for the *WHO-ART* and *COSTART* dictionaries will produce labeling issues because *MedDRA* contains many thousands of additional terms that are more specific ("granular") than the terms they are replacing. For example, *MedDRA* version 3.3 contains over 13,000 preferred terms and 49,000 lower level terms; *WHO-ART* and *COSTART* have 2000 to 4000 preferred terms.

SEVERITY AND GRAVITY OF THE EVENT AND ITS CLINICAL OUTCOME

The prescriber would like to know about the severity of the reaction and/or the consequences and about whether fatal reactions have been reported even if there is only a single case. In general, however, it is not advisable to report specific numbers of cases (e.g., "three cases of fatal fulminant hepatitis were seen") since the label will have to be changed as soon as a fourth case occurs. *Fulminant hepatitis, liver transplant* or *fatal hepatic insufficiency* provide more information to the clinician than a simple mention of *acute hepatitis. Acute renal insufficiency* carries more severity information than *interstitial nephritis.*

RISK FACTORS

Risk factors are worth noting if their mention can reduce or prevent the reaction. The prescriber must have this knowledge to prescribe safely.

RELATIVE OR ABSOLUTE FREQUENCY

If knowledge of the estimated incidence of worldwide cases of a particular AE/ADR is pertinent for the prescriber to decide for or against the use of a particular drug, then this information should ideally be included in the labeling. These data usually are developed from phase III and IV trials and from cohort studies, not from postmarketing spontaneous reporting data, for the following reasons:

> The true and complete numerator is impossible to know. The only data that can be obtained are *reported cases* and this number virtually always underestimates the true number. The quantity of the underestimate is not known, nor is the underestimation necessarily consistent from drug to drug or country to country (see also RULE OF THREES).

> The denominator is impossible to know. The number of tablets produced or sold may be known but not how many were actually used by the patients and how many remained in the medicine cabinet unused. Even if this were known, it is not clear how to determine an actual incidence: is equal weight given to the patient who takes an antihistamine only once a year versus the patient who takes it daily for 6 months during allergy season?

> When the data are good, it is possible to use an estimate of patient-days of exposure. For example, it might be found that a drug was associated with 300 cases of somnolence in 8 billion patient-days of exposure. From this the clinician might conclude that the likelihood of this AE/ADR in a patient or patients is small. More meaningful data must be obtained from controlled clinical trials or comparative cohort studies.

>> *Lamotrigine:* The prescriber who is aware that the risk of a cutaneous eruption leading to hospitalization (Stevens-Johnson syndrome, Lyell's syndrome) is estimated at 1/1000 for lamotrigine should be aware of this information before prescribing this product to an adult (CSM/MCA, *Curr Probl Phamacovigil* 1993;19;3 and 1996;22:12). This ADR is fully labeled by the manufacturer.

In clinical trials, it is very important that the absolute frequencies of serious AEs be incorporated rapidly into the investigator's brochure as soon as the data are obtained. In particular this should occur as one moves into phase III.

LABELING; PRODUCT MONOGRAPH; SUMMARY OF PRODUCT CHARACTERISTICS

REGULATORY

This word is used in two senses. In pharmaceutical regulation area, *labeling* refers to the officially approved monograph, which includes the description of the characteristics of the product, its uses, dosing, contraindications, warning, pregnancy information, drug interactions, and AEs, as well as (in most countries) the packaging, the patient leaflet, and other materials prepared for the marketplace. *Labeling* here is an all-encompassing, global term and refers to the contents as well as the form of the information.

The synonyms used to describe labeling are confusing. Confusion occurs because the terms may actually mean different things in different regions. In the United States, the usual term for this is *labeling* or *product labeling*. In Europe the term used is *Summary of Product Characteristics* (SPC or SmPC). In the United States, the term *SPC* is used by Americans to refer only to the *European* labeling and not to labeling in general. Thus no one in the United States would refer to a "U.S. SPC." In Canada, the term is *monograph*. In other areas, "monograph" may refer to a large document available on request to prescribers that has additional detail on the product with summaries of clinical trials, clinical pharmacology, and other information.

"Labeling" represents the document prepared by the manufacturer and approved by the governmental authorities whose audience is the competent intermediaries (prescribers, dispensers, etc.) using the product. It contains information on the product that is essential for its *safe and efficacious use* such that the benefits are maximized and the risks are minimized. This document represents the official labeling and may appear in the national compendia in the countries where it is sold. It is the reference document used by companies to determine whether an adverse effect is expected or not (*labeled*) for use in reporting expedited AEs (*15 day reports*). It may also serve as the legal basis for advertising and promotional materials. It may also form the basis for reimbursement of the cost of the drug to the patient by insurance companies or the national health service, as use of the drug for unapproved (*unlabeled*) indications may not be covered.

NONREGULATORY: LABEL, STICKER

The more informal and lay use of the term *labeling* refers more narrowly to the sticker attached to the bottle and not necessarily to its contents. That is, "The label is unreadable" would refer to the fact that the writing or printing on the sticker, prepared by the pharmaceutical company, distributor or pharmacist cannot be read because of its size, color, or other characteristics.

LABELING, OFFICIAL

This term describes the wording approved by the pharmaceutical health authority that summarizes the product's characteristics. There are various synonyms, which vary by country or region: *Summary of Product Characteristics* (SPC or SmPC), *product labeling*, *package insert*, or *product monograph*. It includes information on the pharmacologic properties of the drug as well as its packaging, dosing, indications, contraindications, AEs/reactions, warnings, use in pregnant women and other specific groups, drug interactions, and so. In its original sense *labeling* refers to the manner of editing a text, but in pharmacotherapy it is used to designate the text itself. The word *official* is often omitted in talking about the labeling. The official labeling is critical in that it forms the basis for advertising claims for the drug as well as being used to determine whether the indication being treated is a labeled and thus reimbursable ("legitimate") expense in the eyes of an insurance company or government agency. In some countries (e.g., the United States) it also serves as a legal document protecting the company in certain lawsuits.

LABORATORY RESULTS, COMPLETENESS OF

If the results of laboratory tests are relevant in the description of an AE, they should be presented in the case report form. For each relevant lab test the following descriptive elements should be listed:

- The date of the test and, if appropriate, the time of day
- The name of the test and "bodily source" (e.g., serum creatinine or urine sodium level, skin biopsy of arm lesion)
- The units of measurement (e.g., milligrams, International Units, grams per liter)
- The normal values (e.g., 6–40 IU, none, <2 g/l)
- The results

If the test was repeated several times, for example, before, during, and after treatment with the suspect medication, the ideal situation would be to present only the values that are most useful for the evaluation of the causality of the adverse effect:

- The last value before the start of the reaction (*control or baseline value*)
- The first abnormal value (in order to evaluate the time to appearance)
- The most abnormal value (in order to evaluate the severity)
- The last value before stopping of the suspect product (in order to understand the course during treatment)
- The first normal value or the least abnormal value after the stopping of the suspect product (i.e., the value after dechallenge)

When possible, multiple or repeated lab test results should be presented in tabular or structured form. This will most likely be required when electronic transmission of safety data becomes obligatory.

LACK OF EFFICACY

In many regions (e.g., the United States) the failure of a drug to be efficacious in the indication for which the drug is approved and prescribed is considered a reportable AE/ADR.

LACTATION AND DRUGS

A drug that is administered to a woman who is breast-feeding her child can be transmitted to the baby in the breast milk (transmammary transmission). There are two types of AE/ADR reports that can be made (ICH E2B):

> If the AE/ADR affects the baby but not the mother, it is referred to as a *parent-child report* and only a single form (e.g., CIOMS I, MedWatch) needs to be filled out.

If the mother and the child are affected, it is recommended that two separate reports be made, specifying that they are "linked."

LANCET

This medical journal is often in the lead in publishing case reports of ADRs. In a study of case reports published in medical journals, a literature search was made to determine the number of indexed references in the course of a year. The number of case reports was calculated by consulting five major journals of internal medicine, a bibliographic database, and seven pharmacology journals.

The results of published case reports were as follows: *Lancet*, 212; *Br Med J*, 115; *Ann Pharmacother*, 94; *N Engl J Med*, 72; *JAMA*, 59; *Presse Médicale*, 57; and *Thérapie*, 54. This showed that the *Lancet* is a key source for published ADRs. The presence of a large number of case reports in two French-language journals demonstrates that literature investigations for ADRs should not be limited to the English language (Haramburu, *Lancet* 1993;341:1030).

LATENCY PERIOD

The time or duration between the *last* dose of a suspect product and the first manifestation of an ADR . Some authors use this term to designate the (sometimes very long) period between the *first* dose and the appearance of the ADR during continuing treatment with the suspect drug. In order to prevent confusion we do not use this meaning.

The latency period can be quite variable, and its use is usually reserved for intervals that are so long that they play a confusing role in the differential diagnosis of the problem.

As the following examples show, a long latency period can be quite disconcerting:

- If the ADR is a withdrawal or rebound syndrome, there is always a latency period, but it is usually short.
- In teratovigilance, there is usually a delay between the administration of a drug in the first trimester and the diagnosis of a malformation either at the time of birth 6 months or later, or at the time of an ultrasound examination weeks to months later during the pregnancy.
- In the case of retroperitoneal fibrosis due to the beta-blocker practolol, the surgeon would not recognize the lesion until the secondary effect of intestinal or ureteral occlusion occurred.
- In the case of clear cell adenocarcinoma of the vagina due to in utero exposure to diethylstilbestrol, the latency period was about 20 years, the longest in the history of modern pharmacovigilance.

LIFE-THREATENING CONDITION

A medical condition that, in the absence of acute medical treatment, would likely prove fatal. Examples include anaphylactic shock requiring epinephrine, a ventricular arrhythmia requiring defibrillation, and acute hepatic injury requiring a liver transplant. In regulatory terms, a life-threatening condition is one of the criteria of *seriousness* and may necessitate an expedited report of this AE.

LINE LISTING

A computerized tabulation of ADR data associated with a particular product. The columns contain the specific information on the product, the patient, and the AE/ADR and each row corresponds to an individual case.

PREPARED BY THE MANUFACTURER

In a Periodic Safety Update Report (PSUR) as prepared by the manufacturer to be submitted to health authorities, this table summarizes the AEs/ADRs associated with a product. The format has been standardized by the International Conference on Harmonization (ICH) (following the original CIOMS II format very closely) and has been accepted by the European Union (EU), Japan, and the United States. See the safety documents at the ICH website (http://www.ifpma.org/ich5e.html#Safety) particularly E2C (see E2C). It is obligatory for submissions in Canada, the EU, and Japan. Its use in the United States is permitted upon request and is expected to become obligatory soon.

PREPARED BY A GOVERNMENTAL AGENCY

In a pharmacovigilance bulletin or a medical journal, the line listing gives *collective feedback*. In correspondence to reporters of AEs, it may serve as individual feedback. The format has not been consistent from agency to agency.

CIOMS II LINE LISTING

The CIOMS II Working Group has proposed that ADRs be classified by the organ system involved in pharmacovigilance periodic reports, which must also include a narrative section. See the CIOMS website (http://www.who.int/dsa/cat98/zcioms8.htm) particularly E2C (see E2C). The columns of the report are as follows:

- Country
- Source (clinical trial, health care professional, literature)
- Age
- Sex
- Dose
- Time to appearance
- Description of the reaction reported
- Outcome (fatal, recovered, etc.)
- Comments
- Reference number of the manufacturer

LISTED ADVERSE DRUG REACTION

A regulatory term used in regard to the preparation of the Company Core Safety Information (CCSI). A *listed* reaction is one in which the nature, severity, specificity, and outcome are consistent with the information in the CCSI. See the Notice to Marketing Authorizations Holders Pharmacovigilance Guidelines at http://www.emea.eu.int/pdfs/human/phvwp/010899en.pdf (see also LABELED).

LITERATURE SEARCH

In pharmacovigilance this term may include the querying of one or more AE/ADR databases, in addition to a classic review of published (and in some cases unpublished) medical literature. The extent of the search depends upon its objectives.

SEARCHES

There can be three objections :

> **Response to a Clinician's Query**

The query may or may not accompany the reporting of an AE/ADR. The question usually revolves around whether a particular AE/ADR has been seen before, in what types of patients, course, and treatment. The result of the query may increase the likelihood that an individual case should be added to the *signal list* of AEs/ADRs to undergo more intense surveillance.

▶ Signal Investigation

During the course of a pharmacovigilance investigation, the literature must be reviewed and various databases may be searched for this AE/ADR. In a pharmaceutical company, this could include an examination of the postmarketing safety database and the clinical trials database internally as well as Food and Drug Administration's and World Health Organization's (WHO) pharmacovigilance databases.

▶ Review Articles

This investigation may be done in preparation for the publication of a review article or for the preparation of an "expert report" or in response to a query from a health authority.

DEPTH OF THE SEARCH

▶ Summary Review

This can be limited to:

- Reading the latest product monograph and labeling obtained from the company or from a compendium
- Querying the database maintained by the national health authority (if allowed)
- Contacting the local subsidiary of the manufacturer (though not all companies will disclose this information)

▶ In-depth Review

During a pharmacovigilance investigation or in the preparation of a review, the search would be more extensive. In addition to the previous elements, some of the following may prove useful:

- Contact the manufacturer's drug safety surveillance group at the world headquarters.
- Obtain reports from the FDA and WHO databases.
- Review the content of key national pharmacovigilance bulletins such as *Current Problems in Pharmacovigilance* (United Kingdom) and the *Australian ADRs Bulletin* and of course the formidable EMEA and Food and Drug Administration websites.
- Review the key pharmacovigilance bulletins (*Reactions Weekly* is a good start) and websites.
- Review reference dictionaries such as *Martindale* (the most complete), the *AHFS-DI*, the *USPDI*, and *Drug Facts and Comparisons*, and national compendia (e.g., the *Physician's Desk Reference*).
- Review the indexes of the medical specialty journals appropriate to the AE/ADR in question, with the help of *Current Contents*.
- Review the *Side Effect of Drugs Annuals* and the *Meyler's Side Effects of Drugs* when appropriate.
- Review the *Cochrane database* (see COCHRANE COLLABORATION AND LIBRARY) for syntheses of published and unpublished clinical trials.
- Consult internal or external experts in the field.
- Conduct a library search either directly on the Internet (e.g., *National Library of Medicine Grateful Med,* http://igm.nlm.nih.gov/) or with the assis-

tance of the medical library. Although the number of periodicals included in Medline is rather large, it is worthwhile to use *Embase/Excerpta Medica Drugs and Pharmacology.*

Antidepressant: bruxism: After observation of this AE in a 65-year-old man treated with an antidepressant, several pharmacists in Toronto made a Medline search during the preparation of a publication. They found no similar cases (Pin, *Clin Pharmacol Ther* 1996;3:123). This would increase the signaling value of the case as the index case. However, after consultation with expert psychiatrists a speciality publication was found with four similar observations (Ellison, *J Clin Psychiatry* 1993;54:432). Their case thus became the fifth to be published.

LITERATURE SURVEILLANCE

The regular and periodic review of the published literature using one or more of the many databases available to track medical publications. This is required by law for the New Drug Application (NDA) or marketing authorization holders in many countries. Finding cases in the literature then entails the usual follow-up and reporting (15-day-alert reports and/or periodic reporting). It is also a routine practice for national pharmacovigilance centers, at least for those drugs that are *under surveillance* or on the *watch list.*

LOCAL SAFETY OFFICER

An expression designating the person responsible for pharmacovigilance in the national or regional subsidiary of a pharmaceutical company or sometimes in a national or regional health authority. In some situations, the functional head of pharmacovigilance in a company (whether in the headquarters or a subsidiary) is not always the legally responsible person (*Chief Safety Officer*) whose name is supplied to the local health authority.

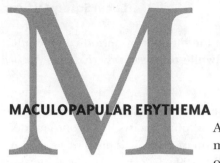

MACULOPAPULAR ERYTHEMA

A frequently seen term in dermatovigilance. A simple, benign eruption whose mechanism is not always clear. Often called a "rash" or "eruption," it constitutes one of the most frequently reported ADRs because of its reporting frequency and because of its visibility. Maculopapular erythema is not always drug-related as there are other causes (e.g., viral). Its frequency is even greater when the reporter is not a health care professional. The issue is even worse if the diagnosis is not reliable (i.e., made by an observer who cannot distinguish among an exanthema, urticaria, dermatitis, febrile eruption, and other conditions).

There is most probably a relative overreporting of cutaneous ADRs compared to more important hepatic and hematologic ones, which occur unnoticed when they are subclinical or picked up only by laboratory examinations. Reported isolated rashes do contribute to the workload of all concerned, sometimes without signaling value. They usually have more signaling value when they are the presenting symptom of a more serious AE/ADR.

MANUFACTURER CONTROL NUMBER

A number given to an AE/ADR case by the manufacturer. A governmental health agency also gives this report a number whether it is received from a reporter directly or via the manufacturer.

The situation is complex, and it is always a challenge to avoid reporting duplicate cases because a single report may have multiple numbers: the manufacturer's subsidiary may assign a local control number; the manufacturer's home office safety group may assign a corporate control number; each health authority receiving the report assigns a (different) number; and if the case is transmitted by a health authority to the World Health Organization (WHO) Monitoring Centre in Uppsala, it is assigned another number there. All of this presents a challenge in keeping track of cases and preventing duplicate counting and reporting. The E2B/M2 Working Groups have addressed the issue of a unique control number for use in electronic data transmission. See the E2B document at the website (http://www.ifpma.org/ich5e.html#Safety).

MARKET WITHDRAWAL

The result of *product discontinuation, delicensing,* and *suspension of the marketing authorization by the authorities.* It may be voluntary or obligatory. Reasons are often but not necessarily safety-related. Nonsafety reasons include portfolio rationalization after a company merger, reformulation (long-acting, new delivery system), reimbursement decisions by governments or insurers, regulatory review of "grandfather drugs," legal reasons (see BENDECTIN), low sales, and obsolescence that results from advances in pharmacotherapy (Sheffield, *Med J Aust* 1985;143:143).

MARKETING AUTHORIZATION (MA)

There are two uses of this term and the related U.S. term New Drug Application (NDA) Approval.

AUTHORIZATION

Permission given by the appropriate governmental drug agency to the sponsor, manufacturer, or patent holder allowing the commercialization of a new pharmaceutical product or a new indication or formulation of an already marketed product. Generic products, as new formulations, also usually require a marketing authorization, but the latter is based mainly on human bioavailability studies.

This permission is given after

■ the submission of the preclinical and clinical dossier (package, submission) accompanying the marketing request and
■ the analysis of the dossier by the health authorities.

Some governments also require pricing approval. The date of the first MA in any country corresponds to the International Birth Date for the new drug (see INTERNATIONAL BIRTH DATE).

DOSSIER

In Canada the dossier is called the *New Drug Submission* (NDS) and in the United States it is called the *New Drug Application* (NDA), and one speaks of an NDS or NDA as being approved. Sometimes the term *NDA* refers to the actual approval and sometimes to the documents ("We submitted the NDA (i.e., documents) last week." "We've had an NDA (i.e., approval) for the syrup formulation for 5 years"). One section of the confidential dossier includes a summary of all of the AEs observed in the course of clinical trials and postmarketing ADRs in countries where the drug is already marketed. Sometimes summaries of the dossier are available after approval. In the United States these are known as *Summary Basis of Approval* documents (SBOAs) and in the European Union as *European Product Assessment Reports* (EPARs).

MARKETING AUTHORIZATION HOLDER (MAH), MA HOLDER, LICENSE HOLDER, APPLICANT, NEW DRUG APPLICATION/NEW DRUG SUBMISSION (NDA/NDS) HOLDER

A company, person, organization who has asked for and received the permission to market a pharmaceutical product. The permission can be for a new drug or a new indication or formulation of a drug already on the market. In the United States the Marketing Authorization is referred to as an *NDA* and the MA Holder is called the *NDA Holder* (see APPROVAL PROCEDURE—EUROPE).

MARTINDALE, THE COMPLETE DRUG REFERENCE

This excellent British reference work (formerly called the *Extra Pharmacopoeia*) is an international dictionary of medications and, in addition, a guide to pharmacotherapy. It is useful to everyone involved in pharmacovigilance or drug therapy. It was first published in 1883 by a London pharmacist, William Martindale, aided by a physician, Dr. Wynn Westcott. "It provides comprehensive & international coverage of drugs & related substances including all U.S. drugs & preparations, names, & manufactures; all information is independent, evaluated, & referenced."

The work is more encyclopedic and more complete than national formularies or drug guides. The latest edition is 2315 pages long and covers 5300 drug monographs and 70,000 preparations, as well as rare substances. It is now available as a CD-ROM and on-line (Parfitt K, Editor. *Martindale: the complete drug ref-*

erence, 32nd edition. London: The Royal Pharmaceutical Society of Great Britain, 1999; see the website, http://www.rpsgb.org.uk/)

MEASURES TAKEN (see ACTIONS TAKEN)

MECHANISM OF ACTION

The mechanism of action is the effect or effects that explain the physiologic perturbations producing the undesirable manifestation in question. It is necessary to distinguish a mechanism of action for a drug-induced adverse reaction from a risk factor tied to the administration of the product (such as an overdose due to a dispensing error) or from an effect tied to the underlying disease (e.g., renal insufficiency).

MEDICAL ASSESSMENT

In the context of a case report, the *medical assessment* refers to clinical evaluation by medical professionals of information about the patient and his or her history, including the following:

Differential diagnosis of the cause of the AE/ADR, evaluation of alternative, non-drug related causes

Search for risk factors favoring a drug-related cause, which may be

- Related to the suspect drug such as an overdose
- Related to the patient's history, such as a history of a similar reaction to the drug in the past (positive prechallenge)
- Search for risk factors favoring an alternative cause related to the patient's history, such as a negative prechallenge, the presence of disease likely to cause the AE, and/or several prior episodes of the same AE that occurred without exposure to a drug

MEDICAL DEVICE SURVEILLANCE, MONITORING

Surveillance of the undesirable effects of medical devices. Reporting is usually obligatory and, unlike drug reporting requirements, is to be done as soon as a defect is discovered that exposes patients to the risk of serious injury or death even if no incident has yet occurred. Sometimes called *materiovigilance.*

Unfortunately there is minimal harmonization among countries of device reporting. The definitions are different, as well as the forms used, the reporting times and so on. Similarly, there is minimal harmonization among countries and even within countries between drug and biologic adverse effect reporting and device reporting.

Finally, it is not always clear how to classify and report devices that contain drugs (e.g., syringes prefilled with medication). In some countries these may be considered drugs, in others devices, and in some cases both. This can produce double reporting and confusion in what to report and local expertise in each country is required. Sometime the AE results from an interaction between a device and a drug.

MEDICAL DICTIONARY FOR DRUG REGULATORY AFFAIRS (MEDDRA)

Medical terminology destined for international communication of matters involving regulatory affairs. It was begun by the Medicines Control Agency in Great Britain and was probably the best dictionary of its type; it contained a thesaurus of adverse effects, a list of diseases (International Classification of Diseases (ICD)) and a list of medications. One of the major movers in its creation was Dr. Sue Wood of the Medicines Control Agency (Wood, *PEDS* 1994;3:7–13; CIOMS, *PEDS* 1997;6:115). This dictionary was the precursor of the next entry, *MedDRA* (watch the spelling!).

MEDICAL DICTIONARY FOR REGULATORY ACTIVITIES (MedDRA)

The ICH M1 Working Group (*Standardization of International Medical Terminology for Regulatory Purposes*) devoted itself to the international harmonization of medical terminology with a goal of normalization of administrative terminology. *MedDRA* was inspired by the similarly named *MEDDRA* thesaurus (*Medical Dictionary for Drug Regulatory Affairs*) developed by the pharmacovigilance unit in the Medicines Control Agency in Great Britain.

In October 1994 the International Conference on Harmonization (ICH) officially adopted *MedDRA* (called at the time *International Medical Terminology* (IMT)) as the single dictionary to be used for medical information transmission during the entire life cycle of a pharmaceutical product (before and after marketing). Further information is available at the website (www.ifpma.org/ich5m.html).

In November 1997 the Food and Drug Administration officially adopted *MedDRA* version 1.9 for use in its Adverse Event Reporting System (AERS) pharmacovigilance database. Further information is available at the AERS website (www.fda.gov/cder/aers/concept.htm).

The transition to and adoption of *MedDRA* by the governmental health agencies and pharmaceutical companies have begun and will take a significant amount of time, effort and money. Although *WHO-ART* and *COSTART* terms are included in *MedDRA*, it is not always clear that the direct adoption of these terms as *MedDRA* terms is most fitting since *MedDRA* is more *granular* (i.e., has a greater number and more detailed terms) than these two dictionaries and a more appropriate term may exist. The conversion to *MedDRA* will have repercussions in regard to a drug being *fully labeled* for an ADR if the term appears in *MedDRA* but not in *WHO-ART* or *COSTART* at the preferred term level. There are major issues involved as companies and health authorities move to adopt *MedDRA* first for drug safety, then for clinical and medical research (PSURs, clinical trial reports, integrated safety summaries, etc.), and finally for labeling.

TERMINOLOGY HIERARCHY, VERSION 3.3

- System Organ Class (SOC pronounced "sock") $n = 26$
- High Level Group Term (HLGT) $n = 334$
- High Level Term (HLT) $n = 1,653$
- Preferred Term (PT) $n = 13,003$
- Low Level Term (LLT) $n = 49,247$ (actually 36,244 since all PTs are LLTs also and are counted twice in the 49,247 figure)

The three highest levels (SOC, HLGT, and HLT) are used for querying the database and for presentations. The LLTs correspond roughly to *Reported Terms* in *COSTART* and to *Included Terms* in *WHO-ART* and J-ART. The LLTs are to be used for data collection and entry as well as reporting to EU health authories. The PTs are unique medical entities and are to be used for reporting the cases to non-EU health authorities, including the FDA. *MedDRA* is being translated into multiple languages (at the PT level and above but not at the LLT level yet, as it is not clear that jargon and lay terms can be adequately translated into jargon and lay terms in other languages).

Each term in *MedDRA* is represented by a unique eight-digit number, allowing electronic transmission of data as numbers rather than as characters (e.g., Japanese kanji, Greek, and Russian) for the coded terms in E2B.

The major idea behind *MedDRA* is that it can be changed only by the *MedDRA* Service Organization (MSSO) and not by individual companies or health agencies. This limitation eliminates the current system whereby all companies or agencies can add terms to their dictionaries at will. Thus the *WHO-ART* version used by one company is not the same as the *WHO-ART* version used by another. Rather, upon request to the MSSO, new terms will be added to *MedDRA* in biannual updates after careful medical review by the MSSO and agreement that each new term can be fully and adequately translated into the other language versions of *MedDRA*. If it cannot be so translated, it will not be added to *MedDRA*. It is also possible that some terms can change level in *MedDRA* or even be removed from *MedDRA*. This means that after each change to *MedDRA*, it will be necessary for each company and agency to review queries and reports to ascertain whether they also need to be updated. *MedDRA* is expected to be mandated for AE/ADR reporting (especially electronic reporting—E2B) in about 2003. See the MSSO website (www.meddramsso.com/).

MEDICAL LETTER

A bimonthly four- to eight-page bulletin, produced in New Rochelle, New York, by a nonprofit entity independent of the pharmaceutical industry. The *Medical Letter,* founded in 1959 by Harold Aaron and Arthur Kallet, two members of Consumers Union, an independent consumers group, was the first publication of its type in the United States. It reviews newly approved medications in the United States and periodically reviews groups of medications (e.g., antihypertensives, antibiotics). Its opinions are highly respected. Over the years pharmacoeconomic concerns have been added, leading to price comparisons that may help the prescriber in evaluating benefit/cost ratio in addition to risk/benefit ratio (*Medical Letter on Drugs and Therapeutics*, 1000 Main Street, New Rochelle, NY 10801-7537, U.S.A.; website, www.medletter.com/; fax (914) 632-1733).

MEDICAL PRODUCT

Certain health authorities, the U.S. Food and Drug Administration in particular, use this term to include all of those products under their regulatory jurisdiction: drugs, biologics, devices, nutritional products and others. Other agencies, such as the Canadian health authority, prefer the term *therapeutic product.*

MEDICATION ERRORS

There are many causes of ADRs that are related to incorrect administration of medications. Supratherapeutic dosing and frank overdose are the most frequent, but other errors also occur:

- Incorrect route of administration (e.g., intraarterial rather than intravenous; intradermal instead of subcutaneous)
- Incorrect product (e.g., erroneous labeling)
- Inadequate labeling of packaging
- Misuse of the packaging (e.g., blister pack swallowed without removing the packaging)

- Incorrect preparation (e.g., incompatible or incorrect dilution)
- Incorrect patient (e.g., patient of the same or similar name in the next bed)
- Inadequate patient preparation (swallowing a tablet while lying down without water)
- Unclear labeling in regard to preparation instructions for the pharmacist or the patient
- Confusing names (Omeprazole was originally marketed in the United States as Losec®. But to prevent potential confusion with Lasix® (furosemide), the name was changed to Prilosec®.)

A nonprofit U.S. organization that is devoted to the safe use of medications is the Institute for Safe Medication Practices, which has a very interesting website (www.ismp.org) and publishes a newsletter. A book by one of the principals of the organization has been published (Cohen, Michael. *Medication Errors.* American Pharmaceutical Association, Chicago 1999).

MEDICINES CONTROL AGENCY (MCA)

The drug agency in Great Britain. Pharmacovigilance is administered by the Committee for Safety of Medicines (CSM). Its national pharmacovigilance publication is *Current Problems in Pharmacovigilance* (Headquarters, MCA, Market Towers, 1 Nine Elms Lane. London SW8 5NQ, U.K.) They have a fairly extensive and interesting website (www.open.gov.uk/mca/mcahome.htm).

MEDLINE (MEDICAL LITERATURE ANALYSIS AND RETRIEVAL SYSTEM (MEDLARS) ON-LINE)

The computerized system of automated retrieval of medical information from the National Library of Medicine in the United States (www.nlm.nih.gov/medlineplus/medline.html). The most used tool when starting to scan the literature for an AE associated with a suspect product. It should be complemented by a MEDBASE search when a pharmacovigilance investigation is under way, complemented with other databases when appropriate (such as in teratovigilance or vaccinovigilance investigations) (see LITERATURE SEARCH).

MEDWATCH

The name given in 1993 to the American pharmacovigilance program created by the Food and Drug Administration to draw particular attention to the new FDA 3500 and 3500A MedWatch forms to be used by consumers and the industry, respectively, to report an AE, a device problem, or a material or manufacturing problem with a drug. The form allows the description of two or more suspect products; when such is the case, each drug may be acting independently or they may be interacting with each other. Much information is available on FDA's website (www.fda.gov/Medwatch) including detailed information on the MedWatch program, a copy of the 3500 form with instructions and direct on-line submission capabilities, continuing medical education articles, and contents of Dear Doctor (Dear Health Professional) letters sent over the last several years (MedWatch (HF-2), Room 9-57, FDA, 5600 Fishers Lane, Rockville, MD 20857, U.S.A.).

MEYLER'S SIDE EFFECTS OF DRUGS (SED)

This book, published every fourth year, "features contributions from an international team of over 100 specialists." The latest (14th) edition is edited by Dukes and Aronson (Amsterdam: Elsevier, 2000) and has 1850 pages. The current edition covers the last four editions of *Side Effects of Drugs Annual* (See SIDE EFFECTS OF DRUGS ANNUAL). A superb and invaluable source of information on the safety profile of individual drugs from selected case reports and articles in the literature, plus relevant review articles and in depth discussions of drug safety topics.

MIBEFRADIL: WITHDRAWAL FROM THE MARKET

Commercialized in August 1997 and withdrawn 10 months later in June 1998, this calcium channel inhibitor was the ninth approved in the United States. However, the inhibition of hepatic cytochrome P450 isoenzymes led to a significant number of drug interactions, resulting in withdrawal from the market (*FDA Talk Paper,* June 8, 1998 and Dear Doctor Letter, www.fda.gov/medwatch/safety/1998/poscor.htm). It constitutes another example of a *product effect* compared to a *class effect,* of the uniqueness of pharmacovigilance for detecting new drug interactions, and of the efficacy of a speedily conducted pharmacovigilance investigation.

MISUSE

Misuse can occur at any level: that of the prescriber, dispenser, patient or other. Inappropriate decisions and actions made by the prescriber can occur at any step along the road of rational pharmacotherapy: diagnosis, therapeutic objective, therapeutic strategy, drug class, drug product, dosing directions, daily dose, duration of treatment, surveillance of adverse effects, changes in dosing, verification of efficacy, ending of therapy when no longer needed. These decisions must be made in the context of the risk/benefit ratio, remembering that no ADR is acceptable when there is no real indication to prescribe a given medication to a particular patient at a particular time. Similarly, ADRs are unacceptable if there are contraindications that make the risk of treatment too dangerous.

Dispensing errors are related to incorrect labeling, difficulty in reading handwritten prescriptions, drug name confusion, incorrect dilution of syrups, suspensions, and so forth.

Potential as well as *actual* misuse are end points of Medication Utilization Reviews. Others are engaged in the study of misuse of drugs in the context of iatrogenic complications, particularly in the hospital setting. All errors, whether by negligence or accident, that lead to incorrect pharmacotherapy are included in the broad category of misuse.

Finally, misuse by the patient includes dependence, abuse, dangerous nonmedical (recreational, doping of athletes) drug use, suicide, and lesser, but nonetheless unsafe practices such as use of outdated drugs, dispensing of prescription drugs to others, self-diagnosis and treatment with prescription drugs, improper storage of drugs, and failure to read and follow patient instructions. See the website of the Institute for Safe Medication Practices (www.ismp.org).

MONITORED ADVERSE REACTION (MAR)

An old term used by the Food and Drug Administration to designate an ADR that has been placed "under surveillance" during a pharmacovigilance investigation (also called a *safety signal evaluation*).

In the new Adverse Event Reporting System (AERS) this concept has been replaced by *Designated Medical Event* and represents certain adverse effects/ADRs that get very close scrutiny such as seizures, aplastic anemia, liver necrosis, anaphylaxis, and acute liver failure; see the AERS website (http://www.fda.gov/cder/aers/).

MONTHLY INDEX OF MEDICAL SPECIALITIES (MIMS)

In Australia, the national compendium of medications (www.medical.net.au/mims/).

MORBIDITY AND MORTALITY WEEKLY REPORT (MMWR)

A weekly publication of the U.S. Department of Health and Human Services' Centers for Disease Control and Prevention in Atlanta. This publication carries statistics, detection and prevention alerts, regulatory actions and other information concerning vaccinovigilance, maternal pharmacovigilance, toxicovigilance, and occasionally pharmacovigilance. Its primary focus is the global aspect of public health in the United States (Editor, MMWR Series, Mailstop C-08, CDC, 1600 Clifton Rd., N.E., Atlanta, GA 30333; website for the Centers of Disease Control (CDC) www.cdc.gov. Website for MMWR, www2.cdc.gov/mmwr. The electronic version is free and available as an e-mail subscription from their website. For a paper subscription, contact Superintendent of Documents, U.S. Government Printing Office, Washington, D.C. 20402.

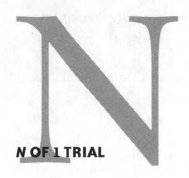

N OF 1 TRIAL

This is a double-blind clinical trial conducted in a single patient in which a randomized sequence of administration of the suspect drug and a control may confirm the causality of an ADR or of a beneficial effect. The idea and designation were first proposed in the 1980s (Guyatt *N Engl J Med* 1986;314:889, and *Can Med Assoc J* 1988;139:497; Strom (2000:615). For an annotated bibliography on single-subject design see the website (http://www.silcom.com/~dwsmith/Critical_Assessment/annobib.html).

BACLOFEN: HALLUCINATIONS
This ADR occurred after the sudden stopping of the product during a blinded trial against placebo (Lees, *Lancet* 1977;I:858).

ZIDOVUDINE: PANIC
An immunodepressed patient experienced panic attacks after each dose of zidovudine. During a double-blind zidovudine/placebo single patient trial done with the patient's complete consent, he panicked after taking both products. When these results were made known to the patient his iatrogenic panic attacks stopped (Levitt, *Can Med Assoc J* 1990;142:341).

NAMES OF DRUGS

The name of the drug used in the course of a case follow-up or of a drug safety investigation must be carefully ascertained as there are many similar sounding drug names. In addition, at times it may be important to ascertain the country of origin of the drug as some products have the same name in different countries but have different active ingredients or excipients.

NATIONAL PHARMACEUTICAL COMPENDIA

These compendia include extracts from the officially approved product monographs or labeling of approved and commercialized products and are incorporated into a single volume. They do not necessarily contain compendia for all products commercialized in a country and rarely cover generic drugs. Most industrialized nations produce such compendia. The products may be grouped by manufacturer, drug class or trade name alphabetically. We are calling such books *compendia* even though they may be dictionaries, formularies, pharmacopoeia, or merely an alphabetical list of drugs in a particular country, for example:

- Australia: *MIMS* (http://www.mims.com.au/.)
- Canada: *Compendium of Pharmaceuticals and Specialties* ("the CPS") (http://www.cdnpharm.ca/pubcps.htm)
- France: *Dictionnaire Vidal* ("le *Vidal*") (http://www.vidal.fr/)
- Germany: *Rote Liste* (http://www.rote-liste.de).
- Great Britain: *Compendium of Data Sheets and Summaries of Product Characteristics* (http://emc.vhn.net/.)

- Sweden: *Farmacevtiska Specialiteter I Sverige*
- United States: *Physician's Desk Reference.* ("the *PDR*") (http://www.pdr.net/)

The manner in which safety information is listed has been and remains an area of controversy. For many prescribers these compendia remain the major source of information on the safety and risks of medications since few physicians make the effort to obtain the product monograph from the manufacturer (when it is available).

The safety data presented do not always meet the needs of the prescribing physician, even though these works usually contain government-approved labeling. Much of the safety information concerns phase III trials with all the limits these data have: homogeneous patients, no concomitant medications or diseases, limited treatment duration, and so on. The postmarketing adverse effects are rarely presented with frequency estimates (though this is rather hard to determine) nor indications of severity. Serious or fatal adverse effects/ADRs may be lost in a sea of other benign or inconsequential events. In addition, evaluations of the likelihood of causality (see CAUSALITY: THREE TYPES) are rarely noted. ("The following events have been seen after marketing. Relationship to the drug has not been determined.")

All of these limitations make the rational determination of a risk/benefit ratio by the prescriber for a particular patient very difficult. In some countries, the national compendium is readily available to the lay public at an inexpensive price. (Even more problematic is the availability of older editions of the compendia at used book sales. The propagation of outdated information can be particularly unsafe.) The interpretation of the information in the compendia by the lay consumer often produces a risk/benefit evaluation at odds with that arrived at by the prescriber.

It would also be useful to note with a logo (such as the British black triangle) a new product that the clinician should pay particular attention to when prescribing, and that would encourage him or her to report serious and unexpected AEs to the pharmacovigilance authorities.

The limitations of the current safety labeling are well recognized by health authorities, the pharmaceutical industry, and the medical community. Sporadic efforts have occurred to change product labeling to make it more user-friendly though to date these efforts have not produced much change. The CIOMS III effort (see CIOMS III) has been one step toward rational and useful safety labeling. In June 2000, the Food and Drug Administration proposed new labeling standards in a guidance draft (www.fda.gov/cber/gdlns/cfadvers.txt).

Also see Litlejohn (*Drug Inf J* 1987;21:63) and Graham (*Drug Inf J* 1991; 25:211), and CIOMS III 1995:8.

NATIONAL PHARMACOVIGILANCE INVESTIGATION

A term used in France (Enquête nationale de pharmacovigilance) to designate a safety signal investigation piloted by one of the Regional Pharmacovigilance Centers. If the signal's origin is spontaneous reports, the center begins by validating the cases found in the ADR database of the national network of centers. The delegation of this inquiry to a regional center in a pharmacovigilance system is unusual in the industrialized world as most systems are centralized in a single national center but it seems to encourage their participation in national investigations.

NATURAL PRODUCT

Most of the products dubbed with this term are medicinal plant products or food supplements. They are usually ineffective pharmacologically and are at times dangerous. However, when they do produce ADRs the risk/benefit ratio is unacceptable because of minimal or absent advantages (see PHYTO-VIGILANCE).

NEW DRUG APPLICATION (NDA); NEW DRUG DOSSIER (NDD) (see MARKETING AUTHORIZATION)

NEW MOLECULAR ENTITY (NME) OR NEW CHEMICAL ENTITY (NCE)

A new molecule that has not been approved for marketing as a medicinal drug product in the past. This term is generally not aplied to biologics, vaccines and diagnostic agents. See the Food and Drug Administration's website for listings of NMEs (http://www.fda.gov/cder/rdmt/default.htm).

NEW PRODUCT

In the regulatory context, the notion of a new product is not only a new active ingredient or new chemical entity; it may also include

- New preparations and presentations: dose, galenic formulation, route of administration
- New indication
- New population approved for use: pediatric, geriatric, or other

In many countries, the use of the word *new* in advertising and publicity is limited to a fixed period after approval or launch (e.g., 6 months). In the context of pharmacovigilance, this is important to know because it is possible that there will be an increase in AE/ADR reporting during this period. This is known as the Weber effect (see WEBER EFFECT).

NOCEBO EFFECT

The nocebo effect is the undesirable equivalent of the placebo effect. It refers to an undesired ADR whose mechanism is psychologic and is based on a mistrust of the product. It is the opposite of the placebo effect, in which a favorable therapeutic effect, also based on a psychologic mechanism, is produced as a result of the confidence the patient has in the medication.

> *Zidovudine and panic*: An immunodepressed patient experienced panic attacks each time he took zidovudine. In the course of a double-blind single-patient clinical trial of zidovudine versus placebo in which he was participating (with informed consent), it was observed that he had suffered from panic attacks after both the zidovudine and the placebo. His attacks stopped after the breaking of the blind in this N of 1 trial (Levitt, *Can Med Assoc J* 1990;142:341).

NONSTEROIDAL ANTI-INFLAMMATORY DRUGS (NSAIDs)

This pharmacologic class of drugs often tops the list for frequency of ADRs that occur in the general population. This is due both to the elevated use of these drugs and to the high incidence of ADRs from NSAIDs. Much attention has been paid to this class of drugs because of the benefits that will result from safer products—particularly those that are less irritating to the gastrointestinal (GI) tract. The new COX-2 (cyclo-oxygenase inhibitor) class of NSAIDs is less irritating for the GI tract but nondigestive ADRs remain a problem, as is the case for COX-1 agents.

Another interesting aspect of this class is the wide disparity of reported ADR incidences among products, such that the safer NSAIDs, which had been at the bottom of the ADR frequency list for several years, became available without prescription. See the websites (http://www.jr2.ox.ac.uk/Bandolier/painres/painpag/nsae/nsae.html; http://www.amcp.org/public/pubs/journal/vol5/num6/feature.html).

NOTICE OF COMPLIANCE (NOC)

Canadian regulatory term denoting a Marketing Authorization.

NUMBER OF PATIENTS NEEDED TO TREAT (NNT) OR TO HARM (NNH)

This concept has become very important in decision analysis, clinical epidemiology, clinical pharmacology, pharmacotherapy, and pharmacovigilance (http://www.jr2.ox.ac.uk/Bandolier/band59/NNT1.html; http://www.acponline.org/journals/annals/01may97/numeric.htm; http://cebm.jr2.ox.ac.uk/docs/nnt.html).

IN PHARMACOVIGILANCE: NUMBER NEEDED TO HARM (NNH)

The minimal number of patients needed to be treated with a medication in order to produce an ADR in *one* of the patients exposed. Calculated by taking the reciprocal of the *risk of the ADR attributable* to the suspect drug. Thus, if the attributable risk of melena in patients on nonsteroidal antiinflammatory drugs (NSAIDs) is $P = 0.005$ or 0.5% per month of treatment, the NNH to produce one case of melena would be 200 patient-months (1/0.005) taking NSAIDs. Dr. Jacques Lelorier has proposed an alternative phrasing of NNH: *number needed to harm one* (NNHO).

IN CLINICAL PHARMACOLOGY: NUMBER NEEDED TO TREAT (NNT)

The number of subjects needed to be treated in order to produce the beneficial effect in *one* patient exposed. This concept was developed at the Division of Clinical Epidemiology at McMaster University in Hamilton, Ontario. It is calculated by taking the reciprocal of the *attributable risk* (of benefit) for the product studied.

NUTRICEUTICS (NUTRITIONALS)

Food supplements prepared by the pharmaceutical industry or others and often sold in pharmacies, supermarkets, and health food stores. They are often not regulated to the same degree that drugs are. In the United States nutritional supplements are not regulated by the Food and Drug Administration.

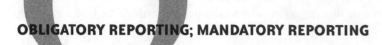

OBLIGATORY REPORTING; MANDATORY REPORTING

REGULATORY AND LEGAL REQUIREMENTS

In most developed countries the manufacturer or sponsor is legally required to report certain AEs/ADRs to the health authorities, usually on specified forms (e.g., CIOMS I, MedWatch in the United States).

HEALTH CARE PROFESSIONALS

In most developed countries the physician, pharmacist, nurse, and other health care professionals are *not* legally obliged to report AEs/ADRs to the authorities. Some countries, in contrast, such as Sweden, Norway, and France, have adopted laws requiring physicians to report AEs; it is not clear, however, that reporting levels have increased to any measurable extent because of this legislation. In practice, the obligation on the health care professional is an *ethical* or moral one, in which the practitioner, as a "privileged and skilled observer" feels compelled to report serious and unexpected events, particularly those that are considered to be unacceptable and preventable (by taking the approrpiate measures).

DEVICE SURVEILLANCE AND VACCINE SURVEILLANCE

In many countries physicians and other health care professionals are obligated to report problems and events associated with devices and vaccines.

OBSERVATIONAL STUDY

This type of study involves the prospective examination of cohorts and/or a retrospective examination of case controls. The data to be collected and the method of collection are decided upon by the investigation, a condition for building a primary database. Observational studies are

- Structured, in contrast to the system of spontaneous reporting, which is not
- Clinical, in contrast to the study of cases in a database, where the information has already been selected and computerized
- Analytic (comparative), in contrast to descriptive studies, which do not contain control groups
- Nonexperimental, in contrast to a clinical trial since the treating physician, rather than the protocol, chooses the treatment each patient receives
- Nonrandomized, as far as the treatment allocation is concerned

ODDS

A ratio formed by the probability of the occurrence of an event divided by the probability of its nonoccurrence. The concept dates back to the 17th-century French philosopher and mathematician Blaise Pascal, but its first use was for betting on horses in the United Kingdom and it is used in the world of gambling.

For example, on average 51 boys are born in every 100 births, so the odds that any randomly chosen delivery being that of a boy is:

N of boys = 51, divided by N of girls = 49 = 1.04

By adding the numerator and denominator the total number of chances is obtained (epidemiologists say that the denominator is the complement of the numerator). The odds can be transformed into a decimal or expressed as a percentage. For example, 8 to 2 odds are equivalent to 8 chances out of 10 chances or 0.8, or 80%.

ODDS RATIO

In pharmacoepidemiology an odds ratio is calculated by dividing the odds in the treated (exposed) group by the odds in the untreated (unexposed) control group. In a classic epidemiologic 2 X 2 table (see TWO-BY-TWO TABLE) it represents the association of exposure to a drug with the occurrence of an event. A good website with some approachable sections on epidemiology and trial methodology is found in Bandolier's evidence based medicine, created by the University of Oxford. See their website section on trials methodology (www.jr2.ox.ac.uk/bandolier/booth/booths/trials.html).

ONCOVIGILANCE

Safety surveillance of anticancer drugs. The domain of pharmacovigilance that consists of the surveillance of unexpected ADRs in cancer patients exposed to new antineoplastic agents. Since cancer patients are usually quite ill and the chemotherapeutic agents used are often quite toxic, the threshold for spontaneous adverse effect/ADR reporting by oncologists is unfortunately fairly high. Their reasoning for reporting only very severe or unusual AEs is that *all* of their patients have AEs and ADRs and some practical selectivity must be used in reporting.

> *Irinotecan*: This anticancer drug, which is a little less toxic than the similarly acting camptothecin, raised some issues in Japan regarding the problem of making public some fatalities associated with the product seen after launch. During the clinical evaluation prior to the Marketing Authorization, 55 deaths occurred in 1245 patients. The product was launched in April 1994; in September 1995, the authorities made public information regarding nine reported deaths associated with the product. Nothing further was said until an oncologist at a cancer center demanded that the health authority make more information public. The authorities subsequently revealed additional deaths associated with the drug, a total of 39 deaths out of 5430 patients exposed. The issues of transparency and what information must be made public were raised by this episode (Akabayashi, *Lancet* 1997;350:124) (see PHARMACO-TRANSPARENCY: DECLARATION OF ERICE).

OPINION & EVIDENCE: DRUG SAFETY, 2ND EDITION

This 208-page book dated March 2000 is produced by Adis Books (Fax, (877)-ADIS-FAX in the United States and 01829 770-330 in the United Kingdom). A spin-off from *Drug Safety* and *Reactions Weekly* from the same publishers, it presents case reports selected for their signaling value (first reports, interactions, overdosing, serious events) and summaries of recent topics, issues, and meetings in drug safety. The guest editor is Professor Ralph Edwards, director of the Uppsala Monitoring Center. A 36-page booklet *Drug Interactions Alert*, is also offered.

ORGANIZATION OF NATIONAL PHARMACOVIGILANCE

A national pharmacovigilance program can be constituted on a large or a small scale. Goals to aspire to may include high visibility and promotion of the program, ease of AE/ADR reporting, flexible and open-minded personnel, efficient and high-quality actions and feedback on an individual and a collective level, efficient computer systems, and transparency of data.

VISIBILITY AND PROMOTION

Promotion and advertising are indispensable to sensitize the medical profession and possibly the public also to the existence of, need for, and procedures involved in pharmacovigilance. Unfortunately, this is generally not done in medical training programs for physicians (France is a welcome exception), though nurses and pharmacists do get some exposure in a few countries.

Various modalities are available to spread the word, including letters, hospital conferences, inclusion in continuing education courses, professional contacts, contacts in the university and hospital settings, articles in widely read journals (e.g., the section "From the FDA" in *the Journal of the American Medical Association*, health authorities websites, and insertion of the Therapeutic Products Program (TPP) pharmacovigilance bulletin in the *Canadian Medical Association Journal.*)

EASE OF REPORTING

The voluntary reporting of AEs/ADRs can and should be made as easy as possible:

AE/ADR report forms with postage-paid return envelopes should be distributed periodically.

Free access to the Pharmacovigilance Center by telephone (a toll-free 800 number), fax (also a toll-free number), e-mail, and so on, should be provided. Phones should be staffed during working hours with rapid pick-up and little or no "holding" time. A voice mail system should be used after hours or access to a poison control center should be made available. Return calls or contact with the reporter should be done quickly and efficiently. The form should be in the local language of the country or region and the report form should be simple.

THE FDA

The MedWatch program can receive case reports in several ways: by fax, by modem, by telephone, by mail using business reply versions of the 3500 form (i.e., fold, seal, mail with no postage needed), and by Internet at their website (www.fda.gov/cder/medwatch).

PERSONALIZED FEEDBACK

If the reporting health care professional has a positive experience when making an AE/ADR report to the health authority or manufacturer (for example, rapid and polite response, nondefensive attitude, little holding time on the phone, feedback), then the likelihood of further reports may be enhanced. If a country is very large, in area or population, or if it has various languages, accents, and cultures, it is clear that in some cases (e.g., France, Canada) decentralization with regional pharmacovigilance units can smooth the contacts with reporters of the suspected ADRs, help validate their observations, and encourage continued reports of other suspected ADRs in the future.

Efficacy and rapid replies as well as a spirit of professionalism and cooperation can strongly and favorably influence the reporter to continue to report suspected

ADRs. Direct and personal communication is also important, as is prevention of ongoing turnover of personnel at the agency. "In our opinion it is preferable that a reporting system be based on direct communication between clinicians and professionals at the monitoring center" (Wiholm in Strom 2000:175).

COLLECTIVE FEEDBACK

A national or regional bulletin of pharmacovigilance is an excellent tool. In the United States, the Food and Drug Administration gives feedback through its publication *The FDA Bulletin* and through its excellent and extensive website (www.fda.gov). The U.S. Center for Disease Control (CDC) in Atlanta, Georgia, publishes information on statistics, alerts, and various vaccinovigilance, maternal pharmacovigilance, and device vigilance in its publication *Mortality and Morbidity Weekly Report (MMWR)*, which is also on the web (http://www2.cdc.gov/mmwr/).

ORGANIZATION OF PHARMACOVIGILANCE: FUNCTIONS

A pharmacovigilance unit in a drug company or a health authority must serve four functions: receipt, collection, evaluation, and information.

RECEIPT

Receipt entails the actions performed when a case is received; it includes proper and immediate triage, date stamping, and assignment to the appropriate person for action within the pharmacovigilance organizaiton (whether governmental or private).

COLLECTION

Collection constitutes timely and accurate data entry into a validated computer system; each manufacturer and each health authority should have one. It includes summarization of the case and accurate and precise coding of the event/reaction. Coding in *MedDRA* (see MedDRA) will likely continue to replace coding in *COSTART* or *WHO-ART* terminology. Usually, follow-up contacts with the reporter, hospital, consultants, and occasionally even the patient are necessary to amass complete information.

EVALUATION

The evaluation includes the detection, analysis, and reporting of a signal when appropriate. It may include the launching of a pharmacovigilance investigation. The analysis, which must be done on a case by case basis as well as on the collective basis of the aggregated data, includes evaluation of the factual reliability of the data, the plausibility, the completeness, the drug's track record (whether it can produce such a reaction, in terms of theoretical and historical data), the causality if appropriate, the signal generating value, and the risk/benefit ratio.

The unleashing of an early warning is the most important and the most scientifically challenging and interesting function of a pharmacovigilance unit. This includes the launching of a safety investigation (also called signal *follow-up, intensified investigation,* or "a full court press"—a colorful sports term referring to aggressive defensive ball playing in basketball and a major effort to accumulate the needed data in a very rapid time frame in pharmacovigilance) when a signal appears to be important, that is, when its confirmation will alter the risk/benefit ratio and require that a series of measures be taken.

INFORMATION

When and to whom a pharmacovigilance unit should communicate their results after analyzing a series of case reports and conducting an appropriate signal investigation can be summarized as "in due time to those who need to know."

ORGANIZATION OF PHARMACOVIGILANCE: GREAT BRITAIN

Britain was the first country to create a national pharmacovigilance system. Professor W. H. W. Inman, known as "the father of the yellow card," referring to the yellow card used in the United Kingdom for reporting, accepted the task of setting up the program. After his success there, he moved on to set up a system of cohort studies, the Prescription Event Monitoring (PEM) system known as the "green card system," in the Drug Safety Research Unit at the University of Southampton. Professor Inman became the first holder of a university chair in pharmacoepidemiology.

The governmental organization that handles pharmacovigilance is known as the Committee for Safety of Medicines (CSM), which is a part of the Medicines Control Agency (MCA) (Waller, *PEDS* 1996;5:363); see their website (http://www.open.gov.uk/mca/csmhome.htm). The CSM can be credited with several successes in signal detection and pharmacovigilance investigations since the 1980s.

ORGANIZATION OF PHARMACOVIGILANCE: JAPAN

Japan has chosen to take a different approach to AE/ADR monitoring, preferring active pharmacovigilance in the hospital setting rather than reliance on passive and voluntary reporting by prescribers. Over 1000 hospitals and several thousand sentinel pharmacies participate in active drug surveillance. This is, in effect, a phase IV study that can last up to 6 years in designated university hospitals. It is not clear, however, that this system is more sensitive than the spontaneous reporting systems of North America and Europe in picking up early signals.

In some cases the authorities release a summary of the clinical dossier (called the *Summary Basis of Approval* (*SBA* or *SBOA*)) that was submitted to the authorities for marketing authorization. This is a model of transparency that other health authorities should consider following (Wiholm, in Strom 2000:175). Recently, Japan has modified its laws and regulations to bring them in line with the spontaneous reporting system described by the International Conference on Harmonization (ICH) though there are still some clear differences from Western systems. See the website of the Ministry of Health and Welfare (http://www.mhw.go.jp/english/).

Japan maintains a National Drug Information Site (www.pharmasys.gr.jp), which includes pharmacovigilance, including "individual ADR case reports from the national pharmacovigilance centre. The case information is provided as line listings, and more detailed description of unusual cases" (*Uppsala Reports* #11 (Jan 11) 2000).

ORGANIZATION OF PHARMACOVIGILANCE: THE UNITED STATES AND THE FOOD AND DRUG ADMINISTRATION (FDA)

Let us look briefly at some historical background and the present organization of the largest national system in existence.

> *Arsenic*: In 1922 the first cases of icterus were seen after arsenic treatment. The Council on Pharmacy and Chemistry of the American Medical Association was formed in 1929.

Diethylene glycol: In 1937 several cases of a severe and unacceptable ADR to a pharmaceutical product raised the public consciousness sufficiently to produce action. Sulfanilamide was launched as a suspension in an organic solvent, diethylene glycol, a congener of which is used as antifreeze in automobile engines. There followed 107 deaths (76 in 2 months) due to hepatotoxicity and nephrotoxicity. Note that this catastrophe was not the result of exposure to the active chemical entity but rather to an excipient that apparently had never been tested in human or animal. This produced the first large scale modern alert in the United States due to a pharmaceutical product (Geiling, *JAMA* 1938;111:919; Temple, *Drug Inf J* 1992;25:1; Lewis, *Drug Inf J* 1993;27:1037).

In 1938, a year later, the authorities reacted vigorously with the passage by the US Congress of the *Food, Drug and Cosmetic Act*. For the first time ever, the producers of drugs were required to conduct tests of animal toxicity and to submit a clinical dossier as proof of new drug safety. Note that proof of efficacy was not required. As with other subsequent changes in the law, these requirements were due to political pressure following a drug toxicity drama which shocked public opinion.

Chloramphenicol: In 1954, the association of this antibiotic with cases of severe or fatal aplastic anemia pushed the Council on Pharmacy and Chemistry of the American Medical Association to create a registry of blood dyscrasias reported by clinicians and small hospitals. This was the first ADR registry in the United States (Erslev, *JAMA* 1962;181:114). It ended in 1970 after the Food and Drug Administration took up this duty.

Thalidomide: In 1961, the thalidomide catastrophe occurred primarily outside the United States as the drug had not been approved in the United States though some samples were distributed. When the FDA began to collect spontaneous AEs/ADRs, the first reports were in university hospitals. The administration reacted rapidly, that is, a year later. In 1962, the legislators passed the Kefauver-Harris Amendment to the Food, Drug and Cosmetic Act. For the first time, manufacturers were required to report to the FDA all ADRs received by them spontaneously or from other sources, such as clinical trials or scientific publications (both domestic and foreign) for their products. This included all products marketed since 1938. The database was computerized in 1965 but was only searchable for reactions reported since autumn 1969. It was named the *ADR Reporting System* (ADRRS). It has since been replaced with a new system, the *Adverse Event Reporting System* (AERS).

In 1985 and 1987 further revisions in FDA regulations were passed (21 CFR 310.305 and 21 CFR 314.80). These rules oblige manufacturers, but not health care professionals, to notify the FDA of certain AEs/ADRs. Two changes reduced the number of obligatory reports by the manufacturers:

- Only cases that met the definition of "serious outcomes" could be submitted, eliminating those that were not serious
- Cases in which a drug cause of the event was excluded did not have to be reported

In March 1992, the *Guidelines for Postmarketing Report of ADRs* were published and updated in May 2000. On 3 June 1993 the FDA modified the name of its national pharmacovigilance program to the Medical Products Reporting Program, known to everyone as the MedWatch Program. At the same time the FDA modified the form on which the event/reaction is recorded, allowing two suspect drugs rather than one (when applicable) and adding a section on medical device problems. The newly devised form is available in two versions: one for health care professionals and consumers (for voluntary reporting), and is designated *form 3500*; the other (for mandatory reporting) for manufacturers, distributors, and institutions, *form 3500A*. The forms are very similar.

Manufacturers may submit reports from outside the United States on CIOMS I forms or on MedWatch forms. Reports from inside the United States must be on 3500A MedWatch forms. These rules also apply to reports on biologics that are submitted to the Center for Biologic Evaluation and Research (CBER) (21CFR600).

Form 3500 (for health care professionals and consumers) is available on-line (https://www.accessdata.fda.gov/scripts/medwatch/) and can either be printed out and filled in or completed and submitted directly on-line. A copy is also available on the last page of the *Physicians Desk Reference* (*PDR*).

The Office of Post-Marketing Drug Risk Assessment (OPDRA), the Center for Drug Evaluation and Research (CDER), and the Center for Biologics Evaluation and Research (CBER) evaluate the MedWatch reports sent to FDA directly and from manufacturers. In CDER the duties of pharmacovigilance were elevated to the "office" level (a higher level) within the FDA. There is now an Office of Post-Marketing Drug Risk Assessment, which is composed of two divisions: The Division of Drug Risk Evaluation I and II. There is an extensive and invaluable website (www.fda.gov) that anyone involved in pharmacovigilance should get acquainted with and consult regularly.

Two excellent summaries of pharmacovigilance in the United States are those by Faich (*N Engl J Med* 1986:314:1589–1592) and Strom 2000 (see the chapter by Kennedy, Goldman, and Lillie). Also visit the updated info on CDER's website (www.fda.gov/cder; www.fda.gov/cder/aers). There follow other useful web sites from the same sources:

- *Federal Register:* http://www.access.gpo.gov/su_docs/aces/aces140.html
- Adverse Drug Experience Index: http://www.cvm.fda.gov/fda/infores/ade96/adeindex.html
- CDER What's New (alert reports, withdrawals): http://www.fda.gov./cder/whatsnew.htm
- Medwatch Important Safety Information: http://www.fda.gov//medwatch/safety.htm
- Medwatch index:http://www.fda.gov/medwatch/index.html
- CBER What's New: http://www.fda.gov/cber/whatsnew.htm
- VAERS: http://www.fda.gov/cber/vaers.html
- Blood products safety surveillance and recalls: http://www.fda.gov/cber/recalls.htm
- Free e-mail notification service: http://www.fda.gov/cder/cdernew/listserv.html
- CDER: http://www.fda.gov/cder/about/default.htm
- CBER: http://www.fda.gov/cber/index.html

These sites should be visited frequently as they are full of useful and timely information. A free e-mail alert service is also available.

ORGANIZATIONS (see PHARMACEUTICAL MEDICINE)

ORPHAN ADVERSE EVENT

A term proposed by the Bordeaux Regional Pharmacovigilance Center in France. It refers to an "isolated and convincing" AE/ADR that is probably associated with the drug but without any meaningful effect on public health or on the risk/benefit ratio of the product. By *isolated* it is meant that the ADR has been reported (and/or published) once, maybe more than once, but very rarely (Haramburu, *Thérapie* 1987;42:63, in French).

An orphan ADR is not seen frequently, either because the product in question is rarely used or because the true incidence of the AE/ADR is low. An orphan ADR does not justify an alert because it has no impact on public health. It is, of course, of critical importance to the individual patient, who should not be reexposed to the suspect product. The event must be kept in the pharmacovigilance database since additional cases could always be reported, making this no longer an orphan.

Thus an orphan is a type of signal that, for the moment, is merely a curiosity but nevertheless could ultimately contribute to the safety picture and help explain the mechanism(s) of the drug's toxicity. On the other hand, should the patient in question experience the event a second time without having taken the suspect drug or should the reporter uncover further evidence that the original observation was not valid, the signal is proved false. Three examples (not taken from Haramburu's paper) follow:

Pemphigus: A rash of an exfoliative pemphigus type occurred in a 73-year-old woman. The seven medications that she was taking were stopped and this *multiple dechallenge* was positive (i.e., the lesion disappeared) 3 weeks later. Readministration of digoxin alone led to the reappearance of the reaction. Cutaneous allergy tests with the seven products showed a positive test only for digoxin. From an epidemiologic point of view, this reaction is not very plausible since it could be said that given the millions of patients who have taken the product since the 19th century it would have been observed already. On the other hand it is hard to ignore a convincing case where a positive rechallenge has produced a very rare event. Thus it is isolated but convincing and one may thus postulate an idiosyncratic immune mechanism specific to this patient (Inadomi, *Eur J Dermatol* 1993;3:33).

Acute pancreatitis: This serious reaction occurred in a young woman after a single oral dose of a nonsteroidal anti-inflammatory drug (NSAID) taken for dysmenorrhea. She had acute abdominal pain radiating to the back. Dechallenge was positive after several days. Blood work showed elevated lipase and pancreatic amylase levels. Whether this is an orphan ADR or a false signal, it is doubtful that anyone would prescribe this NSAID to this woman again (Du Ville, *Am J Gastroenterol* 1993;88:464).

Delayed Cutaneous Reaction: A case of severe cutaneous necrosis was observed at the site of extravasation of an antineoplastic agent 11 days after the end of a 24-hour intravenous infusion. What makes this an orphan ADR is not the nature of the reaction but rather the latency time to onset (Herrington, *Pharmacotherapy* 1997;17:163).

ORPHAN BENEFICIAL DRUG EFFECT

Occasionally the orphan effect is beneficial rather than an AE.

Omeprazole against ulcerative colitis: A 34-year-old male suffering from ulcerative colitis since adolescence had three bloody stools per day along with abdominal cramping. He avoided milk products and was being treated with sulfasalazine. Because of an esophagitis he was prescribed omeprazole for 2 weeks. Four days after he had started omeprazole, his stools normalized and he could now tolerate milk products. Seven days after stopping of omeprazole severe colitis returned. At the request of the patient the omeprazole was restarted and 5 days later the colitis symptoms disappeared. The causality would be graded at level 3 = probable because of the short time to appearance of the effect (4 days), short time to disappearance (7 days), and positive rechallenge in 5 days.

Nicotine against agitation: A 68-year-old Dutch cancer patient in a terminal phase being treated with multiple and appropriate therapies for his disease suddenly stopped smoking his usual 30 cigarettes a day; 24 hours later he experienced pallor, agitation, convulsive movements, confusion, and screaming. Midazolam given subcutaneously was not effective. A nicotine patch considerably improved the symptoms within 3 hours. This case represents an unexpected orphan benefit as well as supporting the diagnosis of nicotine withdrawal syndrome (Krjni, *Lancet* 1995;346:1044).

ORPHAN DRUG

A regulatory term introduced by the Food and Drug Administration to designate a new product indicated for a very rare disease (defined to be less than 200,000 cases in the United States), which is intended to motivate its research and development by the pharmaceutical industry. There are about 5000 diseases that affect only 1 in 1000 people. In order to promote the commercialization of efficacious products, which are often off-patent and for which there are few patients to treat, the Orphan Drug Act of 1983 offers incentives for development. These incentives include a smaller number of patients studied, more rapid review by FDA, and monetary benefits (Affner, *Drug Inf J* 1994;28:495). See the FDA websites: ⟨http://www.fda.gov/orphan/about/odreg.htm and http://www.fda.gov/orphan/about/progovw.htm⟩.

Decreasing the requirements for approval decreases the number of patients studied and treatment duration in controlled clinical trials. This method decreases the likelihood of the detection in phase III trials of ADRs that are rare, have long latency periods, are of type B, or are due to drug-drug interactions. In other words, if the preapproval study of the drug is truncated, the postapproval pharmacovigilance study of the drug becomes even more critical. In such cases, health authorities may impose certain phase IV postapproval requirements such as cohort studies of the first patients exposed after approval, as was the case with zidovudine for acquired immunodeficiency syndrome (AIDS).

OUTCOME

The outcomes or consequences of an adverse effect are recorded on most notification forms (e.g., CIOMS 1, MedWatch). The choices differ from form to form and generally include variations on the following categories: death, recovered, and not yet recovered. Note that *recovered* really is not a description of seriousness and that *not yet recovered* really denotes incomplete information either because the physician rapidly reported an ongoing case or because follow-up information has not yet been obtained or cannot be obtained.

OUTCOME SERIOUSNESS

Thanks to the efforts of the World Health Organization (WHO), International Conference on Harmonization (ICH), the Council for International Organizations of Medical Sciences (CIOMS), Food and Drug Administration, and the health authorities of the European Union and Japan, the criteria for *serious* have been standardized and harmonized. Seriousness centers around three criteria: death, hospitalization and incapacity complemented by several more specific categories. If an adverse effect or ADR meets one or more of these criteria it is considered "serious." If it does not, it is considered *nonserious*. If the outcome is unknown, it is considered nonserious until shown to be serious. (This benefit of the doubt for the drug may change. Some health agencies are contemplating a regulatory change making all AEs or ADRs serious until shown to be nonserious.)

Note that for devices, it usually is sufficient that a product problem be considered life-threatening even if no patient has yet experienced this event. Examples include the unexpected shortening of battery life in a pacemaker or a mechanical problem in a prosthetic heart valve that has not yet caused a clinical problem.

There are several serious criteria for drugs.

DEATH OR A LIFE-THREATENING CONDITION

> **Death**

Death is not an AE or ADR in the strict sense. It is the outcome of one AE/ADR or several indirect, secondary AE/ADRs. There is an implied double-causality link involved in a death: first, the link between the suspect drug and the AE/ADR; second, the link between the AE/ADR and the death. Some report forms recognize this distinction and note three classes: death probably related to the drug, death possibly related, and death unrelated. In certain cases, however, when the patient is found dead (e.g., "found dead in bed"), death may be listed as both the outcome and the AE/ADR for want of further information.

> **Life-Threatening**

This is a more controversial criterion. A life-threatening event is one (usually in the short term) that represents an immediate risk to survival if no intervention occurs. Examples include anaphylactic shock, severe hemorrhage, and respiratory or cardiac arrest. It does not include such medical conditions as an infection or chronic hepatitis that might be life-threatening at a later date without treatment.

HOSPITALIZATION

By convention, most health authorities do not consider a visit to a hospital emergency room an *admission* to a hospital for reporting purposes, though if the patient stays overnight in the emergency room (ER) some might consider that a hospitalization. Also some patients may remain overnight in the ER for the simple reason that in-patient beds are not available.

The *prolongation* of a hospitalization occurs when a patient is already in the hospital (on the inpatient service) and the AE/ADR causes the hospitalization duration to be increased whether for treatment or for observation.

There are two exceptions to this situation: If a hospitalization is scheduled, as for chemotherapy or dialysis for a known condition, it is possible, particularly in clinical trial reporting, to obtain a waiver and not consider these admissions as criteria for AE/ADR reporting. Less clear is whether to report a hospitalization due to a clear intercurrent but definitely unrelated event such as an auto accident in which the patient is a passenger.

In Japan, the threshold for hospitalization is much lower than it is in Europe and North America. Patients there may be admitted for observation or testing that would be done in the outpatient setting elsewhere. Hence in Japan, hospitalization was not a criterion for seriousness until recently. However, now that Japan has adopted the ICH consensus definition, hospitalization and prolongation of hospitalization are serious criteria.

DISABILITY

A disability may be either temporary or permanent. A stroke or transient ischemic attack after use of oral birth control agents from which the patient recovers fully would be temporary even if the stroke did not abate for several weeks. An example of a permanent disability would be a stroke from which the patient did not fully recover, loss of vision with antimalarial therapy, or loss of hearing after an aminoglycoside antibiotic. Disability need not be medically severe to qualify. ICH and the FDA have adopted the concept of *medical intervention being required to prevent a disability or a permanent incapacity.*

OTHER CATEGORIES

▶ **Congenital Malformation**
Though congenital malformations might be considered disabilities, the FDA and many other agencies consider all congenital malformations (whether severe or not) to be automatically classed separately as a serious outcome in some countries.

▶ **Cancer**
Although cancer might fall into one of the other categories, its presence, even if a "minor" one such as a localized basal cell cancer of the skin, is considered to be automatically serious in some countries.

▶ **Overdosage or Misuse**
An overdose is really a misuse of a medication—whether voluntary or accidental—and is a risk factor for the occurrence of an ADR. Many agencies consider this to be a serious outcome not only because it might lead to severe medical consequences but also because it is important in the global safety evaluation of a drug to understand which AEs occur with higher doses (overdosage) of the drug with regard to the dose consumed, the mode of administration (e.g., misuse if a tablet is crushed, dissolved, and injected intravenously by a drug addict), the clinical presentation, the treatment given, and the response to the treatment.

▶ **Withdrawal Syndrome**
This is not an ADR per se but rather is a pharmacologic mechanism (at the receptor level). Some health authorities require that these AEs/ADRs be considered serious.

▶ **Medically Significant (or Important) Event**
This is a "catch-all" category introduced by CIOMS and adopted by FDA and other agencies to include AEs/ADRs that a clinician considers are important

and worth reporting but do not fall under the other categories of seriousness. This is not always an easy determination, and one observer may consider an event to be significant and another observer may not. In general, for regulatory reporting purposes, most agencies advise that one err on the conservative side and report "controversial" events.

Examples include a drop in the platelet count to a level (e.g., from 250,000 to 75,000 platelets/mm^3) that is not yet low enough to produce bleeding but is very important to note in the safety profile of a drug. Some pharmaceutical companies have attempted to create lists of important events as a guide to determine what to report to health authorities under this category.

OUTSOURCING PHARMACOVIGILANCE

This expression is used in the pharmaceutical industry to designate the practice of delegating the pharmacovigilance function to an outside company (generically called clinical or contract research organizations (CROs)). Thus it is said that a company can *"outsource ADR reporting to a CRO."* CROs that are now being created perform only pharmacovigilance (both pre- and post-approvalvigilance) and not clinical research, thus making the term *CRO* a bit of a misnomer.

Outsourcing may be limited to drugs in the preclinical phases of development (phases I–III) or it may be done for products already on the market (phase IV). This practice is usually done out of necessity by small companies that cannot afford to develop and maintain a department to deal with AE/ADR reporting. Large multinationals are now also looking at this idea when they are working on small and limited projects and do not wish to create a clinical research team that will have no function after the completion of the clinical trials or are working on very large projects (*megatrials* of 10,000+ patients) and cannot create a team and infrastructure in the timeframe required. On the other hand, outsourcing decreases the company's direct control over the project, giving it to others whose skills, capacities, and viewpoint may or may not be equal to those of the outsourcing company. The bottom line is that outsourcing of this responsibility to a CRO does not relieve the originating company of its legal and ethical responsibilities.

PACKAGE INSERT

This term is used in two ways, which can produce some confusion.

Package insert, particularly in the United States, refers to the official product labeling (equivalent to the product monograph or SPC in other terminologies) and is written for health care professionals. It may or may not be dispensed by the pharmacist with the product upon presentation of a prescription in the United States.

Another usage refers to the written notice given to the patient when a prescription is dispensed. It may be given in the original box as prepared by the manufacturer or may be given with a bottle or vial of the medication after repackaging by the pharmacist. That is, if the pharmacist purchases the product (branded or generic) in bulk, he or she can give the notice to the patient at the time of the initial or refill dispensation of the medication. The notice may be prepared by the pharmacy, the manufacturer, or a third party. In some cases, it is synonymous with the patient information leaflet.

It is clear (unfortunately) that patients are rarely conscious of the potentially serious ADRs that their medication may produce. Yet important ADRs that are identifiable by the patient must be clearly described and accompanied by instructions on their prevention and detection as well as the course the patient should follow if one should occur. This situation has not yet been solved.

PACKAGING

BROAD DEFINITION
The actual packaging (box, container, bottle, etc.) plus the galenic formulation (capsule, tablet, gelule, injection, suspension, inhalation product, etc.) and the labeling.

NARROW DEFINITION
It is the most common usage, designating the primary and secondary presentations. The primary presentation concerns the actual container (bottle, blister package, watertight container). The secondary presentation includes the packaging (outer box, label, accessory for administration such as an eye dropper or a metered dosage aerosol). Packaging problems can lead to administration errors that can lead to ADRs. For example, there are numerous instances of unclear reconstitution instructions for the preparation of suspensions from powders. Such instructions can produce suspensions that are too potent (overdose) or too dilute (underdosing and lack of efficacy).

In examining packaging during a pharmacovigilance investigation, it is necessary to keep in mind that there may in fact be three (or even more) packagings to consider:

> The *trade packaging,* which is the container that the manufacturer ships out, for example, bottles of 500 or 1000 tablets destined for the pharmacy or wholesaler.

The *pharmacy packaging,* which is the packaging the pharmacy uses at the retail level, for example, transfer of 30 tablets to a small vial that is given to the patient.

The *patient packaging,* which is the container the patient uses in his or her home or travels, for example, by transferring a few tablets to a small pill-box or tissue for use later that day. Each time the drug is moved from one package to another, storage conditions are altered and the potential for stability problems arises with drug products that may lead to misuse, loss of efficacy, and so on.

PARADOXICAL EFFECT

This term is used to describe an ADR that represents the opposite of the desired pharmacologic or therapeutic effect. It provides an outstanding example of an undesirable effect that is almost impossible to relate to the drug under study in a clinical trial. Often it is not even suspected of having produced this effect. Sometimes a controlled clinical trial is required to prove or disprove the suspicion. The reaction may be pharmacologic when the observed pharmacodynamic effect is opposite to the expected effect. The paradox may be therapeutic when the product causes a reaction opposite to the desired clinical effect. Several illustrations of paradoxical pharmacodynamic or therapeutic effects follow.

FIAU in the treatment of hepatitis B producing hepatic damage: Fialuridine (FIAU), a pyrimidine nucleoside analogue, was studied in the early 1990s as an antiviral treatment for hepatitis B. In 1993 a clinical trial was stopped by the investigators when it became apparent that patients might have suffered liver damage due to the drug. Of 15 patients treated, 8 experienced minor or no adverse effects, but 7 patients developed progressive hepatic failure and 5 died. The conduct of the trial produced much controversy (Saag, *J Clin Res Pract* 1999;1:21). The paradox here is that the drug apparently worsened the patients' liver status rather than improving it. The diagnostic difficulty revolved around the question of whether the worsening liver test results were due to the worsening of the underlying liver disease (hepatitis) or to the drug.

Type I anti-arrhythmics: fatal cardiac arrest: Encainide and flecainide provide typical paradoxical effects. In the course of the phase III clinical trials, the investigators noted that fatal cardiac arrhythmias were occurring. However, since the goal of the study was to prevent or reduce fatal cardiac arrhythmias in survivors of cardiac arrest after a myocardial infarct, it was practically impossible to attribute the cardiac arrest to the drugs since this group of patients was indeed at significant risk for this very complication. Only after the large scale comparative clinical Cardiac Arrhythia Suppression Trial (CAST) was done was this issue resolved. The paradoxical effect here is both pharmacologic (more frequent arrhythmias) and clinical (more frequent sudden deaths).

Corticosteroids: Paradoxic allergy: The ADRs in question here are immediate, and sometimes serious, cutaneous or respiratory allergic reactions. They are produced by the active moiety, usually when given intravenously, and appear from several seconds to several hours after dosing, thus suggesting that the corticosteroids being injected are the cause. It is unpredictable and very rare. This ADR should be noted in the patient's records since a rechallenge would provoke the same response in half of the cases. This reaction is paradoxical since the corticoid is being used as a treatment for allergic phenomena. However, it is not paradoxical when used in patients with autoimmune diseases.

Earlier total mortality rate: a fibrate. Clofibrate was one of the drugs used to treat hyperlipidemias in a trial—The Coronary Drug Project (CDP)—whose aim was to reduce coronary deaths. However, it was observed that total mortality rate from all causes as well as noncardiovascular mortality rate increased. Since the CDP was a controlled primary prevention trial in men who had no coronary disease on entry, the increase in mortality rate was particularly unacceptable. In a prevention study in healthy subjects the increased noncardiac mortality rate was not acceptable. This signal was not confirmed over the years but is presented only for its paradoxical therapeutic nature (*Br Heart J* 1978;40:1069; *Lancet* 1980;2:379).

Sublingual dihydropyridine: controversial efficacy in hypertensive crises: What should be done when significant ADRs follow the use of a product for an indication that had never been approved? A health authority cannot withdraw approval of an indication that it never approved. Such a situation occurred in the United States when immediate-release nifedipine was being used to treat hypertensive crises. Four elements came into play:

- The indication was unapproved.
- Serious AEs, sometimes fatal, occurred.
- Pharmacologic activity was not in question.
- No therapeutic benefit had ever been shown.

Although the Food and Drug Administration had never approved this indication, emergency room physicians were using nifedipine for hypertensive crises, reasoning that this antihypertensive agent given sublingually might prevent hemorrhagic complications (Winkler, JAMA 1996;276:1342 and 1997;277:790).

Pharmacologic Effect: A rapid fall in arterial pressure, particularly if too rapid, can increase the risk of reflex sympathetic stimulation. The immediate hypotensive effect is used as an immediate efficacy criterion that must be distinguished from the ultimate clinical and therapeutic benefit, which is the prevention of cerebral hemorrhage or cardiac failure due to the hypertensive crisis.

Complications: Significant hypotension after the use of the sublingual capsules could produce pulmonary edema, myocardial infarct, cerebrovascular accident or even death. An article by Grossman (JAMA 1996;276:1328) began an investigation of this issue in the literature. The authors believed that 11 deaths may have occurred because of this treatment. Another paper, by Semplici (JAMA 1997;277:787), reported 34 serious ADRs in 3792 patients treated.

Warfarin: thrombosis: Cutaneous necrosis produced by oral anti–vitamin K anticoagulants can result from the thrombosis of peripheral venules and capillaries after a rapid fall in the coagulation inhibitor protein C. Warfarin has been implicated in more than 300 published cases since 1943. The loss of a limb, a penis, one or both breasts, and other organs testifies to the serious ADRs this drug may produce. The suspicion of a drug effect was not the immediate reaction after the first publication by

Flood (*N Y State J Med* 1943;43:1121), since the second report did not occur until 11 years later (Verhagen, *Acta Med Scand* 1954;148:453). These ADRs were not fully recognized until two other cases were described 18 years after the first publication (Kipen, *N Engl J Med* 1961;265:638).

Thalidomide for toxic epidermal necrosis: During a double-blind placebo-controlled clinical trial for this new indication, the mortality rate in the experimental group was 83% and that in the control group, 30%. The trial was immediately stopped. This trial demonstrated that both for safety and efficacy reasons the use of this product for this indication was not appropriate. The paradox is that the intended therapeutic effect of saving lives in patients with toxic epidermal necrosis (TEN) was replaced by a different threat to their lives (Wolkenstein, *Lancet* 1998;352:1586).

PASSIVE REPORTING

A synonym for the spontaneous reporting system, as opposed to intensified reporting, called *active pharmacovigilance*, aimed at a specific product or AE and usually part of a pharmacovigilance investigation.

PEDS (see PHARMACOEPIDEMIOLOGY AND DRUG SAFETY)

PERIODIC SAFETY UPDATE REPORT (PSUR)

A regulatory term. PSURs are safety reports that manufacturers must submit periodically to regulatory authorities for marketed drugs. It is the key document used by the health authorities to evaluate the safety profile of a marketed drug over time.

The reports, often hundreds of pages in length, may vary in content from country to country. However, under the impetus of CIOMS II and the International Conference on Harmonization (ICH), there is increasing harmonization of form and content. As of early 2001 the European Union, Canada, Japan, and other nations have adopted this format. The U.S. Food and Drug Administration has not yet adopted the harmonized format and content but is expected to do so. It will upon request accept PSURs currently.

The major goals of the harmonization are to allow the manufacturers to prepare one report for one drug to be submitted to all authorities around the world where a drug is approved and to allow all regulatory bodies to see the same data at the same time. In practice, this has turned out to be rather difficult.

Standardized PSURs now generally contain the following:

- Regulatory information (e.g., approval dates in various countries, label changes made, regulatory actions taken)
- Sales volume or patient exposure (e.g., patient-years, patient-days)
- Tables (known as *CIOMS line listings*) of serious and some nonserious AEs/ADRs reported to the manufacturer as well as literature reports, results of phase IV studies done by the sponsor, and other information
- Analyses of pertinent cases
- Recommendations for safety changes in labeling (i.e., new ADRs, warnings, etc.)
- Special sections as requested by health authorities (e.g., consumer reported AEs, pregnancy listings, special subgroups such as the elderly, and children)

LANGUAGE

The language of the report is generally English. Some countries require parts or all of the report to be translated.

FORMAT OF THE TABLES

The tables list the AEs/ADRs by body system and include the event or reaction, demographic data on the patient, and additional clinical information:

- Country where the event was reported
- Source (e.g., clinical trial, health authority, spontaneous report)
- Age and sex of the patient
- Dose and, if pertinent, route and formulation
- Treatment duration
- Nature of the event: standard medical terminology is usually used (e.g., *WHO-ART*, *MedDRA*, *COSTART*). It is expected that everyone will move to *MedDRA* (see MedDRA) over the next few years. The most severe or medically important event is usually listed first and, where possible, a syndrome or disease is listed rather than its components (e.g., myocardial infarction rather than chest pain, diaphoresis, abnormal electrocardiographic (ECG) result)
- Outcome, which is based on the regulatory definition of "seriousness" (see SERIOUSNESS CRITERIA)
- Case comments: other pertinent information, such as comedications, risk factors, and challenge/dechallenge; the manufacturer may also indicate its opinion on causality here
- Manufacturer's reference number

FREQUENCY OF SUBMISSION OF PERIODIC REPORTS

The usual reporting intervals are every 6 months for 2 years, yearly for 3 years, then every 5 years. The clock starts with the approval of a new drug or a new indication or formulation for an old (i.e., already marketed) drug.

BIRTH DATE

This is still a controversial and unresolved issue (see INTERNATIONAL BIRTH DATE). The birth date of a drug determines the frequency of submission of PSURs and varies from region to region. It is based on one or more of the following criteria:

- The date of first approval anywhere in the world (international birth date) or date of first approval in a particular region (e.g., first approval in an EU country: "European or EU birth date")
- Date of commercialization in a particular country
- Approval of a new indication
- Addition of new components or excipients
- Approval of a new route of administration

One of the major areas of controversy concerns the time lag in approvals from country to country. To take only one example, if a drug was approved in country A five years ago and is thus now on an every-five-year PSUR schedule, it is unlikely that country B, which is only now first approving the drug, will wait five years for its first safety report on a newly approved drug.

THE REGULATIONS

The contents of the PSUR were first proposed and fixed by the CIOMS II Working Group in 1992 (*International Reporting of Periodic Drug-Safety Update Summaries.*

Geneva: Final report of CIOMS Working Group II, 1992). The International Conference on Harmonization (ICH) adopted this recommendation with some changes and published it in its E2C document. The E2C document has been officially adopted in many countries, though with some changes in some countries (see ICH EC2 and CIOMS II).

PERSON-YEARS

This epidemiologic concept is used as a measure of patient exposure to a suspect product. It is used in the denominator in the calculations of the frequency of an AE/ADR when spontaneous AE/ADR data are used. Similar terms include: *person-days, person-months, patient-years,* and *patient-days.* The terms *man-years,* and *man-days* are now out of date (see FREQUENCY OF AN ADVERSE EVENT/REACTION).

PHARMACEUTICAL EDUCATION & RESEARCH INSTITUTE (PERI)

Founded in 1989, this nonprofit U.S. corporation teaches pharmaceutical medicine. It is dedicated to the continuing education of scientists in the pharmaceutical industry and offers more than 100 three- to four-day courses in conference centers and hotels, usually in the area around Washington, D.C. (and the Food and Drug Administration) but sometimes in other major U.S. cities. PERI is under the direction of pharmacoepidemiologist Dr Judith Jones (PERI 1616 North Fort Myer Drive, Suite 1430, Arlington, VA 22209; website: www.peri.org).

PHARMACEUTICAL MEDICINE

The medical field devoted to the research, development, surveillance, and transmission of information regarding drugs, biologics, and devices produced by the medicopharmaceutical industry. Pharmacovigilance is part of this field. Most people engaged in this field are in the pharmaceutical industry and, to a lesser extent, health authorities and academe.

There are a few organizations for health professionals in the field:

- The Drug Information Association, the largest organization in the field (http//www.diahome.org/index.htm), which administers a vast program of education in pharmaceutical medicine
- The American Academy of Pharmaceutical Physicians, a fairly new organization for medical doctors in the field in North America covering the industry, government, and academe (http://www.aapp.org/)
- Faculty of Pharmaceutical Medicine, in the United Kingdom with members worldwide (http://www.f-pharm-med.org.uk/)
- L'Association des Médecins de l'Industrie Pharmaceutique (AMIP), an association for physicians in the industry in France
- The International Society of Pharmacovigilance (formerly called the European Society of Pharmacovigilance (http://www.pharmacoepi.de/esoporg.htm)

There are a few publications in the field, such as:

- *International Journal of Pharmaceutical Medicine* (http://www.socpharmed.org/)
- *Pharmaceutical Medicine*
- *The Drug Information Journal* (http://www.diahome.org/English/dhp5a.htm)
- *Pharmacoepidemiology and Drug Safety (PEDS)* (http://www.pharmacoepi.org/jpeds.htm)

PHARMACEUTICAL PRODUCT

A galenic formulation containing an active ingredient and excipients. It may be a branded product or a generic product.

PHARMACOBEZOAR

This term refers to the localized accumulation of an orally ingested pharmaceutical product that has mixed with digestive secretions to form a mass. It can produce an obstruction anywhere along the digestive tract as well as causing pain, ulceration, or bleeding, particularly in the stomach. There is also the danger of sudden release of the active ingredient, which can produce a drug overdose.

Bezoars can also consist of hair (trichobezoars) or vegetable material (phytobezoars). Although endoscopy may be used to remove the latter types of bezoars when located in the stomach, surgical removal may be necessary, particularly for pharmacobezoars, because sudden release of excess amounts of the active ingredient is a risk (Korenman, *JAMA* 1978;240:54; Townsend, *N Engl J Med* 1973;288:1058; Stack, *Dig Dis* 1995;356). The following is an example of a mass formed in the first portion of the digestive tract:

> *Guar gum*: This hydrophilic compound was sold as a weight loss product. In 1989 a 39-year-old male patient entered the emergency room noting that several hours after ingesting three tablets he was no longer able to swallow his saliva. Rigid esophagoscopy was required, but the esophagus was torn during the procedure, requiring surgical repair. Several days later the patient died of a pulmonary embolus. Examination of the Food and Drug Administration database revealed 17 other cases of esophageal retention, though none serious. The product was withdrawn from the market (FDA, *Desk Guide,* March 8, 1998). (www.fda.gov/medwatch/report/desk/casestud.html).

A related problem is swallowing a blister pack. In the examples that follow the ADR is related to the immediate packaging rather than the result of the formation of a mass:

> A 63-year-old female hospitalized on the psychiatric service was given a tablet of acetaminophen that was not removed from its blister pack and was placed on her bedside table. She ingested it without removing it from the blister pack and the next morning exhibited abdominal pain and signs of shock. Echography and upper endoscopy did not reveal a cause and the patient underwent a laparotomy, which revealed a tear of the gastric artery, perforation of the stomach, a splenic lesion, a perihepatic hematoma, hemoperitoneum, *and* the blister pack! (Lurton, *N Engl J Med* 1997;348:754)

> A blind 80-year-old man living alone normally took his daily tablet of phenylacetic acid after its removal from the blister pack by someone else. One day the visitor forgot to remove it from the pack; it was ingested by the patient, who suffered a fatal perforation of the distal ileum caused by a corner of the blister (Norstein, *Lancet* 1995;346:1308; Fulford, *Lancet* 1996;347:128)

PHARMACODEPENDENCE

Dependence on a pharmaceutical product can be considered a type A ADR, behavioral in nature. Benzodiazepines and narcotics are well known for this ADR.

Pharmacodependence is part of the background ADR knowledge of a drug. Clinicians take into account this information by prescribing narcotics only to those whose pain is truly intense, so as to preclude the potential for dependence.

The antecedents of dependence such as genetics factors, the social environment, and addiction to other substances constitute *risk factors* specific for the patient. For example, codeine is avoided in patients who are known to have dependence on other substances.

Dependence on a medication is, by definition, caused by the medication. In this case, causality is established by definition: that is, the behavioral AE *dependence on codeine* is definitely caused by codeine! The same may be said of nicotine.

PHARMACOEPIDEMIOLOGY

A medical science applied to interactions between marketed medications and the population. From the Greek *pharmakon,* "poison"; *epi,* "concerning"; and *demos,* "people." This definition corresponds to that cited in the chapter in Strom 2000 "What is Pharmacoepidemiology?", a well-written chapter worth reading. Pharmacoepidemiology applies the methods of classic and clinical epidemiology as well as the technologies of modern communication to those of clinical pharmacology and pharmacotherapy. The first use of the term in a medical journal dates back to 1984 (Lawson, *Br Med J* 1984;289:940). It represents the last phase in the evaluation of a medication in development and is absolutely essential to complete the picture of a new product to ensure *effective, safe, rational,* and *cost effective use.* There are four general areas in pharmacoepidemiology:

- *Benefit,* obtained by evaluation of efficacy and efficiency
- *Safety,* obtained by pharmacovigilance
- *Use,* obtained by utilization review of drugs
- *Value,* obtained by pharmacoeconomics

PHARMACOEPIDEMIOLOGY

Pharmacoepidemiologist Dr. Brian Strom edited a recommended book on the subject, useful to anyone involved with drug safety in the industrial, governmental or academic setting. The 78 contributors have written 45 chapters with numerous tables and a glossary (Strom BL, Editor. *Pharmacoepidemiology.* 3nd Edition. Chichester: Wiley, 2000; Abbreviated Strom 2000 in this book).

PHARMACOEPIDEMIOLOGY AND DRUG SAFETY (PEDS)

This journal was created in 1991 and, since 1994, has been the official journal of the International Society for Pharmacoepidemiology and of the International (formerly European) Society of Pharmacovigilance. This journal, published in the United Kingdom, is recommended to all those involved in pharmacovigilance. It is available electronically (www.interscience.wiley.com) as well as in its printed version.

In each issue there is an excellent bibliography, "Current Awareness," which contains the titles of recently published articles related to pharmacovigilance. In addition a supplement containing abstracts of communications from the annual international conference is published each year.

PHARMACOKINETICS

The study of the actions of the organism on the medication (ADME): **a**bsorption, **d**istribution, **m**etabolism (biotransformation), and **e**limination. The study of these properties for new formulations and new products is started during phase I of the clinical evaluation.

PHARMACOLOGY

The biomedical science applied to molecular entities used as medications. It describes and explains their interactions with the living organism.

PHARMACOTHERAPY

A therapeutic approach based on the use of pharmaceutic products that cause a pharmacologic effect, as opposed to other modes of therapy, such as radiotherapy and psychotherapy.

PHARMACOTRANSPARENCY

The question of transparency in regard to data collected in the course of pharmacovigilance has been discussed at several European meetings on pharmaceutical information and access to data submitted by companies to governments in support of Marketing Authorizations:

- Monitoring Centre Conference on Pharmacotransparency, Uppsala (Sweden), 24 September 1996, leading to the Uppsala Declaration (see PHARMACOTRANSPARENCY: DECLARATION OF ERICE) (http://www.who-umc.org)
- Erice (Sicily) Conference on Pharmacotransparency, September 1997 (www.who-umc.org)
- European Medicinal Evaluation Agency (EMEA) Workshop on transparency and access to documents, London, 10 October 1997 (http://www.eudra.org/emea.html)

The need for greater transparency in making public the results of clinical evaluations of drugs—in order to protect public health—has been taken up by a growing number of groups and organizations. The editors of various independent medical journals (*Prescrire International*, International Society of Drug Bulletins, etc.) and consumer advocate groups (Health Action International, MaLAM, Public Citizen's/Health Research Group in the United States, Consumers Association in the United Kingdom) are all in agreement on this point.

The director of pharmacovigilance of the Uppsala Monitoring Centre considers that transparency in the communication of data on the risk/benefit ratio of drugs is of paramount importance in the continuing medical and pharmacotherapeutic education of professionals as well as in the education of consumers on the nature of drug therapy (Edwards, *Drug Saf* 1997;17:216).

The U.S. Food and Drug Administration has made available for many years the Summary Basis of Approval (SBOAs) of many drugs it has approved, although the safety data are often given in insufficient detail; see the website (http://www.fda.gov/cder/drug/default.htm). The EMEA has also been making public *European Public Assessment Reports* (EPARs); see their website (http://www.eudra.org/humandocs/humans/epar.htm). However laudable these efforts are, there remains a long road to cover since it is estimated that as little as 1% of the total information contained in submissions for marketing authorization is made public, according to Abassi (*Br Med J* 1998;317:898) and ISDB Assessment of Nine EPARs (Paris: ISDB, 1998).

Individual U.S. MedWatch forms (redacted to remove reporter information) are available at minimal charge but through a laborious procedure from the

FDA under the U.S. Freedom of Information Act (http://www.fda.gov/foi/foia2.htm). So far the FDA databases contain over 1 million such reports. In addition, the FDA has put much of this information on its website as well as making it available with periodic updates on CD-ROMs (www.fda.gov/MedWatch).

There nonetheless has been a lively debate on what and when data should be made public. This debate is centered around whether AE/ADR data should be released when still in the "signal stage" or when the relationship of the AE to the drug in question is dubious. For example, releasing two case reports of torsades de pointes whose causality in regard to the drug in question is unclear is a vexing question. If it turns out that these cases are drug-related, then indeed this information should be released as soon as possible. On the other hand, if it turns out that other causes are far more likely, making this preliminary information public prematurely may push patients away from a drug that is, in fact, safe in this regard.

PHARMACOTRANSPARENCY: DECLARATION OF ERICE

This document summarizes the conclusions of the International Conference on Developing Effective Communication in Pharmacovigilance held at Erice, Italy, on 24–27 September 1997 and organized by the Uppsala Monitoring Centre and the University of Verona with the assistance of the International Union of Pharmacology (IUPHAR), Ettore Majorana Centre and the WHO. Participants from 34 countries attended; see the website (www.who-umc.org).

Their conclusions are summarized in the following five points (*Lancet* 1996;348:908 and 1997;350:1041):

- Drug safety information must serve the health of the public.
- Education in the appropriate use of drugs, including interpretation of safety information, essential for the public at large as well as for patients and health-care providers is vital.
- All the evidence needed to assess and understand risks and benefits must be openly available.
- Every country needs a system with independent expertise to ensure that safety information [. . .] is adequately collected, impartially evaluated and accessible to all.
- Emergent problems must be promptly recognized and efficiently dealt with, and information and solutions are effectively communicated.

PHARMACOTRANSPARENCY: EMEA WORKSHOP

The European Medicinals Evaluation Agency (EMEA) held a workshop in 1997 on the transparency of clinical dossiers submitted for marketing approval by pharmaceutical companies and the rationale behind the regulatory decisions made in regard to these dossiers. The workshop stressed European problems related to which drug data should be made accessible to the public. The first was for the extension to European countries of Freedom of Information (FOI) laws similar to those already in existence in the United States. The second was the need for broader publication of *European Public Assessment Reports* (EPARs) for products approved at the national level. These reports are currently published and available on the Internet by the EMEA for drugs approved at the European level (Scrip, 1997;2283:2); see the website (http://www.eudra.org/emea.html).

PHARMACOTRANSPARENCY: UPPSALA DECLARATION

This document was the result of an international working group that met in September 1996 on the transparency and public control of official decisions concerning drugs; see the website (http://www.who-umc.org).

It was supported by Health Action International (HAI) and the Dag Hammarskjold Foundation. They noted that "reports concerning the AEs of medications . . . remain totally inaccessible" to health care professionals because of the secrecy that surrounds the clinical dossiers submitted by the manufacturers in support of their request for marketing authorization.

A summary of this workshop has been published (*Int J Risk Saf Med* 1996;9:211–217). The declaration is also available in French, Spanish, and Portuguese from Health Action International; see their website (http://www.haiweb.org/pubs/sec-sta.html); HAI-Europe has headquarters in the Netherlands (Jacob van Lennepkade 334-T, 1053 NJ Amsterdam, Netherlands).

PHARMACOVIGILANCE

NARROW DEFINITION

A clinical science whose objectives are the surveillance, evaluation, and signaling of the undesirable effects of pharmaceutical products (drugs, biologics, medicines) used for medical therapy and whose major sources of new information are spontaneous notification and reporting of such effects. Pharmacovigilance also includes the diffusion of this information and the regulatory measures taken to prevent future ADRs, to ensure safer use of drug products as well as an improvement in the risk/benefit ratio.

Synonyms for pharmacovigilance include: *drug surveillance, drug safety surveillance, drug safety monitoring/reporting, pharmaceutical surveillance, pharmaco-surveillance, postmarketing surveillance* (PMS), and *spontaneous reporting system/scheme (SRS)*.

BROADER DEFINITION

A more global definition of pharmacovigilance includes a larger array of tools, products, contexts, and objectives. The term *pharmacoepidemiology* is sometimes used to describe this broader concept of marketed drug surveillance.

▶ **Methods**

Although the major tool remains the system of spontaneous reporting of AEs/ADRs followed by pharmacovigilance investigations of signals, other epidemiologic approaches are possible and useful. These include observational (case controls, cohorts, etc.) and linked-database epidemiologic studies (of data already collected and computerized). Pharmacovigilance and pharmacoepidemiology can work in a complementary manner to resolve vexing safety issues.

▶ **Products**

The products under surveillance can be extended to include medical devices (materiovigilance), blood products (hemovigilance), biologics, human immunodeficiency virus (HIV) medications, cytotoxic antineoplastics (oncovigilance), vaccines (vaccinovigilance), and medicinal plants (phytovigilance).

▶ **Context: Misuses and Patients**

The context can be extended to include dependence and abuse, poisoning by overdose, and various misuses and errors related to prescribing, dispensing, and self-medicaton. Also included may be the special categories of patients: embryo/fetus (teratovigilance), pregnant/lactating mother (maternal pharmacovigilance), children, and elderly adults (gerontovigilance).

▶ **Objectives**

The objectives can be extended to include drug utilization reviews in order to keep prescribers and users under surveillance, and pharmacoeconomic studies to evaluate costs incurred and costs avoided.

PHASE I

A clinical trial of a molecule that has already passed all or most of the preclinical requirements. Phase I trials aim mainly at determining the maximal tolerated dose in healthy normal volunteers. If the drugs are known to be toxic or have predictable serious ADRs, these studies are often done in patients with the disease to be treated e.g., cancer chemotherapy or antiviral therapy in acquired immunodeficiency syndrome (AIDS) patients; in other words, phase I is conducted in phase II patients for obvious ethical motives. Patients are often housed for these studies in special Clinical Research Centers run by academic medical centers or clinical research organizations (CROs).

The risk of serious AEs/ADRs and death remains very low in phase I trials. Even back in 1978 the risk of a severe event was found to be 1 in 9602 patient-days. A more difficult issue arises when a volunteer purposely hides a disease or risk factor in order not to be excluded from the trial—usually for monetary reasons (Apseloff, *Clin Pharmacol Ther* 1996;60:353). Here follow two examples that proved fatal:

- A 23-year-old American female nurse omitted to mention two previous episodes of cardiac arrest one of which was followed by coma for two days (Kolata, *Science* 1980;209;475).
- An Irish volunteer had omitted to mention that the day before receiving an injection of the antiarrhythmic eproxindine, he had received an injection of depot flupenthixol, an antipsychotic. Asystole occurred 1 minute after the beginning of the 5-minute perfusion of 400 mg of eproxindine. An interaction between the two medications at the site of plasma protein binding was suspected (Darragh, *Lancet* 1985;I:93).

PHASE II

Clinical trials of a substance that has successfully passed through (all or parts of) phase I and preclinical trials. Phase II trials are aimed mainly at determining a minimal effective dose on the basis of either a pharmacologic criterion that serves as a surrogate outcome, such as arterial pressure, serum cholesterol levels, viral load, or bone density, or an actual therapeutic benefit such as pain relief by an analgesic.

DRUG RELATED DEATHS

It is very rare that the first patients who volunteer to be exposed to a new drug at this very early stage of development die of it. The following tragic example, however, describes how fialuridine led to hepatic failure:

> This new molecular antiviral was used to treat chronic hepatitis B and was responsible for severe hepatic failure with some fatalities in the course of a phase II trial. Fifteen patients were affected. Seven had very severe hepatic failure after 0 to 13 weeks of treatment. Five died and two others survived as a result of emergency hepatic transplants. The mechanism of action appeared to be due to a mitochondrial lesion. The

study was due to last for a total of 6 months but was immediately stopped after the occurrence of the first fulminant hepatic failure in a patient dosed for 13 weeks. Six other patients had been dosed for 9 weeks or more and for them it was already too late. This catastrophe provoked a major review of the safety measures for phase II trials of new products (Honkoop, *Drug Saf* 1997;17:1; Saag MJ, *Clin Res Pract* 1999;1:21). Various ethical questions, including that of the informed consent, were also raised.

PHASE III

The phase of study of a drug after it has passed through stages I and II. The major method in this phase is the comparative controlled clinical trial that compares the new drug with a placebo or a reference medication. As in phase II, the end points of the study can be either surrogate markers or actual therapeutic end points. These studies are generally larger and longer than phase II trials. The goal is to amass sufficient efficacy and safety data to gain marketing authorization in at least one indication.

PHASE III CONTROLLED TRIALS: WHY THEY ARE NOT SUFFICIENT TO FIND ALL ADRs

The very nature and structure of these trials do not permit the capture of certain ADRs. The usual structure is that of a double-blind, controlled trial against placebo or a standard treatment with evaluation of safety and efficacy. Treatment duration is usually fairly short, and the patients are carefully selected and relatively homogeneous. There are few or no comedications or comorbidity permitted and the number of patients studied is relatively small. There is limited follow-up after treatment is stopped (Faich, *J Clin Res Drug Dev* 1997;1:75). The time frame of treatment is usually fairly short—even for chronic diseases such as hypertension, diabetes, arthritis, or cardiac disease. In other words, the experimental context is artificial and not very pertinent to, representative of, or transferable to the real-life clinical world seen after the drug is launched and used in the general population. The history of pharmacovigilance has confirmed that pre-marketing clinical trials are not sufficient to flesh out a product's safety profile fully.

INSUFFICIENT NUMBER OF PATIENTS STUDIED

The absence of an ADR in the first series of patients exposed to a drug does not mean that the ADR will not occur later. The number of patients needed is a function of the frequency of the ADR's occurrence in the treated group and and of the baseline rate in the comparative group. Tables for determining number of patients needed may be found in pharmacoepidemiology textbooks such as Strom 2000.

In submissions to health authorities for marketing authorizations, the usual number of patients studied is below 2500. The mean number of patients studied in phase III trials for a nonsteroidal anti-inflammatory drug (NSAID) in 1994 was 2128 patients in Europe, 2732 in the United States, and 1651 in Japan (Homma, *Drug Inf J* 1994;28:413). If an ADR is not seen in 2500 patients studied, then there is a 95% probability that its true frequency is less than 1/833 and a 99% probability that it is less than 1/543. It is rare that the number of patients studied is above 5000. In Great Britain in the course of phase III trials for products introduced between 1987 and 1989 the median number of patients studied was 1529 (Rawlins, *Bull R Coll Physicians* 1991;302:223).

Beginning in the mid-1990s several drugs were studied in megatrials that studied 10,000 or more patients. In some of these trials, however, only serious adverse effects were collected as a result of logistic difficulties. Nevertheless, these trials gave an arguably more complete safety picture than those of drugs whose study population numbered only a fraction of this figure.

QUALITATIVE ASPECTS OF THE PATIENTS
They are not representative of the population at large.

▶ Heterogeneity
The targeted population is more heterogeneous than the study population. The population exposed to the product after marketing differs considerably from that studied in phases II and III. This difference is not an accident but the inevitable result of the structure and methodology of clinical research. Collet and coworkers have distinguished six populations in the therapeutic domain (*Eur J Clin Pharmacol* 1991;41:267). The population studied is extremely restricted because of the many explicit and implicit inclusion and exclusion criteria.

▶ Sex
Women represent 52% of the world's population and live longer than men but are often insufficiently represented in clinical trials save those for drugs studied for reproduction, menopause, and gynecologic oncology. In cardiovascular prevention studies, women have often been excluded from major trials. However, they are major consumers of antihypertensive and hyperlipemic agents. This situation was so serious that in 1993 the Food and Drug Administration lifted its ban on participation of women of childbearing age in clinical trials.

▶ Indication
The indication in a clinical trial is often very narrow both qualitatively (only a single disease) and quantitatively (only a single level of severity).

▶ Age
Clinical trials do not include babies and infants and usually do not include adolescents and elderly adults. However, fully a third of the world's population is below age of 15 and 6% of the population is above age 65. Yet the elderly consume much more medicine than the young. The exclusion of these populations has led to difficulties in determining the proper doses to be used as these groups often require smaller doses than those in the middle of the age spectrum. Hence the old may be functionally overdosed in routine pharmacotherapy as result of the lack of clinical trials in these groups to determine the most appropriate dosage.

▶ Concomitant Morbidity
Concomitant pathology (comorbidity) is usually an exclusion criterion in clinical trials. However, in the real world of the practicing clinician, patients have arthritis, diabetes, heart disease, hypertension, acquired autoimmunodeficiency syndrome (AIDS) and other conditions. In addition, they may be obese or anorexic or consume alcohol or be heavy smokers.

▶ Nonpharmacologic Interventions
Other factors can influence the pharmacodynamics and pharmacokinetics of a product such as surgery, radiotherapy, hyperalimentation, special diets, malnutrition, dehydration, drinking, convalescence, sun exposure, and heat or cold exposure.

▶ Physiology
Certain physiologic states are exclusion criteria that eliminate potential sub-

jects from clinical trials: pregnant women, newborns, women of childbearing potential not on birth control, women who are breastfeeding, growing children and others. This method excludes major patient groups who will use drugs after marketing but who are not studied before marketing.

QUANTITATIVE ASPECTS OF THE DRUG TREATMENT

▶ Duration of Treatment

In clinical trials, exposure is almost always too short: several weeks to several months at most. Some ADRs only appear after months or even years of continuing treatment, and others require a cumulative dose not attained in phase III trials.

▶ Dose and Mode of Administration

After marketing, the product is prescribed and used at varying doses, including massive overdoses taken in suicide attempts, children's use of adults' medications, and doubling or tripling of doses by patients ("If some is good, more is better"). A drug may be taken by a different mode of administration (e.g., misuse or abuse by addicts who crush and dissolve tablets and inject them with dirty and contaminated needles). An underappreciated problem is that errors occur in writing prescriptions, in filling them in a pharmacy, in delivering them in the hospital, or in timing administration. There is little work done in the field of dosing and diurnal rhythms (chronopharmacology).

▶ Compliance

Fidelity to treatment in the general population is certainly less than that seen (and required) in clinical trials. This is even more pronounced in asymptomatic diseases such as hypertension. This is an expected phenomenon ("the human condition") and experienced physicians are usually resigned to this fact of life. However, lower compliance can result in lower efficacy (and fewer AEs).

CHARACTERISTICS OF THE ADVERSE EVENT

▶ Latency Period

If the ADR occurs several months (e.g., practolol) or several years (e.g., diethylstilbestrol (DES)) after the end of treatment, it is difficult, if not impossible, to detect these reactions during the limited duration of follow-up in most clinical trials.

▶ High Frequency in the Reference Population

For an AE/ADR that is common in the general population or in the population with the disease being treated, it may be very difficult to determine whether the drug is producing such a problem. Even the spontaneous reporting system may be inadequate to detect this, and only a structured study with sufficient power aimed at this specific event will be adequate. Type C (chronic use) events such as thromboemboli associated with oral contraceptives or hormonal replacement therapy require epidemiologic trials. Paradoxical ADRs such as arrhythmias due to antiarrhythmic drugs require comparative therapeutic trials.

OUTCOME MEASURES

The outcome measures used to evaluate efficacy in clinical trials are not necessarily the same as those that would be chosen if the trial were aimed primarily at evaluating safety data. For example, an echocardiogram has not traditionally been part of a protocol for the evaluation of a new weight-loss drug (Amery, *PEDS* 1999;8:61).

LESSONS FROM THE BEGINNINGS OF ORGANIZED SURVEILLANCE

In the United Kingdom where pharmacovigilance began with Inman's yellow card system, Rawlins has indicated that national programs have contributed substantially to the public health and have been of crucial importance in the surveillance of marketed products and that spontaneous reporting has detected the majority of ADRs that have led to marketing withdrawals in Great Britain since 1972 (Rawlins, *PEDS* 1995;4:5). According to Venning (*Br Med J* 1983;286:458), of the new ADRs discovered since pharmacovigilance became an organized endeavor, the majority were found as a result of spontaneous reporting.

Dr. Faich, then director of pharmacovigilance at the Food and Drug Administration, has commented on the value of the spontaneous reporting of AEs/ADRs (*N Engl J Med* 1986;314:1589). Among the labeling changes made in the United States in 1970, 24% were suggested by reports submitted spontaneously by U.S. physicians to the FDA and 68% were reported by pharmaceutical companies from spontaneous reports submitted to them totaling 92% that were due to spontaneous reporting (Health Canada, *Can ADR Newsl, Can Med Assoc J* 1995;153:63).

PHASE IV

A regulatory term applied to pharmacoepidemiologic studies (often of a single cohort group) done after marketing approval. These studies, when made for safety reasons, may be a condition and requirement for the marketing approval or they may be made after the identification of an alarming safety signal. Such safety studies should be contrasted to some phase IV trials that are done for marketing aims (*seeding studies*) without proper control measures to prevent biases, for example, studies comparing the drug against competitors or the study of a subgroup of the approved population (the elderly or another subgroup).

Phase IV safety studies are never undertaken lightly by the manufacturer. The first patients are enrolled and followed for a certain length of time. The size of the cohort depends on the level of use in the population and can reach as many as 10,000 patients for a product that is widely used (e.g., an acid suppressor used for heartburn or ulcers). The length of surveillance of each patient is a function of the average duration of a course of therapy. If this phase IV study reveals or confirms a safety issue, the drug may be restricted in use. Phase IV is discussed in Strom 2000 and in Stephens 1999.

PHENFORMIN: WITHDRAWAL

This oral biguanide hypoglycemic produced very rare cases of lactic acidosis of which nearly half were fatal. The actual number of such cases was not very high since the frequency was estimated at 1 per 2500 patient-years of exposure. Phenformin was withdrawn from the market in 1977 after a petition from a U.S. consumers group, the Health Research Group. The market withdrawal of this drug as a result of a petition was unusual; in most instances, a restriction on usage or a change in labeling is imposed rather than a market withdrawal. The reason for the withdrawal was that several other oral hypoglycemics that were available on the market did not produce lactic acidosis. Had this been the only oral agent on the market, the risk/benefit ratio would have most likely favored a labeling change or restriction rather than a market withdrawal.

A linked database study done in the Canadian province of Saskatchewan showed that the incidence of lactic acidosis with metformin was 1 per 1110 patient-years and that the nine cases that had been reported were due to misuse by the prescribers since all nine patients had contraindications to the use of metformin (Stang, *Can J Clin Pharmacol* 1998;4:53).

PHENOLPHTHALEIN: WITHDRAWAL

Phenolphthalein, a base of many over the counter (OTC) laxatives, was reclassified by the Food and Drug Administration in 1997 from category I (safe and effective) to category III (more safety information needed) in response to animal toxicology data that were not confirmed in humans. Later the FDA decided to withdraw this product. In December 1997, the Committee for Proprietary Medicinal Products (CPMP) in the European Union published an unfavorable report on this product. In Japan, the health authorities announced the "voluntary" withdrawal of this product, and in Italy the authorities opted for a forced withdrawal.

This situation illustrates the market withdrawal of a product that was based entirely on the carcinogenic potential seen in animal toxicology studies (mouse) without any clinical support of this signal. The apparent reason for this is that agencies believed that the theoretical risk/benefit ratio had been altered with these results. As a result of minimal clinical benefit, availability of other pharmacologic and nonpharmacologic modalities of constipation treatment, the balance tipped against the product.

PHOCOMELIA

A congenital malformation (dysmorphology) that affected thousands of babies born in the early 1960s after in utero exposure to thalidomide (see THALIDOMIDE). The almost total absence of the upper limbs gave the impression that the victims had seallike flippers (hence the name derived from *phoque*, "seal," and *melos*, "limb," in Greek). This drama triggered the formation of national pharmacovigilance units within national health agencies. In many countries the laws protecting the public from unsafe drugs were strengthened in response to the catastrophe.

PHYSICIAN'S DESK REFERENCE (PDR)

An American drug compendium. The counterpart in Canada is the *Compendium of Pharmaceuticals and Specialities (CPS)*, in France the *Dictionnaire Vidal*, and in Germany the *Rote Liste*. The *PDR* contains the Food and Drug Administration approved labeling for most of the major drugs available on the U.S. market. It is a good source to examine to see whether an ADR is labeled though it should be kept in mind that the threshold to be considered labeled is lower in the United States than elsewhere. For some drugs, *all* adverse effects seen in clinical trials are included; for others postmarketing AEs may be listed with a disclaimer noting that they have been reported but causality has not been established (i.e., they are AEs and not necessarily ADRs). The U.S. labeling provides a more conservative listing than most other nations' labeling. The U.S. labeling is said to include "treatment emergent" AEs while EU labeling includes "treatment related" ADRs.

PHYTOVIGILANCE

From *phuton*, "plant" in Greek. Surveillance of the AEs seen with plant-based products (also known as *herbal medicines*). Although a plant product may be perceived as benign, "natural," and harmless by the public, major sequelae and even deaths are reported. Phytovigilance is being recognized as an area well worth medical attention.

■ The Monitoring Centre in Uppsala has engaged the services of an expert in phytovigilance and has published an article on the topic ("Consumer protection and herbal remedies," *WHO Drug Information* 1998;12(3):141). Also see Farah (*PEDS* 2000;9;105) and the European Medicinal Evaluation Agency (EMEA) website (www2.eudra.org/gendocs/general/hmpwg.htm).

■ In October 1998 the European Scientific Cooperative on Phytotherapy (ESCOP) organized a symposium in London on phytomedicine and the protection of consumers (*Uppsala Rep* 1998;8).

■ The EMEA has done extensive work in this field through its Herbal Medicinal Products Working Party; more than a dozen final documents were issued in 1999 (www2.eudra.org/gendocs/general/hmpwg.htm).

■ The FDA has devoted extensive time and resources in the more broadly defined field of dietary supplements, which includes plant products. In January 2000 federal regulations were issued (21CFR101). See the FDA website (www.fda.gov under foods).

Here are a few examples:

■ A study on toxicovigilance done by the Poison Control Centre of Guy's Hospital in London revealed 1297 spontaneous reports of adverse effects associated with so-called natural products (Shaw, *Drug Saf* 1997;17:342). The *New England Journal of Medicine* felt compelled to publish a cautionary editorial on the subject (Angel, *N Engl J Med* 1998;39:839).

■ *Aristolochia species involved:* Another study reported a case series of serious nephrotoxicity (105 cases of renal failure, of which 43 were very severe) in female patients consuming *Aristolochia fangchi* (actually mislabeled as *Stephania* and *Magnolia*); if this was not enough, 18 cases of carcinoma of the urothelium were detected and appeared dose-related (Nortier, *N Engl J Med* 2000;342:1986). Again the *New England Journal of Medicine* felt the need in an editorial (by Kessler) to denounce the absence of quality control of medicinal plant products in most countries.

■ Hypertension has been associated with use of ginseng and renal insufficiency (sometimes fatal) with use of Chinese plants (ADRAC, *Aust ADR Bull* 1993;12(3):11; *Can ADR Newsl* 1994;4(2)).

■ Medicinal plant extracts sold in Austria under the guise of homeopathic products produced anaphylactic reactions (De Smet, *Drug Saf* 1995;13:81).

■ *St. John's Wort*: This product used for depression was cited by the FDA (www.fda.gov/cder/drug/advisory/stjwort.htm) and the EMEA (http://www.eudra.org/humandocs/PDFs/PS/632100EN.pdf.) for producing an interaction with various acquired immunodeficiciency syndrome (AIDS) medications.

■ *Royal jelly: death*: This product of bees contains allergenic proteins that presumably are responsible for contact dermatitis (Takahashi, *Contact Dermatitis* 1983;9:452). In addition, severe anaphylactic reactions, of which two were fatal, were reported in Australia (Drew, *Med J Aust* 1997;166:538). The first death reported occurred in an 11-year-old female asthma patient after her third exposure to the product (Bullock, *Med J Aust* 1994;160:44). These investigations illustrate the growing importance of phytovigilance.

There are three types of risk associated with herbal medicines:

■ The first risk concerns medical care. When confidence in the plants results in a delay in seeking proper medical *diagnosis* and advice, it can be of tragic proportions if the disease (e.g., cancer) can be successfully treated by orthodox medicine when detected early.

- The second risk is that of ADRs associated with the *active* ingredients of the plants (intrinsic effects) either by direct action or by interaction with orthodox medicines also being taken.

- The third risk is that of ADRs associated with *excipients* or with *contaminants* (extrinsic effects) introduced by "involuntary" errors or even by "voluntary" errors whereby various active ingredients are added. These may be "real drugs" such as nonsteroidal anti-inflammatory drugs (NSAIDs), benzodiazepines, or corticosteroids. They may also be other, more dangerous plants (Nortier, *N Engl J Med* 2000;342:1686).

Other areas of concern in regard to herbal and plant medicines include quality control during manufacture and claims for efficacy and safety. The term "natural" may be misleading and does not by any means guarantee harmlessness. In most countries (the United States, for example), there is little or no governmental regulation of these products, especially if no medical claims are made in regard to specific diseases.

Hepatitis associated with certain herbal products sold in "natural health" stores and pharmacies has begun to tarnish the reputation for innocuousness that these products have enjoyed until now.

ADRs can be classified as *intrinsic* (type A or B, associated with the active ingredient) and *extrinsic* (associated with a material problem or defect due to faulty manufacture). These ADRs are rarely noted in the product labeling, which is often rudimentary at best (Drew and Myers, *Med J Aust* 1997;166:538).

EXTRINSIC EFFECTS

- Contamination with arsenic, cadmium, mercury, heavy metals, microorganisms, lead, pesticide residues, toxic metabolites, radioactive materials, thallium, and other materials.

  > *l-Tryptophan*: This product had much notoriety, particularly in the United States, as a result of the eosinophilic myalgia syndrome associated with it. By May 1990, the FDA had already received 1500 reports of cases of which 23 were fatal. The eosinophilia is pronounced, with levels greater than $10^9/l$, and accompanied by myalgia and other signs such as rash and fever. A contaminant was suspected in the U.S. cases since this syndrome was associated with the product of one manufacturer in particular. The contaminant was a dimer of L-tryptophan. In contrast, no cases were seen in Australia (Adrac, *Aust ADR Bull* 1990;Aug:4). See also the August 2000 warning by the FDA (www.fda.gov/ora/fiars/ora_import_ia5404.html).

- Faulty identification or inadequate or fraudulent labeling. The existence of four different terminologies for each plant poses continual difficulties for poison control centers (But, *Lancet* 1993;341:637).
- Absence or insufficient amounts of the active ingredient. This may be intentional or unintentional, the result of quality control problems. A study of 50 different brands of ginseng in 11 countries revealed that the concentration of ginsenoside varied from 0% to 9% (Cui, *Lancet* 1994;344:134).
- Substitution with another plant.
- Substitution with active pharmacologic substances (hormones, NSAIDs, psychotropics, etc.).

■ Inappropriate dosage or galenic preparation.

INTRINSIC EFFECTS

Intrinsic effects are less frequent. ADRs may be of type A or B and due to the plant in question.

■ *Yohimbine and adrenergic antagonism*: This alkaloid of the bark of *Pausinystalia yohimbe* possesses an antagonist activity to alpha-2-adrenergic receptors and can produce type A, dose-dependent hypertension and anxiety and type B bronchospasm (Landis, *Chest* 1989;96:1424; Desmet, *Br Med J* 1994; 309:958).

The following examples are associated with severe AEs/ADRs and death.

■ *Aristolochic acid: interstitial nephritis*: This component of the medicinal plant *Aristolochia fangchi* can be nephrotoxic. This phytovigilance signal was first recognized after nine young Belgian women developed interstitial nephritis. There had been 80 cases described already in 1993, half of which ended in fatal renal failure (Vanherweghem, *Lancet* 1993;341:387 and 1994; 343:174).

■ *Aconitine: intoxication*: This plant contains very toxic alkaloids that must be markedly reduced during preparation by boiling. An Australian publication described eight troublesome clinical problems associated with the Chinese preparations of *Aconitum species* (Chan, *Aust N Z J Med* 1993;23:268).

■ *Chapparal: hepatotoxicity*: A medicinal plant capable of producing an acute toxic hepatitis, including irreversible hepatorenal insufficiency. This signal surfaced with the notification of the Food and Drug Administration of the first case in August 1992, followed by four additional cases 4 months later. A phytovigilance investigation was begun. Five American and three Canadian cases were examined in detail. A request for stimulated reporting by physicians was made by the Center of Disease Control (CDC) in Morbidity and Mortality Weekly Reports (*MMWR*) 30 October 1992 (2 months after the first case) and in the Journal of the American Medical Association (*JAMA*) 20 January 1993, 1 month after the first irreversible case. This was followed by the highly unusual publication by the FDA of a message aimed at discouraging the use of chapparal as a nutritional supplement. Of note is the exceptional rapidity with which this investigation was conducted (Nightingale, *JAMA* 1993;269;328).

PLACEBO EFFECT

A desirable effect produced by a medication, of psychologic origin, and whose mechanism, not linked to a pharmacologic effect of the active ingredient, is rather due to *confidence in the product* by the patient. This confidence can be strengthened by similar positive feelings of the physician and pharmacist as well as by publicity in the media, popular belief, and personal experience with the product. In comparative therapeutic clinical trials, the placebo effect, which is not always desirable in these settings, can be reinforced by the surroundings and ambience, as well as by the attention and enthusiasm of the research team.

PLANT, MEDICINAL (MEDICINAL HERB, BOTANICAL MEDICINE)

A plant extract used as a medication for therapeutic purposes. Risks exist with the use of these products and the surveillance of these risks is known as *phytovigilance*. (See PHYTOVIGILANCE).

PLASMA (SERUM, BLOOD) LEVEL

IN CLINICAL MEDICINE

The plasma (or serum) level of a drug and/or its metabolites is considered in the surveillance of patients in pharmacotherapy, particularly when there is a very narrow therapeutic window. This is also known as *therapeutic drug monitoring*. The goal is to produce plasma levels sufficiently high to obtain the desired pharmacologic effect while avoiding levels that are too high and would be toxic. Therapeutic drug monitoring is thus a means of *preventing* dose-dependent ADRs rather than a means of detecting such reactions.

IN CAUSALITY ASSESSMENT

When an ADR is tied to a supratherapeutic dose or to a frank overdose, the plasma level of the drug or its metabolites can turn out to be very useful in many cases. It is used routinely in poison centers and during autopsies done for forensic reasons. Ideally, the blood is drawn just as the undesirable reaction is beginning. In causality assessment, a high blood level of the suspect drug is a risk factor in favor of a drug cause; in probability terms it modifies the *general prior odds*, leading to higher *case-specific prior odds*.

PLAUSIBILITY

The term *plausibility* is used here in the sense that it is a necessary condition and a validity criterion for a reported case. An adverse effect that is suspected of being an ADR must be *reasonable* or *plausible* on biologic and epidemiologic grounds. If it is not, a causality tied to the suspect drug would be very unlikely or even ruled out. Similarly, the timing (*chronology*) of the occurrence of the AE and the extent of exposure to the suspect drug must be analyzed as certain values also make drug causality very improbable if not excluded.

BIOLOGY

An event whose occurrence "is in conformity with known scientific and medical facts and theories" is said to have *biologic plausibility*. An AE that is not plausibly related to the biologic, physical, chemical, pharmacologic, immunologic, or other properties of the suspect product is unlikely to be related to or caused by the suspect product. For example, it is more biologically plausible that an esophageal ulcer would be caused by a large, irritating tablet, swallowed without water while lying down, than by a syrup taken under the same conditions. Another example would be metastatic malignancy discovered one month after the patient started a new medication.

EPIDEMIOLOGY

An easily detectable AE that has never been reported with an old drug that has been administered to millions of patients over many years and is now reported in a single patient would be very unlikely to be related to the drug. Exceptions to this generality about old drugs would be drug interactions with a newly approved product or the administration of the old drug to an entirely new group of patients (e.g., infants) who were never previously exposed to it, or to patients with a new indication or comorbidity.

When an isolated AE has a convincing association (causality) with a drug based on a solid clinical picture (e.g., positive rechallenge), even though its biologic plausibility and epidemiologic characteristic may be borderline, it is referred to as an *orphan AE/ADR*. It is likely a very rare idiosyncratic reaction in a very special patient.

CHRONOLOGY: TIME TO ONSET

An AE is not likely to be associated with a drug if the time between exposure to the drug and the appearance of the event is either too short or too long or is negative.

▶ **Unlikely or Impossible Timing**

After clinical details of a suspected ADR have been obtained, it may become clear that the event occurred before the exposure to the drug. In this case it is easy to exclude the drug as a cause of the event. A surprising and interesting apparent exception are the nausea and vomiting in some cancer patients that occur before receiving doses of chemotherapeutic agents that had caused these reactions in these patients after previous administration of these drugs. This "anticipated ADR" is actually a nocebo effect.

▶ **Interval That Is Too Short**

In some situations, investigation may reveal that the event occurred too quickly after exposure to the drug—usually by a nonparenteral route. This analysis is complex, and it is necessary to examine the absorption, metabolism, elimination, mechanism of action, and other factors before excluding the drug as the cause of the event. An example would be a hemorrhage that occurs 5 minutes after the first dose of an oral anticoagulant. However, certain reactions (e.g., anaphylaxis) indeed occur in a very rapid manner after exposure. ADRs associated with drugs given by the parenteral route may occur very rapidly whether of type A or type B.

▶ **Interval That Is Too Long?**

As with too short an interval, prudence is required in evaluating an AE before excluding a drug as a cause. ADRs may appear after long intervals:

After first dose: time to onset: a time to appearance (or its detection by a lab test or from a complication) of an AE after the first dose of an ongoing treatment may be very long. There is a natural bias among clinicians against reporting an AE that first occurs after months or even years of a continuing drug treatment. This explains why it took some time, for example, to identifiy the association of visceral angioedema with use of angiotensing converting enzyme (ACE) inhibitors or retroperitoneal fibrosis with use of practolol.

After last dose: latency: a delay in the appearance of an AE after the last dose of a treatment may be very long. The pharmacokinetics of the drug in the particular patient plays a major role in this situation. The longest delay known is that of vaginal adenocarcinoma, which appeared 20 years after in utero exposure to diethylstilbestrol. In some situations it is possible to determine a time after exposure beyond which an AE is unlikely to be related to the drug. For example, with acute hepatitis, the latency time (unless the product is metabolized very slowly) is usually less than 15 days for cytolytic lesions and usually less than 30 days for cholestatic or mixed lesions (Benichou 1994).

CHRONOLOGY: TIME TO DISAPPEARANCE

Also known as *time to offset*. Even if a dechallenge seems positive, it can occur too rapidly or too slowly to be plausible.

Too short: When the ADR is of type A and the half-life of the product is very long (e.g., amiodarone), the disappearance of the event within hours after the last dose does not support a drug related causality.

Too long: When the ADR is of type A and the half-life is very short, the disappearance of the ADR many weeks or months after the last dose also does not support a drug-related causality.

PNEUMOVIGILANCE

The area of pharmacovigilance concerned with ADRs that affect the lungs and the respiratory system. The Council for International Organizations of Medical Sciences (CIOMS) has supported a consensus conference on the definitions of pulmonary ADRs (CIOMS, *PEDS* 1997:6:115).

POISON CONTROL CENTER

A clinical service group whose goals are providing information and assisting in the diagnosis and treatment of toxicity produced by chemicals, overdoses of pharmaceutical products, and drugs of abuse. These centers are usually directed by physicians who are clinical toxicologists. They play a major role in the pharmacovigilance of new drug products since phase III trials do not study overdoses—particularly massive overdoses. The functions of these centers include the following:

- Recognizing the first cases of accidental or suicidal overdose
- Determining the blood levels of the suspect product
- Recommending or testing antidotes or treatments of overdose
- Recording in detail the course of the overdose manifestations and treatments for it
- Notifying promptly the appropriate health authorities, pharmacovigilance centers, or manufacturers of cases of overdose *with* AEs and even of overdoses *without* adverse effects
- Serving as the after-hours call center for pharmaceutical companies and health agencies to receive and respond to calls from physicians, consumers, and others about the company's products during nights and weekends

If the consequences of an overdose are medically serious, the information on the early cases should be published/reported rapidly along with the nature of the treatment or antidote (if known) so that other poison control centers and the medical community at large are fully aware of the treatments needed.

PRACTOLOL: MARKET WITHDRAWAL

This beta-blocker commercialized in the United Kingdom caused a mucoocular-cutaneous syndrome now known as the *practolol syndrome* that had the following major clinical manifestations:

- An ophthalmopathy characterized by corneal drying leading to blindness
- Retroperitoneal fibrosis producing intestinal and uretheral occlusion
- Lupus erythematosus syndrome and psoriasis

TIME TO ONSET
The relatively large number of patients who suffered from this problem was due to difficulties in associating the adverse effects with the drug because of the long period before the appearance of symptoms after the first dose (while therapy was continuing) and the long and variable periods (*latency period*) after the last dose. As a result of this problem, Professor W. H. W. Inman developed the Prescription Event Monitoring (PEM) system, also known as the *green card* system in the United Kingdom.

This syndrome was not seen in the preclinical animal toxicity trials, which were begun after the synthesis of practolol in 1964; nor during the phase III clinical trials, which started in 1966; nor during the first years after market launch in 1970. By 1972 there were 80 AEs reported. The first cases of lupus erythematosus were noted in 1972 and psoriasis, sclerosing peritonitis, and deafness in 1974. The first case of the muco-ocular-cutaneous syndrome was not suspected until June 1974.

The first call to physicians for reporting was done in 1972 with a Dear Doctor letter sent by the manufacturer. This was immediately followed by more than 200 reports of ophthalmopathies including corneal ulceration and permanent blindness. Three warning letters were sent by the manufacturer as well as two informational letters and a letter from the Committee on Safety of Medicines (CSM) in 1975 and 1976. In July the product was restricted to hospital use only, and in September it was entirely removed from the market.

A delay in appearance of 18 months was noted for the eruptions, 23 months for the ocular problems, and 34 months for the peritonitis. In retrospect, the sclerosing peritonitis proved to be the most difficult result to detect because it was seen 3 years after the last dose—a very disquieting latency period. The risk/benefit ratio was also tilted against the drug because it was used as a prophylactic treatment and multiple other antihypertensive agents were available on the market. Interestingly, this problem was not discovered in other countries where the drug was sold. An estimated 1 million patients were treated with practolol (Wright, *Br Med J* 1975;1:595; Editors and Wright, *Br Med J* 1975;2:577).

PRECHALLENGE

IN PHARMACOVIGILANCE

Previous administration of the drug in question. This information is a component of the past medical history and is an important part of the information supplied in a spontaneous report.

IN PHARMACOTHERAPY

A conscientious physician who prescribes a product must inquire as to whether there were prechallenges (previous administrations) and whether any adverse effects were associated with them. This should be noted in the patient's chart and on the AE report. The following is an example of prechallenges as risk factors for halothane hepatitis:

> Fatal hepatitis has been reported with this anesthetic gas. Between 1985 and 1995 fifteen reports of hepatotoxicity requiring liver transplant were reported in the United Kingdom. This product illustrates how the examination of *case series* of spontaneous reports in national databases revealed specific risk factors. This knowledge can thus prevent additional cases. See the website (http://www.usyd.edu.au/anaes/lectures/hepatotox_clt/hepatotox.html).

- *Prechallenge*: a previous exposure to this anesthetic increases the risk of hepatotoxicity.
- *Recent prechallenge*: a recent exposure to this anesthetic also increases the risk of hepatotoxicity. Of the 15 British patients, 4 had received halothane within the preceding 30 days. Some experts recommend that at least 3 months pass between exposures if halothane is to be used again.
- *Positive prechallenge*: a febrile reaction or jaundice after a previous halothane exposure is an absolute contraindication to its reuse (Ray, *Br J Anaesthesia* 1991;67:84; CSM/MCA, *Curr Probl Phamacovigil* 1997;23:7).

NEGATIVE PRECHALLENGE

The absence of the AE/ADR during a previous administration of the suspect product. On a spontaneous report form this information should be included in the past drug history. Several points must be kept in mind:

A negative prechallenge is not always an absolute argument against a drug cause of for the AE/ADR. If the mechanism of the event is immunologic, the (negative) prechallenge may have played a sensitizing role and is thus an argument in *favor* of drug cause and not an argument against it.

A negative prechallenge done with a low dose of the drug does not exclude the drug as the cause of the AE/ADR if the mechanism is dose dependent, type A.

A negative prechallenge when the drug was given by mouth does not exclude the possibility of an ADR when the drug is given by another route (e.g., intravenous).

A negative prechallenge with a product containing the same active ingredient but manufactured by a different company or by the same company but in a different formulation (e.g., tablet instead of capsule) does not exclude the possibility of an ADR. When a different brand or formulation with the same active ingredient is administered, an ADR may be caused by an excipient in the new product.

POSITIVE PRECHALLENGE

The occurrence of an AE/ADR during a previous administration of the suspect product. On a spontaneous report form this information would be included in the past drug history. A positive prechallenge may be *specific* (same drug, same ADR) or *nonspecific* (similar drug, similar reaction). In case causality assessment a positive prechallenge is a risk factor for that specific patient and supports a drug cause of the AE. For the pharmacotherapist, a positive prechallenge to halothane (fever, jaundice) is an absolute contraindication to its reuse.

SENSITIZING PRECHALLENGE

This term can be applied to a negative prechallenge if it is believed that the mechanism of the ADR that occurs on the next exposure is immunologic. This phenomenon is seen in particular in vaccinovigilance: Cases of arthritis have appeared after the second or third vaccination of hepatitis B vaccine as reported by Pope (*J Rheumatol* 1998;25:1687). Prechallenges with halothane are also in this category.

PRECLINICAL PHARMACOVIGILANCE

This expression, which is the equivalent of *preclinical safety assessment of new drugs,* is sometimes used instead of the expression *pre-clinical toxicology* which really refers only to classic animal toxicology studies (e.g., acute, subacute, chronic, survival, liver, kidney) but has been extended to include teratogenicity, oncogenicity, and mutagenicity trials. Overlaps in terminology are likely to continue.

PREFERRED TERM

In a coding dictionary such as *MedDRA* or *WHO-ART,* medical words describing an AE/ADR. These terms are more inclusive than lower level or verbatim terms but less inclusive than higher-level terms. For example, *blood clot in the leg* may be a verbatim term, *thrombophlebitis* may be the preferred term, and *venous disease* may be the higher-level term. Preferred terms are the usual level of reporting of AEs/ADRs to health authorities on MedWatch or CIOMS 1 forms and in line listings. However, the EU has indicated it desires lower-level terms in *MedDRA* to be used for reporting, not preferred terms.

PRESCRIPTION EVENT MONITORING (PEM)

This is a type of phase IV cohort scheme with a dedicated drug safety database, where each patient serves as his or her own control during and after receiving the suspect product. This system was created by Professor W. H. W. Inman in 1980 in the Drug Safety Research Unit (DRSU) at the University of Southampton in the United Kingdom, after the yellow card system did not produce early detection of the practolol syndrome. It is financed by the pharmaceutical industry in the form of unconditional grants administered by a trust and registered as an independent, nonprofit foundation. Data are taken from the medical charts of general practitioners who voluntarily write them down on a green reporting card. Each drug (usually newly commercialized products) that the DSRU independently chooses to study has a cohort, on the average, of over 10,000 patients. The data collected are *medical events*, not ADRs, abstracted from the patient's record by the practitioner.

The functioning of the system is as follows: As soon as a patient has a prescription filled at the pharmacy, the surveillance center is notified of it by the Prescription Pricing Authority, which receives the pharmacists' billings, permitting the identification of the prescribing physician and the patient. Six months later the surveillance center sends a letter to the prescribing physician asking him or her to voluntarily complete a "green card" listing *medical events* noted in the patient's chart that have occurred in the previous six months whether they are thought to be related to the drug or not. This is done to capture the *events* that occur in the course of a medical practice and not in the context of the prospective study of ADR*s* in a cohort of exposed patients.

As the majority of patients do not take the medication for the full 6 month period, the period of observation after the cessation of the medication serves as the control period. In addition, the frequency of events occurring during the first month of treatment is compared with the frequency during the subsequent months, independently of whether the treatment is continued or not. These data also allow comparisons within patients (i.e., the patient is his or her own control). They pertain to the entire country, including subsets of patients such as children, women, elderly adults, and pregnant women.

PEM is useful for the estimation of incidence of ADRs; reassurance of users, prescribers, and health authorities; comparison of drug products within a class; and sometimes generation of a signal. The quantification of adverse effects in the real world, especially in subgroups at risk, represents important information for prescribers, and there is unfortunately no equivalent of this system outside the United Kingdom and New Zealand. As Nelson (*PEDS* 2000;9:253) suggests, this aspect of drug safety in most countries is "second rate [. . .] and we still do not know the incidence of known adverse reactions in the different clinical practice situations."

One of the limitations arises from the number of physicians who responded in the 65 studies reported in the 1990s (discussed later): it remained fairly level at 57.6% (range 39.6% to 74.1%). The number responding does not seem to increase because there may be a sort of competition with the usual spontaneous notification system ("yellow card") and with "promotional studies" done by pharmaceutical companies.

The PEM system understandably does not seem to have as much sensitivity as spontaneous reporting in the generation of signals of rare AEs.

> *Cisapride and tachycardia*: In 1992 the SIGNAL Program of the Uppsala Monitoring Centre detected this signal and published it the same year (Olsson, *Br Med J* 1992;305:748). At the same time the suspect product was followed by the Prescription Event Monitoring (PEM), but this method was not able to detect this association (Inman, *Br Med J* 1992;305:1019). Later, however, the signal was confirmed in two clinical studies (Usha, *Indian J Pharmacol* 1994;26:233; Ahmad, *Lancet* 1995;345:508).

Unlike the yellow card system or its equivalent which is used in all countries collaborating with the Uppsala Monitoring Centre, a similar Intensive Medicines Monitoring Programme has only been used in New Zealand where the follow-up period is 4–5 years and the average number of cohorts is 10,228 patients (Coulter, *Br Med J* 1996;313:756). A series of PEM studies appeared in 1993 and others followed in 1998 (Inman, *PEDS* 1993;2:239 and 259; Mackay, *Drug Saf* 1998;19:343). (Read also Stephens, 1999:438.)

PRESCRIRE INTERNATIONAL

An English-language version of selected articles from the independent and respected pharmacotherapy journal *La Revue Prescrire*. It is published six times a year with articles relating only to France removed. Each article is reviewed by at least 25 professionals before publication. This publication gives frank reviews of drugs and of their usefulness, if any, as additions to the therapeutic spectrum. The editorial point of view is above all the protection of the patient and often expresses concern over the ADRs associated with overprescribed new drugs, when their safety profile and risk/benefit ratio are still incompletely known and evaluated.

Selected articles also appear regularly in the *Canadian Journal of Family Medicine*, followed sometimes by lively manufacturer's replies and counterreplies in the form of letters. It is worth reading for a point of view "from the other side of the fence" (Prescrire International POB 459, F-75527 Paris Cedex 11, France; www.hutch.demon.co.uk/prescrire/prescrir.htm).

PREVENTABILITY; AVOIDABILITY

IN PHARMACOVIGILANCE
At the *population* level, an ADR is preventable if the enactment of certain specific measures can prevent or limit the reaction.

IN PHARMACOTHERAPY
At the *individual* level, an ADR is preventable if its occurrence is due to incorrect use or misuse of the product. It should be noted that all ADRs that occur as the result of useless or imprudent prescribing are preventable.

PRIVACY

In 1995 the European Union (EU) issued, "Directive 95/46/EC of the European Parliament and of the Council of 24 October 1995 on the protection of individuals with regard to the processing of personal data and on the free movement of such data" http://europa.eu.int/eur-lex/en/lif/dat/1995/en_395L0046.html. "The Directive establishes new standards for privacy protection and EU member states were to enact conforming legislation within three years of its passage. It also requires firms which engage in the collection of personal data to disclose the actual collection, the purpose of the collection and to identify the intended recipient of the information. The transfer of personal data to a country deemed to have inadequate protection is prohibited" (Carol Morrissey, www.llrx.com/congress/101598.htm). The EU member states were required to enact the directive or its equivalent by 1998. Most member states have done so, though not all as of early 2001. The directive covered all aspects of data (e.g., banking, employment, trade unionism), not only that relating to health care.

In the field of pharmacovigilance, potential effects may be great. It may become necessary that pharmaceutical companies anonymize their data, make them available for review and correction by the patient whose adverse effect is reported, and obtain consent to send the data elsewhere. Data cannot be transferred to countries that do not have equivalent and adequate data protection and privacy laws. This clearly has major implications for nearly all transactions between the EU and other countries (notably the United States). Negotiations between the EU and the U.S. government at ministerial level have produced a "safe harbor agreement" of actions that, if undertaken by U.S. firms, will be considered acceptable by the EU in regard to data privacy and protection (http://www.ita.doc.gov/media/safeharbor731.htm; http://www.ita.doc.gov/td/ecom/menu.html). On December 28, 2000 the U.S. government published a voluminous (nearly 400 pages) proposal on U.S. privacy (65FR 82462) (see www.hhs.gov/ocr/hipaa.html). The implications for drug surveillance and epidemiology could be significant; see the International Society of Pharmacoepidemiology (ISPE) policy statements on data protection (http://www.pharmacoepi.org/publicpol.htm). This is a rapidly changing field, and all those in pharmacovigilance should follow developments closely.

PROBLEM DRUGS

A work published under the direction of Andrew Chetley by Health Action International (HAI), a Netherlands-based association of consumers. This publication consists of several dozen sections covering subjects of concern to both the developed and the underdeveloped world: women, children, elderly, antidiarrheal agents (antibiotics, clioquinol, diphenoxylate, loperamide), antibiotics, analgesics, stimulants and supplements (tonics, vitamins, anabolic agents), pregnancy (diethylstilbestrol), contraceptives, hormone substitution therapy, and psychotropics (Chetley A. *Problem drugs.* Amsterdam: Health Action International, 1996. Their address is: Health Action International-Europe, Jacob van Lennegkade 334T, 1053 NJ Amsterdam, Netherlands).

PRODUCT PROBLEM

This refers to any defect in a lot or batch or formulation. It includes problems in packaging, manufacture, labeling, storage, purity, sterility, contamination, stability, turbidity, and dilution. When labeling is unclear, hard to read, incomplete or misleading, usually the pharmacist is first to know; however, anyone in the chain from the manufacturer of the product to the consumer of the product may discover a product problem. The consequences may include type A or B AEs as well as lack of efficacy. Adverse events that result from material problems are called *extrinsic adverse effects* (see EXTRINSIC EFFECT). In many countries, product problems must be reported to the health authorities and can have regulatory consequences, including recall of the lot, batch, or product in question. The following is an example from the Third World:

> *Contaminated injections*: The parenteral route is more popular in the Third World than in the developed countries for many treatments. In addition to the placebo effect of injections, the past successes of injections of penicillin for yaws and quinine for malaria have remained in the historical medical memory. However, the lack of adequate sterilization and the reuse of disposable needles and syringes increase the risk of transmission of such diseases as human immunodeficiency virus (HIV), hepatitis B, malaria, and dengue fever both to patients and to those treating them (UNICEF, *The Prescriber* 1998;15:1).

PSYLLIUM

A product derived from the plantain, used as a fiber laxative. Its potential ADRs are quite unusual. Hypersensitivity (a type B reaction) can occur in the patient or person preparing the product (nurse, pharmacist), producing asthma (sometimes serious or even fatal) through inhalation of psyllium dust. A pharmacobezoar can occur in the digestive tract (often at the base of the esophagus), producing obstruction, if insufficient fluid is taken and/or if there are gastrointestinal problems (e.g., strictures).

PUBLIC CITIZENS' HEALTH RESEARCH GROUP

Dr. Sidney Wolfe and Mr. Ralph Nader in 1971 founded this group with the goal of protecting U.S. consumers. They publish a book, *Worst Pills Best Pills*, and a bulletin by the same name for the general American public. The group is a member of the International Society of Drug Bulletins and sometimes petitions the U.S. Food and Drug Administration to take certain regulatory measures to restrict the use of or to withdraw a particular drug from the market (Public Citizen, 1600 20th Street NW, Washington, DC 20009; (www.citizen.org/hrg/).

QUALITY CONTROL

In pharmacovigilance, the validation of AE/ADR reports. It includes validation of the facts and plausibility of the case information in addition to validation of the (manual and computer) processing of the data.

RANDOMIZATION: RANDOM ALLOCATION

This term is used in clinical pharmacology and research to designate a procedure done in clinical trials to minimize bias. It aims at evenly distributing known—and most particularly unknown—prognostic factors among the group(s) receiving the treatment drug and the group(s) receiving the control treatment(s). These prognostic factors concern both the pharmacologic and therapeutic effects (benefit) to the experimental drug and the ADRs (unwanted effects); in fact, the latter prognostic factors correspond to the *risk factors* for ADRs from the experimental drug. Randomization is the most powerful tool available for evenly distributing ADR risk factors among the treated and control groups.

A list of random numbers is generated, usually by computer, and used to assign patients to the treatment groups. Usually such trials are double-blinded (i.e., the treatment is not known to the patient, the investigator, and the company's clinical monitors). The codes are usually kept only by the statisticians who create them. Blinded codes are not broken until the end of the trial and may be opened during the trial only in the case of an AE that requires urgent medical attention. Many health authorities (notably the United States and European Union) now require that the blind be broken before a serious, possibly related unlabeled event is sent in an expedited report.

RATE

IN EPIDEMIOLOGY

The ratio in which the numerator is the number of patients with a particular characteristic, the *cases*, and the denominator is the total number of patients capable of having this characteristic. It is given in the form of a decimal between 0.0 and 1.0 or as a percentage between 0% and 100%. In a 2 x 2 table of type *abcd* the rate is the number of cases divided by the total for that row or column; thus, $a/[a + b]$ and $a/[a + c]$ are rates.

IN PHARMACOVIGILANCE

The numerator is the number of patients with an ADR and the denominator is the number of patients exposed to the product and thus capable of having the ADR. When an individual is referred to, rather than a population, the term *risk* is used (see INCIDENCE RATE).

In *case causality assessment,* two rates are of interest and are part of the *general* evidence, allowing the determination of *general prior odds*:

- The rate in those exposed to the drug
- The rate in the population not exposed to the drug: the *baseline rate* (also called *baseline risk* when referring to a given patient)

The *attributable risk* is the equivalent of the rate in the exposed group minus the baseline rate, whereas the *relative risk* is the rate in the exposed group divided by the baseline rate.

REACTIONS WEEKLY

An international pharmacovigilance bulletin, subtitled *Rapid Alerts to Adverse Drug Experience*. This weekly publication (50 issues per year) by Adis (www.adis.com) in New Zealand includes recently published signals, pharmacovigilance studies of serious and unexpected ADRs as well as regulatory measures taken around the world and selected articles published in the literature. In addition, two- or three-page summaries of drug-related conferences and meetings are published.

This tool for staying up to date is indispensable for those with day to day responsibilities in the field. *Reactions Weekly* is available in print and electronically. It is available on CD-ROM, on line in DIALOG (www.dialog.com) and DATASTAR, via Lotus Notes and Intranet (Adis International Inc., Suite F-10, 940 Town Center Drive, Langhorne, PA 19047 U.S.A.; Adis International Ltd., Chowley Oak Lane, Tattenhall, Chester CH3 9GA, U.K.).

REBOUND EFFECT

The manifestation of an undesirable effect that is qualitatively identical to the original problem, sign, or symptom but may be more severe and appears after the cessation of a medication. It is the return, in full force, of the original condition being treated. It is also called a *rebound phenomenon*. The time to onset is calculated from the last dose to the first symptom. It is to be distinguished from a *withdrawal effect* in which the event occurring after stopping the drug is qualitatively different from the condition being treated; this latter effect is due to the sudden stopping of a drug that produces a physiologic dependence at the receptor level.

When a rebound is predictable, the prescriber must inform the patient of three salient points:

- The way in which a rebound effect can be *prevented* (i.e., by the gradual withdrawal of the drug rather than an abrupt cessation, e.g., a beta blocker in a patient with angina and hypertension).
- The way to *recognize* the symptoms of the rebound effect, for example:

    Thiazides: ankle edema: The physician may judge that a thiazide is not indicated for ankle edema when the edema is neither cardiac, renal, nor hepatic, as may occur in elderly adults confined to a chair all day long. If the thiazide is discontinued, the physician should alert the patient that temporary rebound ankle edema may occur (in 23% of cases) around the third week after stopping the treatment (Dejonge, *Br Med J* 1994;308:511).

- The way to *treat* the symptoms: restarting the medication at a lower dosage, substituting another drug, or using a nonpharmacologic approach.

RECALL, PRODUCT

This is a rarely required regulatory measure enacted to prevent ADRs. It may be done on a voluntary basis by the manufacturer or it may be required by the health authority. It may occur for two basic reasons: a reduced risk/benefit ratio, or a product problem. It is part of a market withdrawal.

REDUCED RISK/BENEFIT RATIO
Suppose that new data have emerged that have changed the risk/benefit ratio for the drug. This change might occur for many reasons but is most frequently

seen after a pharmacovigilance investigation and after a newer and better or safer drug has arrived on the market. Such a recall is usually definitive (i.e., it is unlikely that the product will be reintroduced to the market).

PRODUCT PROBLEM

A different situation occurs when there is a *product problem* in manufacturing, production (concerning the active ingredient or excipients), labeling, or packaging or when there is biologic or chemical contamination of a single lot or all of the product manufactured. It is usually related to a specific problem and, after remedy, the product can return to the market. If only selected lots are involved, only these lots are recalled.

Withdrawal from the market is surely one of the most severe actions a company or health authority can take. In extreme cases, the recall may be an emergency and one or more media can be used: television, Internet, radio, and letters to doctors, pharmacists, and patients. Pharmacists and physicians may need to contact their patients if the recall extends to the patient level. Large recalls are exceedingly difficult, expensive, and painful to all concerned. Once a drug has left the wholesaler, it may already have been distributed to thousands of pharmacies in many countries.

The first U.S. recall occurred in 1937 when an elixir of sufanilamide containing the excipient diethylene glycol was associated with the deaths of several children and adults. The first recall done after the Federal Food Drug and Cosmetic Act became law was that of sulfathiazole in 1941, when it was contaminated with phenobarbital (Rumore, *Drug Inf J* 1998;32:65). When the risk is of the highest order, the Food and Drug Administration terms it a *class I recall*. Between 1982 and 1996 a total of 64 class I recalls occurred. The major reasons were as follows:

Inadequate sterility accounted for 41% of recalls. A prominent example involved contamination with the *pseudomonas* organisms.

Packaging or labeling errors, of which 86% were associated with generic products, accounted for 35% of recalls. Examples include an anticoagulant labeled as an antidepressant, a diuretic labeled as a calcium blocker, and an antipsychotic labeled as a cold medication.

Strength or potency problems entailed incorrect amounts of active drug substance in the product which generated 10% of the recalls. Examples include an oral contraceptive in which the row of tablets to be taken during the first week of the menstrual cycle contained placebo rather active drug and an inhalation aerosol that did not distribute the particles adequately.

Toxic or unlabeled active ingredients or excipients accounted for 9% of the recalls. One example was a multivitamin that contained too much vitamin D.

ADRs: This accounted for 6% of the recalls. These reactions were unpredictable; an example was an injectable preparation that produced mycobacterial injection site infections.

Cyanide in acetaminophen: In a very well known case in the United States, after criminal tampering (producing fatalities) with a well-known brand of acetaminophen, all the bottles of this brand were rapidly withdrawn from the U.S. market.

Fragments of glass: A 5-ml bottle of diphenhydramine suspension contained glass fragments produced by a problem during manufacturing. This problem was revealed when the bottle was shaken. Because of the potential intestinal problems that the glass could produce, all the bottles were rapidly recalled and no ADRs were noted.

Metal cable. The FDA reported the story of a metal cable attached to a crank on a motorized hospital bed that had become frayed and posed the risk of a short circuit. As soon as this was signaled by a nurse, the manufacturer recalled 33,155 cranks. Although this episode relates to a medical device, it serves to show that even the *potential* for an adverse occurrence can precipitate major actions in the interest of the public health (FDA. *Desk Guide* 1996).

RECHALLENGE

Readministration of the suspected product at a dose and via a mode of administration capable of reproducing the AE/ADR. This is a critical criterion used in the determination of causality.

NEGATIVE RECHALLENGE

In causality determinations, a failure of the AE/ADR in question to reappear in the same or nearly the same manner after reexposure to the suspect product. The rechallenge must be performed by using a mode of administration and dose of the drug capable of producing the undesirable event in question and without prophylactic treatment aimed at preventing the recurrence. If the ADR is an allergic reaction, a negative rechallenge with the product might occur, however, if the challenge acted as a desensitizer.

POSITIVE RECHALLENGE

The reappearance of the AE/ADR (medically confirmed) in question in the same or nearly the same manner after reexposure to the suspect product. For a type A (pharmacologic) reaction the readministration should be comparable in terms of dose and mode of administration, whereas for an allergic reaction a trace may suffice if the patient is sensitized.

In an allergic reaction, the positive rechallenge may produce a more severe reaction with a shorter time to appearance than during the original challenge. These characteristics aid in diagnosing and discerning the mechanism of the ADR. Nonallergic type A reactions do not reappear more quickly or more severely after a rechallenge at the same dosage.

Note that cutaneous allergy tests ("skin tests") are generally not considered true rechallenges but rather as laboratory examinations of the immune status of the patient. In this view, a positive skin test result would be looked upon as a risk factor. Allergists often designate these tests *challenge tests.*

A positive rechallenge is one of the strongest diagnostic criteria in favor of a drug causality of the AE. That is, an AE with positive and medically valid rechallenge is almost certainly an ADR.

RECORD LINKAGE; LINKED DATABASE

A type of pharmacoepidemiologic investigation or study done in a secondary database of medical and pharmaceutical information composed of health insurance claims or patient records computerized from doctors' offices. These databases contain (broadly speaking) the following:

■ A file of AEs (diagnoses)
■ A file of drugs prescribed or filled at pharmacies or in hospitals

■ A file of patient identification data allowing the linkage of the drug and the event

This linkage permits a case-control, nested case-control, or cohort study. It is used primarily for the evaluation of the rationale, the consequences, and the utility of prescribing a particular medication (Drug Utilization Review), but it can also be used for quantifying the frequency of an ADR or detecting or evaluating a signal. The databases used are primarily those of private insurers such as health maintenance organizations (HMOs) in the United States and public insurers such as the Canadian provincial insurers. Dedicated databases are also used, such as those that contain patient office records provided by participating physicians; a good example is the General Practice Research Database (GPRD) (http://www.bu.edu/bcdsp/gprd.htm), formerly known as Value Added Medicinal Products (VAMP) in Great Britain.

Physicians' charts, hospital charts and morbidity and mortality statistics can serve as the source for the adverse effects (the numerator). The pharmaceutical records; the sales figures, both wholesale and in sentinel pharmacies; and the number of prescriptions written, filled, or billed can provide usage data (the denominator).

RECOVERY; RECOVERED

This term describes one of the possible outcomes in a spontaneous adverse effect report. It refers to a cure or a return to the patient's baseline or original condition before the event occurred. Recovery can occur with or without sequelae.

REGIONAL PHARMACOVIGILANCE CENTER

A pharmacovigilance center that serves a particular region within a country. It does not exist, for example, in the United States where pharmacovigilance is centered at the Food and Drug Administration in Rockville, Maryland, outside Washington, DC, or in the United Kingdom where it is centered in London at the Medicines Control Agency (MCA)/Committee for Safety of Medicines (CSM).

A regional center can request AE/ADR safety reports from practitioners in addition to collecting and validating the reports it receives. It can circulate safety information *internally* to other regional centers in its network and to the national center or *externally* to clinicians and consumers. It fulfills a double function: facilitating the collection of spontaneous reports and serving as a source of much needed continuing medical education in pharmacotherapy. This formula is being tried in a few other countries (Spain, Canada, Sweden, Poland, and elsewhere) and appears to offer the promise of improving both pharmacovigilance and pharmacotherapy by providing an efficient and user-friendly, local "one-stop shopping" facility.

FRANCE

The concept of regional pharmacovigilance centers was born and developed in France, where 31 regional centers fill the triple role of pharmacovigilance monitors, drug information centers, and therapeutic advice consultants. Each center is associated with a faculty of medicine department of pharmacology, or clinical pharmacology. Occasionally they are associated with a poison control center. Some centers publish periodic bulletins and/or have a website (www.chu-rouen.fr/pharmaco/crpv.html).

The five regional centers are financed by the federal government, managed by pharmacists, and associated with drug information centers.

REGISTRY

In epidemiology, a continuing collection of cases in a geographically defined population. Ideally, the registry should contain *all* the cases with exhaustive detail. Registries been maintained for many decades on congenital malformations, twin births, infant deaths, human immunodeficiency virus (HIV), cancer, and other topics.

In drug safety, registries are used for the evaluation of rare AEs/ADRs in order to evaluate their frequency in the population (secular tendency) as a function of drug use in the population (by volume of sales, number of patients exposed, and other factors). If the registry is able to provide good data on drug use in patients with the AE/ADR as well as in those who did not experience the AE/ADR, this information may be used for a case-control study to evaluate the relative risk. In 1955 the American Medical Association began an iatrogenic blood dyscrasia registry. More recently the Food and Drug Administration has published guidelines on pregnancy registries (www.fda.gov/cber/gdlns/pregnancy.pdf).

INCREASE IN FREQUENCY
If a registry shows that after the launch of a new product, the AE in question increases in frequency, this information can support a drug cause of the AE (i.e., it is an ADR). As an example, it was through a registry in Great Britain that the incidence of thrombophlebitis was noted to increase in women after the launch of birth control pills.

DECREASE IN FREQUENCY
Similar reasoning suggests that if a registry shows a decrease in frequency of an AE after the withdrawal of a product from use (market withdrawal), the case for a drug cause of the AE is strengthened. This phenomenon would constitute a *collective positive dechallenge*. Three examples:

- *Clioquinol*: The frequency of subacute myelooptic neuropathy (SMON) decreased to baseline after the withdrawal of clioquinol from the Japanese market.
- *Low dose estrogen*: The incidence of thromboembolic phenomena decreased after the introduction of low-dose estrogen in Great Britain.
- *Thalidomide*: Phocomelia dropped to its minimal frequency after thalidomide was withdrawn from the market.

REGULATIONS

Regulations are rules that an administrative body promulgates on the basis of a law passed by the government (e.g., a congress, parliament, or national assembly). In the United States, the Congress may pass a drug law, which the president signs, giving the Food and Drug Administration power to make regulations without further consent of Congress or the president. In pharmacovigilance the term is used a bit more loosely and thus in the context of drug safety, *regulations* constitute the body of requirements (laws, rules, and guidance) that govern pharmacovigilance and the conduct of pharmaceutical companies, health care professionals, hospitals, consumers, and others. The goals of these regulations are the protection of public health and the "safe" and "efficacious" use of pharmaceutical products. These requirements may and often do differ from country to country. In addition, within a particular jurisdiction, it is possible to be subject to more than one set of regulations. For example, in the European Union, member states are subject both to pan-European regulations and national regulations.

In many countries, drug laws and regulations are extensive; in others they are rudimentary.

REGULATORY AFFAIRS

IN THE PHARMACEUTICAL INDUSTRY

The unit within a company responsible for the application of the laws and regulations governing the research, development, and registration for marketing of drugs, biologics, and devices in order to ensure safe and efficacious use of these products. It is usually separate from the Legal Department.

IN THE GOVERNMENTAL REGULATORY AUTHORITY

The governmental structure responsible for the application of the laws and regulations governing pharmaceutical products with the goal of protection of the public health and safe and efficacious use of these products.

REGULATORY COMPLIANCE ("COMPLIANCE")

This term can apply to the conduct and behavior of *a pharmaceutical company* in following the laws and regulations that govern its actions. It is always the goal of the company and the governmental agency to assure 100% compliance with all regulations and laws.

This term can also be used to refer to a specific *document* or *procedure* to indicate that it is in conformity with the applicable laws and regulations (e.g., "Our AE reporting procedures are in full compliance with the law").

REGULATORY REPORTING REQUIREMENTS

Although the reporting requirements are promulgated locally in each country, they are tending to become more uniform as a result of the efforts of the Council for International Organizations of Medical Sciences (CIOMS) and the International Conference on Harmonization (ICH). See "Notes on Implementation in the Three ICH Regions" at the ICH website (www.ifpma.org/ich5e.html).

Regulatory reporting requirements vary as a function of certain criteria:

- Validity (usually four criteria: a patient, a drug, an adverse effect, and a reporter)
- Source (consumer vs. health care professional)
- Expectedness (whether previous reports of this AE have been made: labeled vs. unlabeled)
- Seriousness (death/incapacity/hospitalization/others)
- Causality (possibly related/unrelated)
- Geography (domestic/foreign)

An AE that corresponds to the reporting criteria for an *expedited report* (*alert report, 15 day report*) must be submitted, in most countries, within 15 calendar days to the health authority by the manufacturer. Direct submission by clinicians to the health authority is voluntary, and hence there is no time limit. The manufacturer, on the contrary, must report AEs to the health authority and must use a specific form. The CIOMS 1 form is accepted in many countries though some have a different form (sometimes in the local language) for domestic reports. Foreign reports are usually accepted on CIOMS I forms. In the United States, domestic reports must be on MedWatch (3500A) forms (www.fda.gov/medwatch/index.html) whereas non-U.S. cases may be submitted on MedWatch or CIOMS 1 forms. Most countries now accept some or all reports in English.

Reports that are not expedited reports (most of the expected serious reports and all of the nonserious reports) are usually submitted to health authorities in batches or listings (CIOMS line listings) at specified intervals in a Periodic Safety Update Report (PSUR), using the standards originally described by the CIOMS II Working Group and modified slightly by ICH. In the United States, at this time, the Food and Drug Administration is still requiring submission of NDA Periodic Reports, whose format and content are quite different from those of PSURs. The FDA is committed to using E2B and PSURs and is expected to move to this standard (with some modifications).

If a manufacturer does not conform to the national regulatory requirements concerning the reporting of expedited AEs/ADRs or periodic reports, the manufacturer is said to be (in pharmacovigilance jargon) *out of compliance* and has committed a reporting requirement *irregularity*. Such a situation is a very serious matter and is looked on with severe disapproval by the authorities. In the United States periodic, unannounced audits by the FDA are done to verify that the appropriate reporting is being done. The FDA has also audited non-U.S. companies located outside the U.S. doing business in the United States. U.S. law provides for fines up to $250,000 for individuals and $500,000 for corporations as well as a maximum of 3 years of imprisonment for those who have acted with the intention of committing fraud (FD&C Act section 303).

The European Medicinal Evaluation Agency (EMEA) has established an auditing section and other national health authorities either have started pharmacovigilance audits or are planning such audits.

Many, if not most, countries now require that expedited reporting include foreign reports in addition to domestic reports. For practical purposes, this means that any serious AE from any country in the manufacturer's (plus its licensees' and distributors') worldwide sales territories may be an expedited report in one or more of its sales territories. Thus, in practice, the manufacturer must set up a system to capture and process all AEs on its marketed products, particularly if it is selling in a country or region that has strict reporting regulations (i.e., the United States, Canada, Europe, Australia, and Japan).

RELATIVE RISK; RISK RATIO

The incidence rate of an event in the exposed population divided by the incidence rate of the event in the unexposed population. This term refers to the increase (or decrease) in risk of a particular AE in those exposed to a drug product compared to those not exposed. If subjects exposed to nonsteroidal anti-inflammatory drugs (NSAIDs) run a four times higher risk of gastrointestinal hemorrhage compared to people not taking NSAIDs, the relative risk is 4:1.

REPORTABILITY (OF AN ADVERSE EFFECT OR SUSPECTED ADVERSE DRUG REACTION)

This refers to the obligation, whether ethical or regulatory, to report the observation to the competent authorities.

FOR THE CLINICIAN IN HIS DAILY PRACTICE

Unless the reporter is a researcher (clinical investigator) in a clinical trial in which reporting is obligatory, the reporting of an AE or suspected ADR is voluntary, and the determination of whether to report or not is the clinician's. A health care professional is a privileged witness: it is his or her sense of duty that provides the impetus to the observer of an AE/ADR, representing a potentially important signal, to report it to the manufacturer or health agency. There are few countries that make such notification a legal obligation, and in those countries the law does not seem to be applied with any force or regularity. In France, reporting rates did not significantly increase after the passage of such a law in 1984.

FOR THE MANUFACTURER

In most countries in North America and Europe as well as Japan, Australia, New Zealand, and elsewhere, AE/ADR reporting is mandatory and well established in law and regulation. Severe penalties are applied for persistent failure to report.

MEDICAL DEVICE SURVEILLANCE AND PRODUCT PROBLEMS

Notification is usually mandatory for the manufacturer, the distributor, an institution, a clinician, or a paramedical person when a medical device is defective and presents the risk of a serious or fatal event for the patient, technician, or any other person.

REPORTABILITY CRITERIA FOR HEALTH PROFESSIONALS

To help professionals reply to the question, What do I report? some health authorities publish bulletins and directives concerning reportability. Briefly summarized here are the reporting criteria in a few countries.

AUSTRALIA

The directives presented in the *Australian ADRs Bulletin* are listed in the following. They concern the products and the seriousness of the events and now include pharmacoeconomic aspects.

▶ **Products**

Top priority on the list of products goes to "*Drugs of Current Interest,*" new medications, and those with possible drug interactions. Also reportable are AEs/ADRs associated with herbal and traditional products and alternative therapies because ADRs here are unacceptable as these products have no officially confirmed beneficial effects.

▶ **Serious Outcomes**

Death, life-threatening situations, required or prolonged hospitalization, incapacity to perform productive activity, and congenital malformations are considered serious outcomes.

▶ **Costs**

Increased investigational or treatment costs are included.

CANADA

Instructions from the *Canadian ADR Newsletter* are as follows.

▶ **Products**

The Therapeutic Products Programme (TPP) receives reports associated with all types of products (except vaccines, which are sent to a different unit) including prescription and over the counter (OTC) products, biologics, blood products, radiopharmaceuticals, alternative medicines, and plant medicines. It is suggested that all AEs/ADRs associated with a "new product" (i.e., less than 5 months on the market) be reported. This is difficult since the monographs of the *Compendium of Pharmaceutical and Specialties (CPS)* (see COMPENDIA), the national compendium, do not include the date of initial marketing and thus the clinician cannot readily know when this period begins and ends.

▶ Reactions

The TPP accepts all reports of ADRs associated with risk factors such as abuse, overdose, and drug interaction as well as reports of unexpected therapeutic failure (lack of efficacy).

▶ Criteria

It is recommended that all serious, expected, or unexpected ADRs as well as all unexpected ADRs that are serious and nonserious be reported. The definition of serious follows the usual criteria (death, incapacity, hospitalization, and congenital malformations).

UNITED STATES

Reporting of AEs is obligatory for manufacturers and distributors and holders of New Drug Applications (NDAs) (i.e., marketing authorizations); see the *U.S. Code of Federal Regulations* 21CFR600.80 and 21CFR 314.80 (www.access.gpo.gov/cgi-bin/cfrassemble.cgi?title=200021). See also the Food and Drug Administration's document Enforcement of the Postmarketing Adverse Drug Experience Reporting Regulations (www.fda.gov/cder/aers/chapter53.htm). This document gives FDA auditors guidelines on what to examine during a safety audit.

The reporting requirements are tighter for the development phases of a product's life span (phases I–III) than after commercialization. We discuss here only those requirements in the postmarketing (NDA) context of AE reporting.

▶ Criteria

All AEs that are serious and unlabeled (unexpected) must be reported to the FDA or the manufacturer/distributor as expedited reports. The usual definition of serious applies as well as the International Conference on Harmonization/the Council for International Organizations of Medical Sciences (CIOMS)/(ICH) concept of *medically important* or *medically significant* referring to those AEs that are considered by the reporter worthy of reporting but that do not fall into the classic criteria for seriousness. This gives discretion to the reporter (and the manufacturer) to use their clinical judgment in reporting "arguable" cases. FDA, as do many other health authorities, prefers that reporters "err on the conservative" side and report cases when in doubt.

There is no requirement that the AE necessarily be associated with the drug in question. That is, unlike the requirements for clinical trial AE reporting, in which a suspicion of a possible causal relation to the drug must exist, the requirements for spontaneous, postmarketing reporting do not require this link. In the jargon of the trade, all spontaneous AEs are suspect ADRs.

FDA has made clear (June 1997) that "elicited AEs" for marketed drugs must meet the clinical trial criteria to be reported. That is, AEs that are received from outreach programs, follow-up surveys, patient satisfaction surveys, and others, when the reports are not spontaneously received by the manufacturer, must be serious, unlabeled, and possibly associated with the drug in order to meet the criteria for expedited reporting. See *Guidance for Industry* by FDA (www.fda.gov/cber/gdlns/advexp.pdf).

REPORTING AND EVALUATION

This is one of the major functions of pharmacovigilance units that collect and evaluate spontaneous adverse effect reports. For example, the Food and Drug Administration collects and evaluates MedWatch forms received directly from health care professionals and consumers and indirectly from pharmaceutical companies.

Many elements must be considered in the course of the validation and evaluation of an AE report or a series of reports. A report that would be submitted and acted upon prematurely instead of being validated and analyzed appropriately would be a misuse of pharmacovigilance. It represents, at best, a loss of time for all concerned and, at worst, incorrect changes to a drug's labeling and use or perhaps even withdrawal of the drug from the market—all to the detriment of patients.

Validation (quality control) must examine and verify the medical facts themselves and the completeness and plausibility of the event. The evaluation must include the medical history of the patient, the "track record, background knowledge" of the suspect drug(s), the causality (whether the drug is likely to have produced the event), the value of the signal (whether the event is worth spending significant time analyzing), the outcome of the event, its acceptability compared to benefits from the drug, and its reportability. Ideally, every organization or publication that receives such case reports must try to evaluate these characteristics; this includes governmental agencies, corporate pharmacovigilance units, medical journals, and academic and professional organizations. However, as Nelson (*PEDS* 2000;9:253) indicates "only a few . . . have sophisticated methods [. . .] to assess their subset of important spontaneous reports properly."

REPORTING BY A CLINICIAN

This action presumes that the clinician has gone through three steps:

- *Noticed* an AE after a questionnaire or examination or noticed an abnormal result (e.g., elevated liver enzymes level) after a laboratory procedure
- Shrewdly *suspected* a drug to be a possible cause, after reviewing the patient's "pharmacy list"
- Conscientiously completed and sent a *reporting form* to a competent authority

This action is voluntary and unsolicited and is not part of any particular study or structured protocol in which the clinician may be participating. The clinician can notify a governmental agency, the manufacturer, a regional program, or a professional organization (e.g., hospital, poison control center, teratovigilance center, pharmaceutical information center) involved in pharmacovigilance.

REPORTING FORM

A form used for the collection of pertinent information on the case report of an AE/ADR. The form is to be distinguished from a causality algorithm. A form may be considered *universal* if it can be used for all reactions for all products. Examples of standardized collection forms are: CIOMS 1 form (1990), Roussel Uclaf form (Benichou 1994), and FDA's MedWatch (3500 and 3500A) forms (1996). More specific forms exist in many countries for other product categories such as vaccines, medical devices, and blood products. Others have developed forms by organ system (e.g., a renal form, a hepatic form, a dermatology form) for data collection and reporting. Special forms are used in teratovigilance and maternal surveillance centers.

REPORTING FORM: AUSTRALIA

The Australian form is a blue card that is foldable, self-sealing, preaddressed, and postage-paid. It includes the following elements.

Patient: initials or chart number, age, sex, weight, height, pertinent history, allergies, prechallenges, concomitant medications (the relevance of always recording height is not apparent)

Suspect products: brand name, daily dose, route of administration, start date, end date, indication (a table permits the entry of a maximum of six suspect or concomitant products; the duration of treatment can be calculated from the start and end dates)

AE: description, start date, treatment of the event, follow-up, death and date of death, sequelae (yes/no/describe), recovery (yes(date)/no/unknown), (the duration of the adverse effect may be calculated from the start date to the recovery; the form lacks questions on temporary disability and on hospitalization. The title of the form calls for the notification of congenital malformations)

Reporter: name, address, signature, date of notification

REPORTING FORM: THE COUNCIL FOR INTERNATIONAL ORGANIZATIONS OF MEDICAL SCIENCES (CIOMS)

Strongly influenced by the Food and Drug Administration reporting form, this form was proposed by the CIOMS 1 Working Group. It was originally destined for industry, to report foreign serious unexpected reactions to local authorities. Over time, it has become the key tool for the communication of serious or unexpected reactions, both domestic and foreign. It is used for expedited reports and in periodic safety reports. The language of the form is English. In the United States, it can be used only for 15-day expedited reports from outside the United States instead of the MedWatch form; our comments follow in parentheses.

▶ **Patient**

Initials: (used for patient identification only and to prevent duplicate reports)

Country: (useful in international databases)

Birth date: using the U.S. order of day/month/year; the alphabetic abbreviation of the month is requested instead of the number (i.e., JAN instead of 01 (the birth date is used to help identify the patient and help validate the age and is important in the calculation of the age of a newborn)

Age: (useful for patient identification and for causality evaluation in risk factor evaluation; e.g., some ADRs are more frequent in the aged; produces small problems if the age and birth date are both given and are markedly different and breaks the basic rule of data collection, "Never collect the same piece of information twice")

Sex: (useful for patient identification and for evaluation of risk factors; e.g., some ADRs are more frequent in women)

▶ **Concomitant medications**

Dates of administration excluding those used for the treatment of the adverse effect (the generic name of the active ingredient should be used; this list can be helpful in evaluating drug-drug interactions or other alternative causes; concomitant medications can complicate the interpretation of a dechallenge if they are stopped at the same time as the suspect product)

▶ **Other relevant history**

For example, diagnoses, allergies, pregnancy with last menstrual period noted (this information can be useful by suggesting risk factors and alternative causes)

▶ **Suspect product (or products)**

Suspect product(s): include generic name

Daily doses(s): route of administration

Indication(s): (may be useful in evaluating possible alternative, nondrug causes of the AE)

Treatment dates (start and finish)

Treatment duration

Reaction improved after stopping the product? (check appropriate answers)

   Yes: positive dechallenge

   No: negative dechallenge

   N/A: not applicable, or unknown or dechallenge not done, or outcome unknown or inconclusive

Reaction reappeared after reintroduction of the product (check appropriate boxes)

   Yes: Rechallenge was positive

   No: Rechallenge was negative

   Not applicable: (The rechallenge is unknown or was not done or the outcome is unknown or inconclusive)

▶ **Adverse Event**

Reaction onset (day, month, year) (an essential element for the calculation of time to onset of the event)

Describe in English the reaction(s) including relevant lab tests and results

▶ **Outcome**

Check off the appropriate responses

   Patient died

   Required or prolonged hospitalization

   Persistent or significant disability/incapacity

   Medically significant

▶ **Report: Manufacturer notification**

When the manufacturer is the party submitting the expedited report:

   Name and address of the manufacturer

   Manufacturer's case number, control number

Date received by manufacturer

Comment

This information is important to be sure that the manufacturer is following the appropriate time frames for the transmission of the case to the health authorities; this is an aspect of *manufacturer compliance*. This field may, however, be very difficult to fill in. For example, the initial report is a headache and is nonserious. Follow-up data received 3 weeks later reveal that the event was, in fact, a cerebral hemorrhage and thus serious. Which date should be entered? Most observers believe that the date the event was first noted to be serious should be entered here. For a literature report in a foreign language with no English language abstract, should the date the article is received be entered, or should the date the translation is received be entered?

▶ **Source of the information**

Study (clinical trial, epidemiologic study, etc.)

Literature (include the reference)

Health care professional

▶ **Type of Report: helps prevent duplicate reporting**

Initial report

Follow-up report

REPORTING RATE

In discussing reporting rates of AEs/ADRs it should be kept in mind that the number of reports actually sent to pharmacovigilance agencies and units is rather small even for serious, fatal, and unexpected cases.

DEFINITIONS

The numerator is the number of spontaneous reports (voluntary notification of cases) of suspected ADRs. The reporters of these events are practitioners (physicians, nurses, pharmacists, dentists, and other health care professionals). Physicians include those who have inpatient and outpatient (hospital-based) practices and those who are generalists or specialists. In some countries (the United States and Canada notably) consumers are also encouraged to report suspected ADRs (see RULE OF THREES).

▶ **Numerator**

The numerator is quite variable. Not all cases that occur are reported, and the level of nonreporting is not consistent. That is, some suspected ADRs and some drugs are more likely to engender reports than others; however, this is done in an inconsistent and unpredictable manner. Thus, for spontaneous reporting, the numerator is always less than the total number of cases that have occurred and there is no way to know the true degree of underreporting.

In addition to the number of suspected ADRs reported, it is also possible to calculate the *rate of reporters* in a profession. This question was studied in Great Britain. The percentage of physicians who made at least one report of a suspected ADR during a particular period was 35% for the whole of the country from 1992 to 1995. It was 55% for hospital-based physicians (Belton, *J Clin Pharmacol* 1995;39:223). In Ireland, the percentage of hospital physicians in

Dublin who reported at least *one* case was 45% (McGettigan, *Br J Clin Pharmacol* 1997;44:98). A more recent estimate of physicians who have sent in at least *one* case in their career is 60% (CSM/MCA. *Curr Probl Phamacovigil* 1997;23:6). Few countries can boast such a high rate.

▶ **Denominator**

The denominator is also quite variable. Many choices are available:

The number of *actual cases occurring in a hospitalized cohort*; the true number of cases could theoretically be obtained by examining the hospital charts of the patients

The number of *actual cases that occurred in the practice of a group of physicians* who are selected as reporters

The number of *physician prescribers* in a particular area

The number of *units of drug sold*; this can be used as the crude figure or transformed into daily doses (defined daily dose, (DDD)) (see DEFINED DAILY DOSE (DDD))

The number of *tons (kilograms)* of product manufactured/sold

The number of *inhabitants*

The number of *patients exposed*; this is a crude estimate; for example, it can be the number of units sold divided by number of units per prescription. The number of units sold can be known with some precision, though the number of units actually taken by the patients cannot be known. The number of units per prescription is, at best, an estimate.

None of this is easily done as it is necessary to obtain the mean number of tablets written on each prescription as well as the prescribed daily dose and then make the presumption that all the patients took all the tablets prescribed. In addition, renewals must also be factored in if the number of patients actually exposed is desired.

The following example is based on actual cases that occurred in a hospital cohort:

The American insurance company Intermountain Health Care followed a cohort of 36,653 hospitalized patients for 18 months. A total of 731 ADRs were found by examining the computerized medical records of these patients. Only 9 of the ADRs were spontaneously reported, giving a reporting rate of 1.25%. It is estimated that these ADRs were responsible for a mean increase of 1.5 days of hospitalization per patient at a daily cost of about $1000 (Hannan, *Austr Prescriber* 1997;20(4):84).

REPORTING RATE DETERMINANTS

The reasons for the admittedly low rate of reporting of spontaneous adverse effects can be grouped into categories linked to the clinician, the reporter who has the AE, the manufacturer, the AE/ADR itself, the pharmacovigilance program, and the suspect product.

▶ **Factors tied to the clinician**

Many factors can be described:

Is the report reimbursed (i.e., paid for): The influence of being paid for each AE report has been studied in the setting of hospitals in Ireland. Reporting by physicians quadrupled when they were paid for the reports and returned to baseline when the reimbursements ceased. The problem here is that the increase in reports represented cases that were of little use in pharmacovigilance signaling. The receipt of minor AEs/ADRs does not correspond to the objectives of the spontaneous AE/ADR reporting systems, in which the goal is to receive cases of strong signaling value, that is, cases of unlabeled serious events that may alter the risk/benefit ratio (Feely, *Br Med J* 1990;300:22).

Practice of medicine: fee-for-service basis versus salary: In European countries where general practitioners are paid a salary as employees of health departments, the level of suspected ADR reporting would appear superior to that in North America, where physicians are reimbursed on a fee-for-service basis. Interestingly, salaried hospital-based pharmacists have an increasing reporting rate and may in fact be supplanting physicians as primary ADR reporters.

Lack of interest: Professor W. H. W. Inman used the polite term *lethargy* to summarize the lack of interest, time, remuneration, and other excuses for failure to report suspected ADRs (McGettigan, *PEDS* 1995;4:355 and *Br J Clin Pharmacol* 1997;44:98).

Uncertainty about causality: The clinician may be uncertain that the drug caused the event. In a study of British physicians, it was found that the lack of confidence in the role of the drug in producing the event is an inhibitory factor in AE/ADR reporting (Belton, *Br J Clin Pharmacol* 1995;39:223).

Awaiting a second case: The phenomenon of publishing more than one case at a time is not unusual; two or three cases of the same ADR may be published together by a single reporter. Why should clinicians refrain from publishing a first case report until they have a second or third case in their practice? One answer may be, "No suspicion, no ADR report." It is only after the second case occurs that the clinician's threshold of suspicion is reached so that he or she is compelled to report. This phenomenon is an important source of delay in the publication or reporting of important signals, particularly when the second case occurs a year or two after the first. An analysis of five journals revealed 297 articles containing a total of 384 AEs, which means an average of 1.29 observations per publication. Thus as many as 87 authors apparently waited for a second case (our interpretation) before submitting their reports for publication (Haramburu, *Lancet* 1985;2:550). The explanation seems to be that the previously low level of suspicion of a drug causality has increased a notch or two in the mind of the clinician. Although the desire for scientific validation with a second case is very understandable, the clinician is requiring that the second case occur in his or her own practice, although it could, in fact, be seen and thus validated by a different observer somewhere else. The failure to report to the health agencies or the manufacturer can delay the appropriate analysis and actions (e.g., a call for additional cases) of a serious signal.

Belief in the innocence of the drug: A potential reporter may have an exaggerated confidence in the safety of a drug. This is the incorrect belief that the phase III development of a drug reveals its entire safety profile. This may be a form of scientific naiveté, assuming that "only safe drugs are marketed" (McGettigan, *PEDS* 1995;4:355). This credulity has many causes, including the promotion of the drug, which may stress efficacy at the expense of safety issues.

Fear of being sued: This fear seems to be most present in the United States. In Ireland only 4.1% of those studied cited this reason (Feely, *Br Med J* 1990;300:22); in France, of 507 physicians in private practice interviewed, only 1% were concerned about legal liability (Pierfitte, *Thérapie* 1995:50:171, English abstract): differing cultures, different rates.

Ambition: Among specialists and academics in medical schools and university hospitals the desire to publish and enlarge one's curriculum vitae may override the desire to notify the government health authority. This attitude is unfortunate since the author could use the date of notification to prove that he or she was the first to make the observation. The journal *Thérapie* accepts for publication only case reports that already have been submitted to the pharmacovigilance authorities (Inman, *Br J Clin Pharmacol* 1996;41:434).

Prescriber guilt: There exists the entirely understandable impression in the prescriber that he or she has given a patient a medication that has produced harm. In a study of Irish physicians, 7.6% expressed this idea (Feely, *Br Med J* 1990;300:22).

Fear of appearing foolish: The fear of being ridiculed for having sent to a pharmacovigilance unit "an effect that everybody is already aware of" and is "of little or no signaling value" was cited by Irish physicians in a study as a reason to hesitate about reporting a suspected ADR (McGettigan, *PEDS* 1995;4:355).

Profession: In 1993, the FDA examined the AEs/ADRs submitted as a function of the reporter's profession: 55% pharmacists, 16% physicians, 8% nurses, 11% other health care professionals, and 10% other individuals. After adjustment for the numbers in each field, the reporting rates were 1/90 pharmacists and 1/900 physicians. Similar results were seen in Québec, Canada (Horton, *Lancet* 1994;343:285; Biron, *Thérapie* 1996;51:578, English abstract).

Fear of revealing an off-label prescription: If drug was used for an unapproved indication, the prescriber may not wish to call attention to this.

Loss of anonymity: The reporter may not want to supply privileged details even if anonymized, along with his or her name and address, to governments and manufacturers.

Religion: Protestant countries seem to have a higher level of reporting than Catholic countries even where there are large populations of both religions such as Belgium, Germany, and Ireland. The reporting rate in Protestant Denmark before 1986 was 1/3850 inhabitants compared to 1/200,000 inhabitants in Catholic Italy, yielding a reporting ratio of 52:1 (Griffin, *Int Pharm J* 1987;1:145). Even within the same city this effect persists: A study in Montreal showed that English-speaking Protestant parents reported more AEs/ADRs seen in their children than French-speaking Catholic parents did (Biron, *J Pediatr* 1987;110:665).

> **The reporter is the victim**

Two situations are possible: the health care professional is himself or herself the patient and user of the drug; a non-medical consumer has a suspected ADR and becomes the reporter of the event.

> *A medical professional suffers from an AE:* When the nonsteroidal anti-inflammatory drug (NSAID) suprofen was launched in the United States, many physicians received samples of the product they used themselves or distributed to their families. Forty percent of the initial reports of AEs were from health care professionals who "benefited" from the samples (Rossi, JAMA 1988;259:1203). Many years ago, some of the victims of the congenital abnormalities produced by thalidomide occurred in the children of physicians whose wives used samples given to their husbands.

> *AE/ADR reports by nonmedical consumers:* The Dutch have compared the suspected ADR reports received at the Dutch Centre of Pharmacovigilance from patients with those received from health care professionals regarding serotonin uptake inhibitor antidepressants. Two years after launch, patients had submitted 120 reports and clinicians had reported 89. The time lag between the first notification of the new ADR by a patient and the first notification of a new ADR by a medical professional also showed a difference: the patients were faster by a mean of 273 days (Egberts, *Br Med J* 1996;313:530).

> **The manufacturer**

Time and effort involved in follow-up: In many countries (e.g., the United States) the manufacturer is obliged by law or regulation to obtain follow-up information on AEs. Conscientious manufacturers contact the reporter by phone, letter and/or fax requesting complementary data, including patient charts, laboratory reports, and cardiograms. This process costs the reporter some time and effort and may cause a physician to think twice about reporting a case to the manufacturer.

Loss of grants: The concern that an academic researcher, a university hospital, or opinion leader might lose a grant or subsidy from a pharmaceutical company is a possible reason for reticence in spontaneous reporting of suspected ADRs observed in regular patients. This does not apply to AEs and ADRs in clinical trials, in which the safety and efficacy profiles of the drug are being actively sought. This issue does not seem to arise in reports to health agencies since there is rarely a question of financing or grants in these cases.

Attitude: The attitude of the company can be closed and defensive or open and welcoming. Remarks like "This is the first time we've heard of this kind of reaction, you are the only person in the country to have reported this" can be daunting and discouraging. This phenomenon, which was seen more in the past, seems to be receding now that the need for safety monitoring is understood and accepted (even by the marketing departments of pharmaceutical companies!).

> **The reaction itself**

Several characteristics of the AE/ADR can play a role in underreporting:

> *The severity:* A more severe AE/ADR is more likely to be reported. A British study suggests that it is six times more likely that an ADR will be reported if it is serious rather than innocuous (Mann, *PEDS* 1992;1:19).

The death rate of agranulocytosis is 10% in cohort studies (Heinpel, *Med Toxicol* 1988;3:449) whereas that of spontaneously reported agranulocytoses in Great Britain is 30%. The seriousness increases the chances of its being reported threefold; in an Irish study, 94.9% considered that seriousness is an important determinant of reportability (Feely, *Br Med J* 1990;300:22; MCA/CSM, *Curr Probl Pharmacovigil* 1993;19).

The natural rarity of the AE/ADR: The rarity, like the severity, of the event raises its visibility. When zimeldine was followed for Guillain-Barré syndrome (very rare and serious, sometimes fatal), it was relatively easy to classify as a signal. The initial series of cases were studied in depth and the drug was withdrawn from the market. Phocomelia produced by thalidomide is easier to recognize as an ADR than a dry cough produced by angiotensin converting enzyme inhibitors.

Visibility on the skin: Cutaneous reactions are reported more often, all features being equal, than noncutaneous reactions, particularly when the reporter is not a physician.

Short time to onset: Suspicion increases with the brevity of the lag between ingestion of the drug and appearance of the AE. This suggests that an increase in reporting rates will follow.

▶ **Pharmacovigilance organization**

Lack of awareness: "What is pharmacovigilance?": In general, very few physicians and health care professionals are aware of the nature of drug development, the (relatively small) number of patients exposed to the drug in phases II and III, and the need for ongoing AE/ADR reporting after marketing to flesh out the safety profile of a product. Few medical schools around the world include pharmacovigilance in their curricula; those that include it do so in a cursory manner. If the medical community is barely aware of pharmacovigilance, the lay community is even less so. Most consumers believe that if a drug were not totally safe and effective, it would not be on the market.

Weakness of the organization: When a national health agency pharmacovigilance program is poorly financed, slowed by a ponderous bureaucracy, stifled by a "let's not make waves" attitude, managed by continually replaced short-term leaders who do not develop any expertise in the field, the level of reporting of AEs that produce important signals diminishes. In addition, interestingly, some national pharmacovigilance units only look at domestic AEs rather than at worldwide AEs/ADRs. It is thus hardly surprising that few or no signals are picked up (see ORGANIZATION OF NATIONAL PHARMACOVIGILANCE).

Lack of regionalization: In Great Britain, after the creation in Wales of a regional program of pharmacovigilance, there was an increase in suspected ADR reporting of 37%, whereas the national increase was only 16% in 1983–1984. This represents a 131% higher level for the regional center. The Welsh center obtained a reporting rate as high as that of the French regional center in Aquitaine (Bateman, *Br J Clin Pharmacol* 1991;31:188).

In the United States, the level of reporting in the state of Maryland before the installation of a pilot regional program was 42 declarations per year per 10,000 physicians; after the program began, the rate was 134 per year per 10,000 physicians, a 3.8-fold increase (Rogers, *Arch Intern Med* 1988;148:1596). In Great Britain, the percentage of physicians who reported at least one suspected ADR during a 4-year period (1992–1995) was 35% for the whole of the country compared to 51% for the sector served by the Northern Regional Monitoring Centre: an increase of 46% for the regional center (Belton, *J Clin Pharmacol* 1995;39:223; CSM/MCA, *Curr Probl Phamacovigil* 1997;23:6). It thus appears that physicians might prefer, in some cases, to report to local pharmacovigilance units when available, rather than to national ones or to manufacturers.

The lack of promotion of reporting: The manufacturers use different media to promote, both directly and indirectly, their company and the specific products that they manufacture. Often the opinion leaders from medical schools take part in this type of communication in one form or another. On the other hand, the opinion leaders (or the pharmacovigilance experts, for that matter) are rarely seen in the media promoting pharmacovigilance of new products.

The age of a pharmacovigilance program: The FDA went so far as to change the name of its aging pharmacovigilance program when it was "relaunched" in 1993 as the MedWatch Program. This proved to be a major success with the number of reports rising dramatically. See the Center for Drug Evaluation and Research's (CDER's) annual report for 1999 (www.fda.gov/cder/reports/rtn99.htm). Also see an older report on MedWatch for the year 1996 (www.fda.gov/cder/dpe/annrep96/index.htm).

The absence of a national bulletin: In Great Britain and Australia, for example, the clinicians are proud of their publications *Current Problems in Pharmacovigilance* and the *Australian Drug Adverse Reactions Bulletin,* respectively. In countries where no such bulletin exists, awareness is lower.

▶ **The suspect product**

Two characteristics of the product itself can play a role in the reporting rates.

The pharmacologic class: Traditionally oncologists do not report to pharmacovigilance units the serious unlabeled ADRs related to chemotherapy in their patients. Rather they discuss them among themselves. It is presumed that the severity of the indication (cancer) makes the severity of the ADRs less unacceptable. It is also assumed by oncologists that all patients in chemotherapy will have AEs/ADRs and that, except for the very unusual or very severe reactions (out of proportion to what they have seen in the past), it is too time-consuming and of little value to report or publish single cases.

The commercial age of the product: It is during the first 3 to 5 years or less after launch that active AE/ADR reporting occurs. This phenomenon, known as the *Weber effect,* has been well documented. In terms of stimulus to AE/ADR reporting, seriousness of the event is the most important factor, followed by the newness of the drug. It is presumed clinicians consider the signaling value in these cases to be greater than in older drugs (see WEBER EFFECT).

REPORTING RATE: SPONTANEOUS (see SECULAR TRENDS)

▶ **General**

The term *spontaneous reporting rate* refers to the level of case reports received by a pharmacovigilance unit and must not be confused with the actual *occurrence or incidence rate,* which is virtually always greater or much greater than the reporting rate, since not all cases are reported. The number of cases received is the numerator. The denominator, however, is tricky and variable, and its variations are enormous: it can be expressed as number of inhabitants, number of physicians, number of prescriptions, sales, patient-days of use, and in other terms (see RULE OF THREES).

▶ Underreporting

Underreporting is the unfortunately widespread phenomenon of the low level of adverse effect reporting by clinicians. The level of reporting is consistently below 100% and often approaches 0%. For instance, in the United Kingdom in 1986–1987 it was estimated that the reporting rate was less than 10% (Bem, *Br Med J* 1988;296:1319). This global estimate, however, is not very useful in any particular pharmacovigilance investigation since the rate of underreporting is apparently not consistent. Many factors are at play in the level of reporting, including newness of the drug on the market and media attention. Nevertheless, underreporting should not preclude risk/benefit decisions in pharmacovigilance. Because of the unknown and variable underreporting of AEs, the use of a calculated reporting rate (AEs reported/usage) to make the case that an AE/ADR is either rare or infrequent is to be discouraged.

▶ Specific

The reporting rate can refer to the rate for a specific AE/ADR associated with a given suspect drug, to an AE/ADR associated with any number of suspect drugs, or to all the AEs/ADRs associated with a particular product. The denominator can be variable. Let us consider three situations:

- A specific ADR, with number of prescriptions used as the denominator

  Mefloquine and depression: The reporting rate of depression seen in the Australian pharmacovigilance system between 1990 and 1996 compared to the number of prescriptions for mefloquine in the country was 148.5 cases per million prescriptions or 1 case per 6734 prescriptions. The true occurrence rate is unknown (ADRAC, *Aust ADR Bull* 1998;17(1):3).

  There are multiple problems with using this number. The level of underreporting of cases of depression in patients receiving mefloquin is unknown. The number of prescriptions does not necessarily equal the number of patients, as it may include renewals of prescriptions. It may also include patients who used one tablet and never took the rest. It is also unclear what the baseline rate of depression is in patients similar to those on this antimalarial drug.

- A specific ADR with an estimated level of occurrence

  A cephalosporin and serum sickness: The rate of occurrence of this ADR seen mainly in children is 1:200 courses of treatment with a specific cephalosporin, according to a prospective trial, whereas the spontaneous reporting rate was estimated elsewhere at 1:38,000 courses, thus permitting an estimation of 1 case reported per 190 cases actually occurring (reporting rate = 0.53%).

- A specific ADR with the denominator as the number of cases estimated by a clinical trial

  Fatal anaphylaxis: A British study estimated the spontaneous reporting rate of fatal anaphylaxis to an antibiotic to be 42% and fatal anaphylaxis to all medications as being 49% (Pumphrey, Lancet 1999;353:1157). Such exemplary high rates are not likely to be observed in many countries.

RESERPINE AND CANCER OF THE BREAST: A FALSE ALERT

This antihypertensive agent, widely used in the 1980s, was wrongly suspected of causing an increased incidence of breast cancer. The false alert was initially triggered by a case-control study and not by spontaneous reports. The pharmacovigilance investigation led to further prospective and retrospective studies using linked databases and showed the signal to be false. Two lessons: case-control studies are subject to numerous biases, and spontaneous reports are not the only source of false signals (Labarthe, *J Chron Dis* 1979;32:95; Horowitz, *Arch Intern Med* 1985;145:1873; Fraser, *Clin Pharmacol Ther* 1996;60:368).

RISK

Usually equivalent to *rate* but often used to designate the likelihood: the probability that a particular event will occur in an individual. In pharmacovigilance it is used in referring to an adverse effect.

RISK ATTRIBUTABLE TO A DRUG

The *attributable risk* of an ADR for a newly approved drug generally is known only when it is frequent enough to be detected during clinical trials; it is poorly known after marketing, even if relatively frequent, unless cohort studies are undertaken. The attributable risk for a particular ADR is the frequency of the adverse effect in those exposed to the drug minus the frequency of the AE in those not exposed to it in a comparable indication and group of patients. When possible it is worth attempting to calculate this figure, as it is a pragmatically more meaningful tool than relative risk in evaluating the risk/benefit ratio.

Analgesics and fatal anaphylaxis: In the course of multiple studies of fatal anaphylaxis associated with nonsteroidal anti-inflammatory drugs (NSAIDs) the weekly excess fatal anaphylaxis for three products was calculated: it ranged from 0.007 per million treatment weeks to 0.016. (CIOMS IV 1998; Van Der Klauw, *Br J Clin Pharmacol* 1993;35:400).

Zimeldine and the Guillain-Barré Syndrome: Zimeldine, the first in the family of serotoninergic antidepressants, was associated with several cases of Guillain-Barré syndrome (acute polyradiculopathy), convulsions, and hepatotoxicity. It was introduced in the United States in December 1981 and in the United Kingdom in 1982, only to be removed from the market in both these countries in 1983. Approximately 200,000 patients were exposed in five countries before its withdrawal (Kaitin, *Clin Pharmacol Ther* 1989;46:121). A pharmacovigilance investigation done predominantly in Sweden found that the underlying baseline risk of Guillain-Barré syndrome was 20 cases per million person-years, whereas in those exposed to zimeldine it was 580 cases per million person-years. These data permitted the calculation of the following:

Relative risk: 29:1 (580:20)

Attributable risk: 560 per million person-years (580 - 20)

Number of patients needed to be treated for 1 year in order to produce 1 case: 1785 (1,000,000/560)

General prior odds (in Bayesian analysis): 560/20 = 28/1

Analgesics and deaths from all causes: A meta-analysis covering the period 1970–1996 calculated the attributable risk for these products as the number of deaths per million short-term exposures. The values varied from 0.03 (95% CI = 0.007 to 0.06) to 14.9 (95% CI = 1.3 to 28.5) (Martinez, *PEDS* 1997;6(suppl 2):S115).

EXAMPLES IN HEPATOVIGILANCE

The literature contains a number of estimates of incidence levels of acute hepatitis and cholestatic hepatitis attributed to medications. If the estimates are based on cases reported through spontaneous reporting systems, the frequency of cases is clearly inferior to the frequency of cases occurring. In addition, the reported frequency varies from study to study. The denominator is also subject to significant inaccuracy and bias. Here are a few examples from the literature presented without confidence intervals, which would be expected to be very wide:

▶ Acute Hepatitis

■ Nonsteroidal anti-inflammatory drugs (NSAIDs): rate = 0.00001 or 1/100,000 NSAID prescriptions according to a linked database study from Saskatchewan of hepatitis requiring hospitalization (Gutham, *Post Marketing Surveillance* 1993;7:204)

■ Ampicillin: rate = 0.00001 or 1/100,000 prescriptions (Gutham, *Post Marketing Surveillance* 1993;7:204)

■ Cephalexin: rate = 0.00002 or 1/49,000 prescriptions (Gutham, *Post Marketing Surveillance* 1993;7:204)

■ Cotrimoxazole: rate = 0.000052 or 1/19,000 prescriptions (U.K. General Practice Research Database, Jick, *Lancet* 1995;345:1118 and *Pharmacotherapy* 1995;15:428)

■ Erythromycin estolate: rate = 0.00014 or 1/7142 prescriptions (Gutham, *Post Marketing Surveillance* 1993;7:204)

■ Methyldopa: rate = 0.00001 or 1/100,000 prescriptions (Gutham, *Post Marketing Surveillance* 1993;7:204)

■ Trimethoprim: rate = 0.000038 or 1/27,000 prescriptions (Jick, *Lancet* 1995;345:1118 and *Pharmacotherapy* 1995;15:428)

▶ Cholestatic Hepatitis

■ Cephalexin: rate = 0.000015 or 1/65,467 prescriptions (Gutham, *Post Marketing Surveillance* 1993;7:204).

■ Cotrimoxazole: rate = 0.000022 or 1/46,480 prescriptions (Jick, *Lancet* 1995;345:1118 and *Pharmacotherapy* 1995;15:428)

■ Erythromycin: rate = 0.000036 or 1/28,000 prescriptions (Derby, *Med J Aust* 1993;158:600)

■ Flucloxacillin: rate = 0.0001 or 1/13,000 prescriptions (Derby, *Med J Aust* 1993;158:596)

■ Oxytetracycline: rate = 0.00002 or 1/49,000 prescriptions (Derby, *Med J Aust* 1993;158:600)

■ Trimethoprim: rate = 0.000015 or 1/66,740 prescriptions (Jick, *Lancet* 1995;345:1118 and *Pharmacotherapy* 1995;15:428)

■ Zomepirac: rate = 0.000042 or 1/24,000 prescriptions (Derby, *Med J Aust* 1993:158:600)

RISK/BENEFIT RATIO

In terms of ADRs this refers to the *acceptability* of an ADR. This "ratio" is based on the importance, frequency, and duration of therapeutic benefits compared to the seriousness, frequency, and duration of the ADRs. Although the mathematical term *ratio* is used, no quantitative measure is really made, and a more appropriate term might be *risk/benefit assessment*. There are four situations in which ADRs must be taken into account, depending upon whether the "ratio" is being calculated on the individual level (in pharmacotherapy) or on the population level (in pharmacovigilance) and whether it is before or after the occurrence of the ADR. In a more optimistic vein, many use the term benefit/risk ratio.

IN PHARMACOTHERAPY

▶ Before Prescribing a Drug

Before prescribing a medication, the prescriber must evaluate the known ADR profile and the expected benefits: the prior risk/benefit ratio.

▶ After Prescribing a Drug

After the occurrence of the ADR in a patient, the prescriber must now reanalyze the risk/benefit ratio in the specific patient as the incidence of this ADR in this patient is 100%. Several choices are possible: stop the drug and use a different one (e.g., switch from a nonsteroidal anti-inflammatory drug (NSAID) for pain to acetaminophen); reduce or modify the dosing or alter the schedule (e.g., an antidepressant that produces sedation could be switched from morning to before bed dosing or decreased in dose); continue the drug because the benefit outweighs the risk (e.g., hair loss from a drug used in cancer chemotherapy or mild diarrhea from an antibiotic).

IN PHARMACOVIGILANCE

▶ Before Marketing Authorization

The risk/benefit ratio is difficult to determine early in the course of development. In fact, in phase I there is usually no benefit to the individual in a trial, particularly for a normal volunteer. Later in development, after some phase II and phase III results are known, it is possible for the investigator to make a more informed judgment. The risk/benefit ratio for the patient is summarized in the informed consent that the patient signs before entry into the trial.

▶ After Marketing Begins

Cirumstances change! Extensive use in a larger and more heterogeneous population than that studied in the trials along with "irrational" use (overdose, misuse, etc.) provides more extensive data and allows more complete evaluation of the risk/benefit ratio.

RISK DIFFERENCE (see ATTRIBUTABLE RISK)

RISK FACTOR

In case causality assessment, a specific "predictive" factor that is looked for

- *After* ascertaining the safety profile and properties of the suspect drug
- *After* learning about the patient's medical history and status
- *Before* knowing about the occurrence of the adverse reaction

In the Bayesian model the *known* risk factors are expressed as *relative risks*. These modify the *general prior odds* and transform them into *case prior odds modified by history*. Remember, however, that many patients experience ADRs without apparent risk factors. It is the *unknown* risk factors that make each patient as unique as his or her genetic code. This is something that clinicians have known and struggled with since the beginning of the profession.

FACTORS ASSOCIATED WITH THE SUSPECT DRUG

These factors are capable of modifying the likelihood of a drug etiology for an AE.

- The pharmacologic class
- The specific characteristics of the product
- The total or daily dose administered, which can be normal or just supratherapeutic, or frankly above normal (overdose: overdoses may be due to error, negligence, accident, or intention)
- The duration of treatment (overly long)
- The route of administration
- The rate of administration (too fast)
- The time of administration (relation to posture, sleep, eating and drinking, dosing intervals, etc.)

FACTORS ASSOCIATED WITH THE PATIENT'S MEDICAL STATUS

The following factors are capable of modifying the risk of an ADR:

- Past history: positive prior challenges ("prechallenges") to the same product or to the same class of products; prior occurrence of the AE when the patient was not exposed to the drug.
- Concomitant morbidity
- Demographics: age, sex, country, race, others
- Physiological conditions: weight, pregnancy status, and so on
- Chronic medical conditions: Immunodeficiency (human immunodefiency virus (HIV)), allergies, renal, cardiac, hepatic, pulmonary insufficiency, others
- Acute medical conditions: shock, dehydration, others
- Concomitant medications: drug interactions
- Concomitant medical or nonmedical interventions: alcohol or tobacco use, exercise, surgery, diet, others

Metformin and lactic acidosis: The risk factors for lactic acidosis with this oral biguanide hypoglycemic agent are well known, constitute contraindications, and are related to the medical status of the patient.

- Past medical history: ketoacidosis with or without coma whether diabetic or not
- Comorbidity: insulin-dependent diabetes mellitus
- Physiologic condition: pregnancy
- Other medical conditions: renal, cardiac, respiratory, or severe hepatic insufficiency (with or without alcoholism)
- Acute medical conditions: Dehydration, severe infection, ketoacidosis (whether diabetic or nondiabetic), shock
- Interventions: radiologic dye use (risk of acute renal insufficiency after angiography, renal exams, etc.), surgery

RULE OF THREES

This term has a special meaning when used in the world of pharmacovigilance:

STATISTICAL POWER

An expression relating to statistical power proposed by Hanley (If nothing goes wrong, is everything all right? *JAMA* 1983;249:1743). If no case of an adverse effect is seen in N patients exposed to a drug, it can be concluded with $(1 - \alpha)$ confidence that the incidence of this AE does not exceed $3/N$ if $\alpha = 0.05$. For example, if 300 patients are given a new nonsteroidal anti-inflammatory drug (NSAID) and there are no cases of fatal gastrointestinal bleeding, it can be said with 95% confidence $(1 - 0.05)$ that the true incidence does not exceed $3/300$ or $1/100$.

From this it follows that, at the 95% confidence level, to say that the incidence of this AE is less than or equal to $1/10,000$, it is necessary to have 30,000 exposed patients without observing the AE.

Thus it is not really possible to prove the negative concept that the incidence of an AE is zero ("This AE does not occur"). Since absolute safety cannot be proved, we must content ourselves with relative safety within certain limits.

The number 3 is derived from Poisson's law, which permits the calculation of the upper end of the confidence interval when the observed number of AEs is zero. The natural logarithm (ln) of the negative value of alpha can be calculated:

For an 80% confidence interval (CI) or a 20% risk of error, $\ln (-0.2) = 1.6$

For a 90% CI or a 10% risk of error, $\ln (-0.1) = 2.3$

For a 95% CI or a 5% risk of error, $\ln (-0.05) = 3$

For a 99% CI or a 1% risk of error, $\ln (-0.01) = 4.6$

From this it follows that, continuing the preceeding example, to have a 99% confidence that the incidence of an AE is less than $1/10,000$ it would be necessary that no cases of the AE be observed in 46,000 patients.

LABELING

It has been proposed that all product labeling should include the three most frequent ADRs and the three most medically severe ADRs.

S

SAFE AND EFFECTIVE; SAFE AND EFFICACIOUS

A term that is widely used to indicate that a drug has been approved by a regulatory agency (as in "This drug was approved by the Food and Drug Administration, and therefore it has been shown to be safe and effective"). This unfortunate shorthand is meant to indicate that the regulatory agency has reviewed the dossier (New Drug Application(NDA), HRD, etc.) and found evidence of efficacy in the proposed indication and that the risk/benefit ratio is acceptable for marketing. That is to say, the concept of "safe" as an absolute does not exist; safety (risk) is always evaluated in terms of efficacy (benefit). The use of this term is misleading, particularly to the lay public, who do not yet fully understand that safety is relative, not absolute. However, its use is widespread and is likely to continue.

SAFETY

This term is used in pharmacovigilance in three closely related ways:

- To designate the character of innocuousness, danger, security, or tolerance of a medication or drug, as in "the safety of a drug"; it includes the concepts of toxicity, intolerance, and risk.
- To designate the surveillance of ADRs (pharmacovigilance), as in "the responsibility of safety reporting, safety monitoring."
- To designate the whole range of undesirable effects, as in "the safety profile, the safety labeling of a drug."

SAFETY ASSESSMENT OF MARKETED MEDICINES (SAMS)

A British expression designating industry-sponsored phase IV studies for purposes of safety assessment. These studies may be controlled trials, a follow-up of a cohort exposed to a new medication, a case-control study, or case surveillance (Stephens 1999:447).

SAFETY SCIENTIST; SAFETY SPECIALIST

A term used in the industry to designate a scientifically or medically trained person responsible for the safety surveillance of drug products

SCANDAL

When certain unacceptable and serious ADRs occur and recur although preventable, a public scandal may ensue if four conditions are met:

- *Enormity*: the damage is clear, unequivocal, and dramatic; its enormity does not allow room for any doubt.
- *Immorality*: the occurrence is incompatible with the moral values and norms of society.
- *Abuse of confidence*: the occurrence was unexpected and responsible people did not act in the manner expected of them.
- *Cover up*: the occurrence was concealed or camouflaged in some form before it became public.

These conditions were met when human immunodeficiency virus (HIV) and hepatitis C–contaminated blood products were transfused into patients in Japan, France, and Canada. The ensuing dramas evolved into the "contaminated blood scandals" (as a result of which some people went to prison).

SECOND-GENERATION EFFECT

A teratogenic AE that results from exposure in utero is considered to be a second-generation effect. The foremost examples are those of phocomelia associated with thalidomide and vaginal cancer associated with diethylstilbestrol ("DES daughters").

SECONDARY OR INDIRECT EFFECT

An event that is the consequence of an initial, primary (direct) event that can produce a cascade of events. The events in the cascade, referred to as *secondary effects,* are produced indirectly by the suspected drug. Product labeling may not reflect secondary effects, which can vary from individual to individual. Usually the primary effects are listed, and the prescriber must use his or her medical knowledge to anticipate the consequences. A high index of suspicion is thus required of the prescriber. A patient's complaint, which is seemingly unrelated to the drug, may be the consequence of a primary, direct ADR that the prescriber must tease out. *Related death,* an outcome found on most ADR reporting forms, is a clear illustration of an event (actually it is an outcome, a consequence) that is always secondary to an AE/ADR.

> *Benzodiazepines: fracture of the hip:* By using a case-control approach in a linked medical-pharmaceutical database in Saskatchewan, an increase in the risk of hip fracture in users of long-acting benzodiazepines has been observed. The primary adverse reaction is a residual daytime depressive effect on the central nervous system, followed by decreased awareness when walking, followed by a fall, followed by a fracture (Ray, *JAMA* 1989;262:3303).

> *Benzodiazepines: aspiration pneumonia:* In the epileptic child, the use of benzodiazepines can produce swallowing problems, followed by aspiration, followed by pneumonia, as manifested by fever and cough (Wyllie, *N Engl J Med* 1986;314:35).

> *Guar gum: esophageal impaction:* Several hours after taking three tablets of guar gum, a very hydrophilic product, a 39-year-old obese male entered the emergency room because he was unable to swallow—even saliva. Rigid esophagoscopy was required to clear the esophagus. However, during the procedure the esophagus was torn and surgical repair was necessary. Several days later a massive pulmonary embolus occurred and the unfortunate patient died. His death was secondary to the embolus which was secondary to the postoperative state, which was secondary to the endoscopy, which was secondary to the obstruction. The primary adverse reaction was a local obstruction at the site of transit in the esophagus. See the Food and Drug Administration website (www.fda.gov/medwatch/report/desk/casestud.htm).

> *Renal insufficiency:* Renal insufficiency may be produced secondary to an embolus, hemolysis, myoglobinuria, or lithiasis due to medication effects rather than to a direct drug effect on the kidney.

Pancreatitis: Pancreatitis may be due to hyperlipidemia. An antiestrogen used in treating breast cancer has been rarely reported to produce a hypertriglyceridemia of sufficient magnitude to produce secondary pancreatitis. Such a case occurred in Japan, where a 36-year-old female who had breast cancer died of pancreatitis secondary to a hypertriglyceridemia of 36.7 g/l after 4 months of treatment (Nogochi, *Br J Surg* 1987;74:586).

There are many other examples and the clinician must always remain on guard for such events:

- A myocardial infarction may occur secondary to anemia produced by a gastrointestinal bleed or by hemolysis due to a drug.
- Syncope may occur secondary to hypotension seen after treatment with nitrates for angina. A death may be secondary to the primary proarrhythmic effect of encainide or flecainide.
- Digitalis toxicity may be secondary to a hypokalemic effect of a diuretic.
- A gastrointestinal hemorrhage may be an immediate or primary or direct adverse reaction due to a drug (e.g., a nonsteroidal anti-inflammatory drug (NSAID)). Secondary or indirect effects that occur as a consequence of the gastrointestinal (GI) bleeding might be anemia or hemorrhagic shock.

SECULAR TRENDS

This phenomenon is also called *temporal bias* and reflects an increase in AE/ADR reporting for a drug or class of drugs following increased media attention, use of a medication by a celebrity, a warning from a health agency, etc. "Overall ADR reporting rates can be increased several times by external factors such as a change in a reporting system or an increased level of publicity attending a given drug or adverse reaction." Sachs and Bortnichak (*American J of Medicine* 81 (supp 5B):49, 1986). It is to be distinguished from the Weber Effect (see WEBER EFFECT).

SEEDING STUDY

A pejorative term applied to a study that has the appearance of a scientific cohort study but in fact is done to promote a product for an approved indication and yields little or no scientific data. The cohort includes

- A large number of physicians carefully spread around the country
- A small number of patients per physician
- A lack of the usual control and monitoring functions seen in clinical trials
- Compensation in excess of the work demanded of the physician

One of the ethical problems that these studies pose is that the prescriber is put in a situation in which there is a conflict of interest since he or she is compensated for exposing patients to a new medication instead of keeping them on older alternative products to which they are responsive and tolerant (Read MCA, *Br Med J* 1992;304:1470; MCA and Stephens, *PEDS* 1994;3:1). In many countries, these studies are now forbidden.

SERIOUSNESS CRITERIA

The seriousness of an AE, along with expectedness (*labeledness*), represent the regulatory criteria for expedited reporting of AEs. The consistency of these reporting requirements is due to the combined efforts of the World Health Organization (WHO), ICH E2A, the Council for International Organizations of

Medical Sciences (CIOMS), the health authorities in the European Union, and Japan, the U.S. Food and Drug Administration, and the pharmaceutical companies in the United States, European Union, and Japan (the International Conference on Harmonization (ICH)).

An AE is classified as serious or nonserious according to several major elements: death or a life-threatening event, (inpatient) required or prolonged hospitalization, disability (incapacity), or a congenital anomaly (birth defect). Note that hospitalization is not a state of health but rather a surrogate marker suggesting that the level of care required to treat the event is significant. As soon as an event has satisfied one of these criteria, it is considered serious. When an event is judged not to be serious, it is termed *nonserious*.

Note that the term *serious* does not necessarily have anything to do with the actual medical condition but, rather, has a regulatory meaning. If a person is hospitalized for observation or for a mild event for whatever reason, this condition meets the criteria for *serious*. If, however, the patient has a non-life-threatening event such as a mild gastrointestinal bleed or a transient ischemic attack (TIA) that does not require hospitalization or produce any residual disability, the event may be considered *nonserious*. Thus in pharmacovigilance, in treating patients who are very ill the adjective *serious* should not be used to describe the actual medical condition; rather words such as *severe, clinically significant, clinically important* should be employed. This situation has produced much confusion because of the arbitrary use of the word *serious*. In particular, translation of medical documents from other languages may produce problems. This distinction is addressed at length in ICH E2A (see ICH E2A).

DEATH

Logically, death should be a seriousness criterion only if it is related somehow to the AE/ADR, that is, only if the causality implicating the drug is not excluded. This notion of *related death* seems to be implicit in the pharmacovigilance regulations. Death per se is not an ADR; it is, rather, an outcome or consequence or complication of the reaction.

When discussing death there are actually two sequential issues involved: the association between the suspect drug and the ADR and the association between the ADR and the death. Certain AE reporting forms (including the Canadian one) distinguish three categories:

- Death probably related—corresponding to causality level 3 (probable) or level 4 (very probable, definite)
- Death possibly related—corresponding to causality level 2 (possible) or level 1 (unlikely, improbable)
- Death unrelated—corresponding to causality level - 1 (excluded, ruled out)

In practice, occasional reports submitted to companies or health authorities describe a sudden, unwitnessed death that no AE/ADR can explain (e.g., patient found dead in bed in the morning). In regulatory terms, the death (or sudden death) is listed as the AE even though it is actually the outcome.

LIFE-THREATENING

A *life-threatening event* is an immediate grave medical problem from which the patient would die if no intervention occurred. In regulatory terms this excludes chronic conditions, which would likely be fatal without intervention over time (e.g., chronic hepatitis) but not acutely.

Examples of life-threatening events include hepatic necrosis when the intervention is a liver transplant, anaphylactic shock when the intervention is resuscitation, and acetaminophen overdose when the intervention is acetylcysteine treatment. With regard to devices, a life-threatening situation may exist even if the event has not yet occurred (e.g., a heart valve whose struts are known to break at a high rate, producing a catastrophic cardiac event, or a cardiac pacemaker with a defective battery).

HOSPITALIZATION

- The patient required a hospitalization
- The patient, already hospitalized, had a prolongation of hospital stay due to the AE

The word *admission,* which is implicit in the definition of hospitalization, requires some discussion. The strict definition of this term is the actual placement of a patient in a hospital room (inpatient admission). More controversial is a situation in which the patient is kept overnight in the emergency room. Some would consider this hospitalization; others would not. Similarly, when a person requires less than 24 hours of treatment in an emergency room for a condition that cannot be treated outside the hospital or from which he or she rapidly recovers (e.g., an acute allergic reaction), such treatment is considered to be *hospitalization* and thus serious by some.

In the United States, the Food and Drug Administration has accepted the concept that actual hospital admission is required to meet the definition of *serious.* Short stays in the ER do not meet the definition.

A way around this controversy is available, however, through the use of the newer concepts of *required intervention, medically important,* and *medically significant.* Under these criteria (discussed later) the actual duration of the stay in the Emergency Room does not matter if the reporter or safety specialist feels the case is "medically significant" or if intervention occurred in the emergency room (as it usually does). The intent of the regulation is to capture these cases as expedited reports; thus if there is doubt as to whether a case is serious or not, the case should generally be considered serious: better to err on the side of reporting.

Note that, interestingly, hospitalization was not always considered a criterion of seriousness in Japan, contrary to the the Council for International Organizations of Medical Sciences/International Conference on Harmonization (CIOMS)/(ICH) definition. The reason for this was related to the very large number of hospital beds in Japan per 1000 patients compared to those in North America or Europe. Many patients are admitted to a hospital in Japan for what, in the other regions, would be outpatient testing or treatment. Japan has since adopted the ICH/CIOMS definition of seriousness and is now consistent with the European Union and United States. It is suspected that as cost constraints play out in Japan as they have in North America and Europe, fewer patients will be admitted to hospitals in Japan.

DISABILITY OR INCAPACITY

The disability or incapacity must be *persistent* or *incapacitating.* An example of a significant incapacity without permanent sequelae is a transient ischemic attack (TIA) that occurs after use of an oral contraceptive (with full recovery in 24 hours). Permanent or persistent incapacity or disability would be, for example, deafness associated with an aminoglycoside antibiotic, retinopathy associated with hydroxychloroquine used in rheumatoid arthritis, or drug-induced seizures with subsequent residual brain damage.

OTHER CRITERIA

▶ Malformations
Even though a congenital malformation may represent a permanent disability or incapacity, the FDA and some other agencies consider all malformations, per se, to be *serious* for regulatory reporting purposes.

▶ Cancer
Although cancer may fall under one of the other criteria of seriousness, some agencies specify cancer per se as a criterion of seriousness. The FDA formerly considered it a criterion of seriousness in the United States, but this was changed in 1997.

▶ Overdosage
Accidental or intentional overdose is not an outcome but rather a misuse of a medication and thus a risk factor for an ADR and often a risk factor for a medically severe ADR. However, many regulations around the world include overdosage as a criterion for seriousness. There are many reasons for this, including the fact that overdoses (particularly massive overdoses) give important pharmacologic clues regarding the body's response to high doses of the medication and, in some cases, allows a correlation with high-dose animal toxicity data. In fact, there usually are no other ways to learn of the effects of very high doses of a drug than by the spontaneous reporting system, especially from poison control centers.

▶ Withdrawal Syndrome
The syndrome of drug withdrawal is not an outcome but rather implies a specific pharmacologic mechanism at the receptor level that produces the syndrome and is precipitated by tapering or stopping dosage too rapidly; in this latter sense it represents a sort of misuse.

▶ Required Intervention
Some health authorities (including the FDA) and ICH include medical events that may require medical or surgical intervention to prevent one of the other serious outcomes including incapacity or a permanent disability. Although this definition seems to be implicit in other criteria of seriousness such as *hospitalization* or *disability/incapacity* it is nonetheless specified explicitly in the definitions used by many health authorities. It is also useful in that this category allows some AEs to be classified as serious that otherwise would be nonserious; that is, it allows the manufacturer to "bump up" the AE to the serious level. An example would be a skin ulcer in a diabetic patient that followed an injection; it is not life-threatening yet but must be treated (not in the hospital) to prevent it from becoming so.

▶ Medically Significant or Medically Important Events
CIOMS and many major health authorities (FDA) have included this category in the definition of serious in order to capture those events that do not quite meet the other criteria of seriousness when the reporter or the pharmacovigilance officer feels a need to raise the attention level that a particular AE/ADR will receive. Examples include neutropenia or a TIA that was not severe enough to be life-threatening or require treatment or hospitalization. This concept is similar to the WHO Critical Events list.

SEVERE EVENT OR REACTION

A clinical term designating the most grave or dangerous state of a clinical condition. In pharmacovigilance, the term *severe* (which is a medical term) must be distinguished from *serious* (which is a regulatory term). Thus an AE/ADR might be severe but not serious or serious but not severe. For example, an urticaria may be severe (generalized on the whole body, much pruritis) but not serious (i.e., requiring expedited reporting). Conversely, a patient may be hospitalized (hence it is serious) for a petit mal seizure that is not severe (see SERIOUSNESS CRITERIA).

SEX RATIO (M:F RATIO, MALE-TO-FEMALE RATIO)

The proportion of patients by sex in an AE database. It cannot be considered a risk factor unless the ratio of patients exposed is also known.

SIDE EFFECT

This term has been used in two different ways.

ADVERSE DRUG REACTION

The use of the term *side effect* to describe an ADR is now outmoded in pharmacovigilance. It is still a frequently used lay term. However, its use in medical circles is to be discouraged.

PARALLEL

An additional, though uncommon, use of the term *side effect* refers to those events that result from the stimulation of *receptors that were not targeted by the drug to produce a therapeutic effect.* They are type A ADRs and represent an extension of the pharmacodynamic properties of the active ingredient acting on receptors nontargeted by the prescriber. These reactions are predictable and dose-dependent.

They are not always undesirable, however. A "side effect" or parallel, type A untargeted ADR can become a desired pharmacologic and therapeutic effect for a different indication:

> *Terazosine:* Terazosine, an alpha adrenergic blocker used in the treatment of symptoms of benign prostatic hypertrophy, can produce undesired hypotension. The same product, when used to treat arterial hypertension, can produce undesired urinary side effects.

> *Minoxidil:* This vasodilator, when prescribed for baldness, can produce a lowering of the blood pressure. However, when prescribed as an antihypertensive, it can produce hypertrichosis.

SIDE EFFECTS OF DRUGS ANNUAL (SEDA)

An excellent annually updated book that presents and discusses the printed literature in pharmacovigilance. The 2000 edition of *SEDA*, volume 23, *A Worldwide Yearly Survey of New Data and Trends.* (Edited by J.K. Aronson, Amsterdam: Elsevier, 2000) contains 50 chapters and 30 special reviews and a discussion of prescribing errors. This series is an invaluable reference for studying individual drugs' safety profiles and to study the evolution of this field over the last decades. Case reports are discussed and major issues are reviewed in depth. The pharmacovigilance community owes much to Professor M. N. G. Dukes who was the founder and editor for many years. Every fourth year *Meyler's Side Effects of Drugs* is published to synthesize the four preceding SEDAs.

SIGNAL DETECTION

A *signal* can be defined as "a report (or reports) of an event that may or may not have a causal relationship to one or more drugs; it alerts health professionals and should be explored further" (CIOMS IV). It may be a new adverse effect or a change in the character or frequency of an ADR that is already known. If it is potentially important, it can lead to a signal (pharmacovigilance) investigation.

A signal can originate from many sources: spontaneous reports, structured studies (usually epidemiologic ones but sometimes clinical trials), experimental toxicology, questions from health authorities, lawsuits, and others. Signal detection is summarized in Meyboom (*Drug Saf* 1997;16:355).

SPONTANEOUS REPORTS

▶ A Case Report

A report that has a very strong signaling value is also designated as the *index case* or *pivotal case*. A single case that is sufficiently strong to create a signal must have a strong suspicion of causality ("probable" or "very probable"). It is usually a report with a positive dechallenge and rechallenge or without any obvious alternatives (e.g., injection site reaction, anaphylaxis within minutes of treatment).

▶ A Series of Case Reports

Even though the causality of any individual case may be dubious or questionable, the causality may become stronger as more cases are reported ("Where there's smoke there's fire"). Each time a new case is reported, the relative risk in the exposed population increases (even if the background incidence is unknown) as well as the attributable risk of the product (which requires a prospective trial).

▶ Increased Frequency

In theory, an increased frequency of a known ADR should be a signal. For many years the FDA required a calculation in each New Drug Application (NDA) Periodic Report comparing the current report's period to the previous report's period to see whether an increase in any serious AEs was noted. This technique periodically did produce signals, but these were usually previously known or related to reporting artifacts. In 1997 the FDA ended its requirement for this calculation. Periodic Safety Update Reports (PSURs) still require mention of increased frequency, but this section is not stressed and no specific calculations are required.

STRUCTURED STUDIES

▶ Clinical Trial

In rare cases, a signal for a marketed drug can originate in a case-control study, a cohort study, or even a controlled clinical trial as the following example illustrates:

Thalidomide for toxic epidermal necrosis: During a double-blind placebo-controlled clinical trial for this new indication, the mortality rate in the experimental group was 83% and that in the control group 30%. The trial was immediately stopped. This trial demonstrated that for both safety and efficacy reasons the use of this product for this indication was not appropriate. It is also an example of a paradoxic therapeutic effect: life-threatening rather than lifesaving (Wolkenstein, *Lancet* 1998;352:1586).

▶ **Databases**

Rarely, a signal can originate from

■ An undedicated secondary database (health insurance claims)
■ A dedicated database (Prescription Event Monitoring)

ANIMAL TOXICOLOGY AND LABORATORY STUDIES

After marketing authorization, animal studies or in vitro or ex vivo laboratory studies can produce signals in toxicology, genotoxicity, or oncology. These must be very carefully evaluated since some signals are species-specific and do not occur in humans.

SIGNAL, EARLY WARNING

This term has been used for signals that are sufficiently strong and alarming to warrant a pharmacovigilance investigation (see following entry).

SIGNAL EVALUATION; SIGNAL FOLLOW-UP; SIGNAL TRACKING; PHARMACOVIGILANCE INVESTIGATION

There is no single English language term that is widely used for this concept, though the not directly translatable French term (*enquête de pharmacovigilance*) seems to capture the sense rather well and we use *pharmacovigilance investigation* throughout this book. These terms, which are synonymous, are meant to convey the scientific evaluation of a potentially important signal (or *potential signal*). The evaluation is *scientific* because causality assessments are used with the aim of obtaining new data on the safety of the product. The source of the signal can be one or more spontaneous adverse effect reports, a new observation from the pharmacology or toxicology laboratory, the results of an observational study (based on primary data), an epidemiologic study on secondary data in a linked database, or a clinical trial.

When the signal is of sufficient importance to warrant such an investigation, that signal may be referred to as an *early warning signal*. A signal is considered important if the evaluation would be expected to lead to a change in the risk/benefit ratio or would require one or more measures to be taken such as addition of a new ADR to the labeling, a new warning, or a change in an indication (CIOMS IV 1998; Meyboom, *Drug Saf* 1997;16;355).

The generation or detection of signals and the pharmacovigilance investigation represent the major functions, if not the raison d'être, of pharmacovigilance units in health agencies and in the pharmaceutical industry. The procedure first involves a confirmation or refutation of the validity of the signal itself (i.e., determination whether the facts and data are correct and verified) regardless of the source or content of the signal or AE reports. The next step involves a search of the appropriate literature, databases, expert consultants, and so forth. These two procedures are done at the internal level whereby the information is limited to the pharmaceutical company and the governmental health authority(ies).

A spontaneously generated signal is considered *qualitative,* whereas a signal generated from an epidemiologic study or clinical trial is considered *quantitative.*

QUALITATIVE SIGNAL

The report of an AE reaches the level of a qualitative signal if new and important data are found in one or more of the following categories:

- The nature of the new AE/ADR (first case of hepatitis)
- The severity of the AE/ADR (first case of fulminant hepatitis)
- The specificity of the AE/ADR (first case of cholestatic hepatitis)
- The definition of a new risk factor (hepatitis in acquired immunodeficiciency syndrome (AIDS) patients, drug interaction for torsades de pointes)

QUANTITATIVE SIGNAL

A quantitative signal, in contrast to a qualitative signal, is defined only as an increase in frequency of its occurrence in a study. For example, in the course of a clinical trial or a cohort study, an elevation in the liver transaminase level in the treatment group is noted, or in a case-control study there is an increase in the use of hormone therapy in those patients with thromboemboli.

If the signal is alarming and seems to pose a serious and immediate risk to the population of patients in question, it is possible to take temporary or interim measures before waiting for the evaluation of the signal to be completed. This procedure is part of the field of crisis management.

PROBLEMS WITH MANUFACTURE, LABELING, QUALITY CONTROL

When the ADR results from a problem that is not related to the active ingredient but rather to factors related to its manufacture, packaging, labeling (Good Manufacturing Practices—(GMPs)), and other conditions, the signal investigation can and must be done very rapidly in order that the appropriate measures may be taken without delay. For example, if several deaths are reported and if criminal contamination with poison is rapidly found to be the cause, the immediate quarantine and recall of implicated product must be done, to be followed by a change in packaging to make the product more secure. Such an issue occurred in the United States several years ago when a particular brand of acetaminophen was tampered with criminally. The manufacturer, invoking crisis management measures, dealt with the problem rapidly and excellently and was able to restore full confidence in the product. Most issues are more mundane and revolve around specifications of a particular lot or batch of product that are out of the accepted range or similar small but not unimportant problems in manufacture that are tied to manufacturing factors. See the recall action on FDA's website (www.fda.gov).

REQUEST FOR INTENSIFIED MONITORING.

If the causality of a signal detected by spontaneous reports is not sufficiently solid or convincing (because of confounding factors), if the literature and database search do not reveal confirmatory evidence, and if the signal is not very alarming, a second stage in the investigation may be started. This stage is a request for intensified monitoring of the specific AE in question by health care professionals. This is a step that is not taken lightly since it involves the mobilization of the entire health care community and may "tar" the product in question. As an example, some years ago the Australian health authorities requested intensified monitoring of cardiac arrhythmia associated with certain antihistamines. When none was found, the signal was considered to be nonvalidated and no further measures were deemed necessary; in other words, it was a false signal.

ANALYSIS OF A SERIES OF SPONTANEOUSLY REPORTED AES/ADRS.

The causality analysis of a series of AEs/ADRs uses the same techniques and principles that the analysis of individual case causality uses, including prior documentation, validity of report, specific risk factors, and temporal and nontemporal characteristics of the event. However, additional elements must be considered:

The consistency and uniformity of the type of AE, of the risk factors (e.g., dose, age), as well as temporal and nontemporal characteristics between cases in the series

The number of actual cases reported, which is important since each new observation adds to the relative risk of the event in the exposed population, independently of the estimated denominator

The number of actual cases reported compared to the number of patients exposed, in order to make a *very rough estimate* of the reporting rate of the AE/ADR, of its relative risk, and, when lucky enough, of its attributable risk (it is often difficult and sometimes impossible to obtain a valid estimate of the number of patients exposed)

STRUCTURED STUDIES

If the intensive monitoring does not bring about results that allow the signal to be clarified, the next step can involve an epidemiologic study:

■ Analytic observational epidemiologic studies (case-control, cohort: epidemiologic methods applied to secondary claims data or to dedicated computerized medicopharmaceutic data from physicians' records)
■ Comparative clinical trials (rare)
■ Toxicology studies in animals (rare)

Signal confirmation will result in the application of appropriate measures to prevent or minimize its recurrence.

SIGNAL GENERATING VALUE

Any spontaneous report can have a signal generating value if it contains new and previously unknown information on a drug and if probability of causality is strong. A measurement scale based on expectedness and causality could be useful for comparing reporting programs (Biron, *PEDS* 1993;2:579).

SIGNAL INVESTIGATION: HOW TO DO IT

Although the operational aspects of a signal investigation can vary according to the nature and the source of the signal, they are usually fairly uniform. The following are some of the major steps:

DESIGNATION OF RESPONSIBILITY

It is absolutely necessary that a person (or persons) be designated to take the responsibility of ensuring that the investigation is carried out in an appropriate manner and that a final written conclusion is drawn up in a reasonable time frame. The person so designated must have the appropriate qualifications in regard to product knowledge and handling of signals in order to lead the investigation. This requirement is equally applicable to industry and to governmental health authorities. In some countries the "responsible person" is formally and legally designated.

PARAMETERS OF THE INVESTIGATION

▶ **Signal**

If the signal is based on a series of reported AEs, it is necessary to characterize and investigate them clearly. It is also necessary to determine whether the signal is considered to be an acute public health hazard, requiring urgent and immediate measures.

▶ Duration

The investigation should have a clearly defined and limited duration. To prevent a delay in initiating whatever preventive measures are ultimately decided upon, the investigation must be done rapidly. It is often useful to set a *data lock point* (when the database is closed and no further information is collected) and a fixed date for a final report.

▶ Extent

It is also necessary to define and limit the scope of the investigation to medically appropriate and relevant conditions. For example, in an investigation of liver problems, should only fulminant hepatitis cases be examined or should all cases of icterus, cholestasis, and elevated hepatic enzyme levels be examined?

VALIDATION OF THE SIGNAL

If the signal is from spontaneous cases, the principles of validation are applied (see VALIDATION). Since health authorities and industry usually collaborate on signal investigation, it is necessary to examine both (or all databases) and eliminate duplicate reports (after having extracted complementary information from all of the duplicate reports to create a single complete summary of the case).

If the signal is from animal toxicology, epidemiologic studies, database studies, or clinical trials, the person responsible for the investigation may need to consult various experts in the relevant medical specialty. Neither the health authority nor industry should hesitate to enlist the help of these specialists in the field (e.g., rheumatologists, psychiatrists, microbiologists), as well as experts in pharmacology, toxicology, clinical pharmacology, and pharmacoepidemiology. It may be appropriate for consultants to sign confidentiality agreements placing disclosure limitations on some or all parties.

DOCUMENTION SEARCH

▶ Published and Unpublished Studies, Confidential Data

Cohort studies, case-control studies, database studies, clinical trials, animal studies, and all other pertinent information must be collected and examined. A careful examination of the experimental toxicology and premarketing approval data must be made. The latter may be difficult if the information is classified as an industrial secret and is unpublished and unavailable for examination. The summaries available over the Internet (European Product Assessment Reports (EPARs) from the European Medicinal Evaluation Agency (EMEA) and Summary Basis of Approval (SBOAs) from the Food and Drug Administration) are usually not sufficient. Unpublished trials may be found in the Cochrane Library (see COCHRANE LIBRARY).

▶ ADR Databases and Literature

Especially when the signal arises from spontaneous reports, the search must be extended to all cases reported to the pharmaceutical company and its licensees; as those cases in large databases such as the Food and Drug Administration and World Health Organization (WHO) must be examined and validated (where possible). In addition, a literature search for published cases should be done.

The number of patients exposed must be estimated on the basis of sales data and information obtained from companies that track sales and usage (e.g., IMS Health, Inc.) This should be done not only in the country in which the signal originated but also in the rest of the world.

The validation of the entire data set is based on the same criteria used in the validation of individual cases: trustworthiness of the case, plausibility (clinical, epidemiologic, and temporal), as well as data quality. If the data quality is not acceptable in the index cases it is necessary to do aggressive follow-up to obtain complete information. This may involve tracking down data from such diverse sites as ambulance companies, outside laboratories, consultants, and pharmacies, all of which must be done within the appropriate legal, medical, and ethical frameworks.

DISCUSSION AND CONCLUSION

The responsible party must consult all the participants: health authorities, manufacturer, and originators of the signal (the clinician, clinical trial physician, toxicologist, other). After the analysis of the hypothesis generated, a final decision must be reached:

- Signal confirmed
- Signal rejected
- No conclusion possible

The appropriate recommendations follow directly from the final decision. At this stage it is necessary to weigh the following:

- The estimated minimal incidence of the ADR (difficult though this may be)
- The likelihood that the ADR will occur when a patient takes the product
- The approved indication(s) and the indication for which the patient actually received the product
- The existence of alternate therapies and treatments
- The natural course of the indication if untreated
- The importance and likelihood of obtaining the benefit attributed to the product in question
- The seriousness and frequency of the ADR

STRUCTURE OF THE FINAL REPORT

The CIOMS IV Working Group in 1998 proposed the following structure for such reports:

- Introduction (including a brief description of the new ADR in question and whether it has been confirmed or rejected)
- Evaluation of the benefits of the product
- Evaluation of the new risk and its impact on the safety profile of the product
- Comparison with other products and treatments available for the same indication including the prognosis without therapy
- Evaluation of the risk/benefit ratio of the product in question and alternate therapies
- Conclusion
- Analysis of options available

ACTIONS (MEASURES) TAKEN

In many countries the manufacturer may undertake a unilateral action for safety reasons without obtaining prior government agreement. This often occurs in cases that are very clear-cut or have immediate and critical urgency. In situations in which there is more time available, the agency may recommend measures that the company accepts "voluntarily" or the company may propose measures and negotiate with the health authority. If no agreement is reached or if the manufacturer refuses to accede to the authority's requests, then the governmental authority can impose mandatory actions on the manufacturer. In some cases the manufacturer has legal appeal procedures. These procedures vary from country to country.

It is quite interesting also to observe that agency responses can vary significantly from country to country. Such an example occurred with a sedative-hypnotic that was withdrawn from the U.K. market after a safety signal investigation but was allowed to remain on the U.S. market.

An area that poses controversy is whether this analysis should be done in secret or not. From the manufacturer's point of view, public knowledge of an ongoing investigation is unwarranted since it may unfairly tar or even kill a drug that is "innocent until proved guilty." If a signal is ultimately refuted, premature propagation of the adverse effects in question will be very difficult to counter after transmission in the media, the Internet, and so on. Patients who might benefit from the drug might be put off using it. From the point of view of others, full disclosure is always a healthy approach to public health with the most conservative path the best (see PHARMACOTRANSPARENCY).

To learn about the major steps in a governmental or pharmaceutical company signal investigation, read CIOMS IV 1998 and Meyboom (*Drug Saf* 1997;16:355).

SIGNAL, QUALITATIVE

An expression proposed to designate a signal based on spontaneous case reports. If the quality (validity), completeness, case causality, and importance of the signal are sufficient, even a small number of cases can justify a pharmacovigilance investigation. By extension, a quantitative signal would be one based on an increase in frequency of spontaneous reports (corrected for usage) or of adverse effects from clinical or epidemiologic trials (Meyboom, *PEDS* 1997;16:355).

SIGNAL, QUANTITATIVE

This term has been proposed to designate a signal that arises from an increase in the number of spontaneous case reports (corrected for usage) or of adverse effects from clinical or epidemiologic trials (Meyboom, *PEDS* 1997;16:355).

SPONTANEOUS REPORTS
Spontaneous reports in pharmacovigilance databases can to some extent be measured and compared. Prior to 1997, the Food and Drug Administration considered that there was an increase in frequency of AEs when

- The frequency in one period is double that of the preceding period for a product (intraproduct comparison) after correction for sales (usage)
- The frequency for a product is greater than that of products in the same family (interproduct comparison) after correction for sales (usage)
- This was a required analysis in New Drug Application (NDA) periodic reports prior to 1997 (However, because few, if any, signals were discovered by this method, it was dropped as a requirement in periodic reports.)

EPIDEMIOLOGIC STUDIES
These are structured studies and differ from the examination of individual

spontaneous case reports in pharmacovigilance databases. Broadly speaking there are two types of epidemiologic studies: the cohort study, in which the frequency of an AE in a group exposed to the medication is compared to that in a group that was not exposed to the medication, and the case-control study, in which the frequency of exposure to a drug in a group of patients who have the AE is compared to that in a group of patients who did not experience the AE.

In the cohorts of the Prescription Event Monitoring system, patients taking a new drug are monitored for the frequency of AEs in the first month compared to that during subsequent months. A potential signal is thought to occur when the ratio is greater than 3:1 (Inman, *PEDS* 1993;2:239).

LINKED DATABASE STUDIES

Various pharmacoepidemiologic searches can be done with computerized insurance claims databases and medical records databases if record linkage is possible. However, these studies must be interpreted with caution because of the many biases that exist with these data that are not collected for pharmacovigilance reasons but rather for insurance reimbursement or other nonsafety reasons. Studies using such databases must be validated by examination of individual patient medical records.

SIGNAL, UNCONFIRMED; REFUTED SIGNAL

When a signal is not confirmed by a pharmacovigilance investigation, it is referred to as a *false signal* or a *refuted* or *unconfirmed* signal. The examples that follow illustrate the process.

MARKET WITHDRAWAL IN SPITE OF REFUTATION BY EPIDEMIOLOGIC STUDIES
The story of Bendectin provides the foremost example (see BENDECTIN).

MARKET WITHDRAWAL IN SPITE OF NONCONFIRMATION IN HUMANS OF A SIGNAL FROM ANIMAL DATA

Phenolphthalein: A signal can be unconfirmed but still lead to market withdrawal. Phenolphthalein, a base of many over the counter (OTC) laxatives, was reclassified by the FDA in 1997 from category I (safe and effective) to category III (more safety information needed) in response to animal toxicology data that were not confirmed in humans. The drug was later removed from the market (see PHENOLPHTHALEIN:WITHDRAWAL).

SIGNAL FROM SPONTANEOUS REPORTS NOT CONFIRMED IN A LINKED DATABASE STUDY

Scopolamine: convulsions: A signal can be refuted (not confirmed). This anticholinergic in a patch formulation for motion sickness was the subject of spontaneous reports of convulsions. The company performed a linked database study to confirm this signal. The study, at first sight, seemed to confirm the signal since the relative risk of convulsions was four times greater in the 1013 persons exposed to the patch than in the cohorts who received four different comparator medications. However, through good study practices, the medical charts of the patients who had convulsions with scopolamine were examined and not a single case was validated. These results refuted the signal. These results also show the methodologic limitations of linked database studies: all such studies should be validated by examination of the medical charts (Strom, *Clin Pharmacol Ther* 1991;50:107).

SIGNAL FROM SPONTANEOUS REPORTS NOT CONFIRMED BY CLINICAL STUDIES

Pediatric use of vitamin K and leukemia: The publication from 1990 to 1992 of reports of tumors and leukemia in infants previously treated with vitamin K as prophylaxis in the disease of hemorrhage in the newborn led to a pharmacovigilance investigation in the United Kingdom. The conclusions from 12 studies were made public in 1998. The risk of solid tumors was rejected and the risk of leukemia was not confirmed. Since intramuscular vitamin K is effective in this indication, since there is no evident mechanism for this alleged toxicity, and since there is no alternative treatment, no preventive measures were recommended (MCA/CSM, *Curr Probl Phamacovigil* 1998;24:3; Passmore, *Br Med J* 1998;316:178 and 184; McKinney, *Br Med J* 1998;316:173; Parker, *Br Med J* 1998;316:189).

SIGNALS ANALYSIS PROJECT, ADVERSE DRUG REACTION

A project created by the Uppsala Monitoring Center, aiming to discover signals of serious unlabeled adverse effects by looking into the World Health Organization (WHO) database for the presence of unlabeled ADRs, and then examining the utilization data compiled by IMS Health Inc. The project began in 1990 and is aimed at transmitting data to national pharmacovigilance centers. The search for spontaneous reports of strong signaling value can be fruitful in this case because the WHO database is the largest in the world and the center is independent of governments and pharmaceutical companies. Among the 248 new associations identified through 1994, 30 were confirmed by the publication of case reports in the literature (Fucik, *Drug Inf J* 1996;30:461). The bulletin *SIGNALS* is sent to national governmental centers.

Seven "successes" follow:

■ Tiaprofenic acid and aseptic interstitial cystitis (Lindquist, *Pharmacol Toxicol* 1997;80:211)
■ Cisapride and tachycardia, a new association detected and published by the WHO in 1992 but not confirmed by Inman (*Br Med J* 1992;305:1019) using Prescription Event Monitoring; supported in 1994 by Usha (*Indian J Pharmacol* 1994;26:233) and in 1995 by Ahmad (*Lancet* 1995;345:508)
■ Gemfibrozil and arthropathy, a signal discovered by the WHO in 1990 and supported by Smith (*Br J Rhumatol* 1993;32:84)
■ Omeprazole and gynecomastia, noted in the WHO database in 1991, published in 1992 and supported in 1993 from France by Durand (*Rev Med Int* 1993;14:1139, in French) and later in Spain by Pedrosa (*Med Clinica* 1994;102:435, in Spanish)
■ Sumatriptan and cerebrovascular problems detected by the WHO in 1994 and supported by Cavazos (*Lancet* 1994;343:1105)
■ Digoxin (Lindquist, *Drug Invest* 1994;8:73)
■ Omeprazole and visual disturbances (Lindquist, *PEDS* 1996;5:27)

SOURCE DOCUMENTS OF A CASE REPORT

Original written documents (actually these are usually photocopies of the original hospital or physician's office documents) of a pharmacovigilance case report sent to a pharmacovigilance center, health authority, pharmaceutical company, or other body. Source documents may include:

■ The notification form (e.g., CIOMS form, MedWatch form) sent by mail, electronically, or fax and signed by the sender (reporter)

- A medical, legal, or pathology report
- Hospital notes or discharge summary taken from the hospital chart
- Laboratory test results
- Original notes from the pharmacovigilance center when the original report was by telephone
- Responses of the reporter to questions sent to him or her by the pharmacovigilance center in the course of obtaining follow-up information on the case
- Questionnaire completed by the patient or health care provider
- Case log kept by the manufacturer documenting the original receipt date of the report, dates of correspondence with the reporter(s), dates of reporting to health authorities (this document is of particular use by auditors, especially from health authorities, during their examination of cases and is updated as necessary

The case report may also contain additional documents:

- A printout of the case after it is entered into the pharmacovigilance center's database
- Documents reflecting the correspondence between the pharmacovigilance center and the reporter
- Consultation reports forwarded by the reporter or obtained directly from the consultant by the pharmacovigilance center (often in the course of following up on a case, particularly a complicated one, multiple medical consultant reports are obtained, producing multiple "reporters" for a particular case)
- Additional documents obtained in the course of the follow-up from specialists, lawyers, health authorities, consultants to the manufacturer; quality assurance reports showing results of testing of returned or retained samples, and other information

The definition of source documents in the "paperless" environment in which remote data entry of adverse effect information is done directly by the reporter has not yet been fully worked out. In this instance there may never be a written source document other than what is on file in the doctor's or pharmacist's office and these records may be protected from inspection under various privacy laws and regulations (see ELECTRONIC SIGNATURE and PRIVACY).

SPECIAL INTEREST GROUP ON ADVERSE REACTIONS (SIGAR)

A British group that has organized an intensive course in pharmacovigilance for pharmaceutical workers in the European Union. A diploma is awarded after the successful completion of 11 modules (Sigar, *PEDS* 1995;4:305). There are now similar courses in the United States and Europe including those organized by the Drug Information Association (DIA) and Pharmaceutical Education and Research Institute (PERI).

SPONTANEOUS REPORTS DATABASE; ADVERSE DRUG REACTION DATABASE; PHARMACOVIGILANCE DATABASE

A computerized and structured collection of information (database) in which spontaneous reports are collected, classified, validated (by quality control), analyzed, queried, and managed. Such a database constitutes the primary source for pharmacovigilance investigations. This type of database can exist at multiple levels: worldwide, national, regional, hospital, and so forth. It can be run by a governmental health authority, a pharmaceutical company, a university, a quasi-governmental authority (e.g., World Health Organization (WHO)), or some other institution. The largest international database in the world is maintained by the WHO in Uppsala under the direction of Professor I. Ralph Edwards. The largest national database is that of the U.S. Food and Drug Administration. For a specific product, the largest database is usually that of the manufacturer.

SPONTANEOUS REPORTING: DISCUSSION

ADVANTAGES

As a method of surveillance, spontaneous reporting presents certain advantages over structured investigations or trials:

- It incorporates all the medications on the market: old and new; pharmacologics, biologics, blood products; inpatient and outpatient, prescribed drugs and over the counter (OTC) drugs, active ingredients, and excipients; medicinal plants and herbs, and nutritional supplements.
- The system is not expensive since the reporters are acting of their own free will, motivated only by their professional conscience.
- It covers all physicians (primary care, specialists, consultants, etc.) in addition to dentists, pharmacists, nurses, midwives, and other health care professionals and in some countries, consumers and patients.
- In well-organized systems, it provides personalized feedback to the reporter, which constitutes continuing pharmacotherapy education
- It allows for early warning of an alarming new ADR (signaling function).
- By use of a bulletin of pharmacovigilance, it allows communication of new data to practitioners at large.

DISADVANTAGE

The fact remains that it still does not allow the prescriber to "know about the incidence of known adverse reactions in the different clinical practice populations" (Nelson. *PEDS* 2000;9:253). A system of prospective cohorts exposed to selected new drugs would lead to more meaningful information in the drug monographs presented in the national drug compendia since prescribers would appreciate being informed of estimates of incidence rates in the practice setting. For further discussions read Strom 2000 and Stephens 1999.

STEVENS-JOHNSON SYNDROME

In dermatovigilance, a severe form of erythema multiforme with bullae in the mouth, pharynx, and anogenital region often seen with drugs. The eyes may also be affected. It is usually less severe than toxic epidermal necrosis (TEN) (Lyell's syndrome).

STRUCTURED STUDY

A pharmacovigilance investigation may lead to the decision to undertake a structured study to confirm, reject (refute), or clarify a signal. This type of study represents an external part of the investigation since outside health care professionals participate in it. Read the appropriate chapters in Strom 2000 including the section by Strom that begins on page 40: "How Should One Perform Pharmacoepidemiology Studies? Choosing Among the Available Alternatives." These studies would be useful when intensified reporting of AEs/ADRs does not or cannot answer the question posed. Given their high cost, length, and complexity, these studies are usually kept in reserve and used only for the testing of very important signals.

Various types of studies are possible.

SECONDARY DATA STUDY

The application of observational methods to secondary data from health insurance databases not necessarily dedicated to safety are a practical, rapid, and increasingly popular means of evaluating a signal. More useful are safety-dedicated medical-pharmaceutical database studies in which selected data from patient charts in a doctor's office are centrally computerized. The Southampton Green Card System (see PRESCRIPTION EVENT MONITORING) represents a cohort-type study based on medical records of general practitioners (GPs) in the United Kingdom.

PRIMARY DATA STUDY

The creation of a registry of cases is sometimes a prerequisite for a case-control analysis. A case-control observational study is more costly and less rapid than the previous method but is indicated if an AE is very rare. It permits the estimation of relative risk.

An observational cohort study is indicated if the AE in question is relatively frequent, but it is more costly than a case-control study and takes more time. It is, however, less biased and allows estimation of the attributable risk as well as the relative risk.

In very exceptional circumstances, a *comparative clinical trial* can be performed. These studies are still more costly than observational ones but do represent the gold standard for the examination of a paradoxical ADR when the occurrence of the event in the target population is relatively frequent. For instance, the Cardiac Arrhythmia Suppression Trial (CAST) study was able to show the paradoxical pro-arrhythmic effect from anti-arrhythmic agents.

In very rare instances, a *toxicology study* in the appropriate animal species may be useful to study a signal.

SULFANILAMIDE WITH DIETHYLENE GLYCOL

This elixir sold in the United States contained the antibiotic agent sulfanilamide, but it also contained a sufficient amount of diethylene glycol (used still as automobile antifreeze) to produce renal insufficiency. In 1937 after the deaths of 107 people, a major uproar occurred producing the first modern drug safety alert in the United States (Geiling, *JAMA* 1938;111:919). The American government responded by passing the landmark Food, Drug and Cosmetic Act. For the first time there was a requirement that preclinical toxicity testing be done and safety data be furnished on drugs. Efficacy data were not yet required. Nonetheless, this was the beginning of the modern age of drug regulation in the United States.

SUPROFEN: RAPID WITHDRAWAL

This nonsteroidal anti-inflammatory drug (NSAID) produced an unusual entity known as the *flank pain syndrome* with urinary microlithiasis and renal colic. The first reports in the United States rapidly constituted a signal and, thanks to the vigilance of the Food and Drug Administration officials, the situation was investigated and the oral product rapidly withdrawn from the market. Interestingly, the product was also commercialized in the United Kingdom and Italy without the signal's being noted.

Several factors explain the rapid recognition of this problem:

■ The first two reports were from physicians who developed the syndrome after themselves trying samples of the drug. Some have half-seriously proposed that all drugs pass through a phase IV-S (S as in *sample*) by physicians before they are launched!

■ The signal was rapidly evaluated by the FDA and the drug rapidly withdrawn because other NSAIDs were on the market and did not produce this syndrome. The risk/benefit ratio evaluation was clear and straightforward (Rossi, *JAMA* 1983;249:2226; Hart, *Ann Intern Med* 1987;106:235; Rossi, *JAMA* 1988;259:1203; Kaitin, *Clin Pharmacol Ther* 1989;46:121; Strom, *Clin Pharmacol Ther* 1989;46:693).

SURVEILLANCE

There are four types of surveillance associated with marketed drug use, and they should not be confused:

■ Surveillance of patients receiving pharmacotherapy, by their physicians, nurses, pharmacists, and other health care givers (therapeutic monitoring)
■ Surveillance of the costs accrued and avoided (pharmacoeconomics)
■ Surveillance of drug safety profiles (pharmacovigilance)
■ Surveillance of prescriptions and prescribing practices (drug utilization review)

SURVEILLANCE LOG

If patients are taking a drug that is suspected of causing serious and detectable adverse reactions and if early detection can reduce the consequences of these reactions, it can be very useful to maintain a surveillance log for each patient. This log would record the medications taken, blood levels of the drug, clinical state of the patient, and any tests performed to detect or track down the ADR. The keeping of such a log may be done after a pharmacovigilance inquiry has been started, or it may be required by health authorities as a condition of marketing approval.

The antipsychotic *clozapine* provides an example: some national health authorities have required that a surveillance log be kept on all patients prescribed this product because of concern over possible agranulocytosis.

SURVEILLANCE OF PATIENTS RECEIVING PHARMACOTHERAPY

Surveillance is the responsibility of the clinician in regard to all patients receiving a drug product. In this context, the goal is not to discover new ADRs but rather to detect, prevent, and treat any ADRs that do occur. Any AEs/ADRs that occur should be noted in the patient record. They must, of course, be evaluated and treated if appropriate. The term *therapeutic drug monitoring* is used when such surveillance occurs in special situations such as in anesthesia during surgery or is done by monitoring blood levels such as with antiepileptic drugs, digoxin, or lithium therapy. The following examples illustrate the distinction between patient surveillance and pharmacovigilance.

NONSTEROIDAL ANTI-INFLAMMATORY DRUGS (NSAIDS)

▶ **Patient Surveillance**
If an arthritis patient does not tolerate an NSAID the clinician may try a different one or switch to a different class of analgesic (e.g., acetaminophen).

▶ **NSAID Surveillance**
Zomepirac was an NSAID that produced slightly more cases of fatal anaphylaxis than other NSAIDs. It was withdrawn from the market because other NSAIDs were available with less risk and equal benefit.

HALOTHANE AND ICTERUS

▶ Patient Surveillance

If an anesthesiologist observes a posthalothane icterus in a patient, this fact should be clearly and boldly noted in the patient's chart and the clinician should explain to the patient verbally and in writing that he or she should never be re-exposed to this product. The patient should also be questioned again as to previous exposures and risk factors (e.g., previous exposure less than 3 months earlier) (Lack, *Br Med J* 1986;293:1436).

▶ Halothane Surveillance

It is well known that the anesthetic gas halothane can, in rare instances, cause a cholestatic hepatitis probably by way of both allergic and toxic mechanisms. The regulatory action taken after this signal was picked up and confirmed was to change the product labeling rather than to withdraw the drug from the market since the reaction is rare and alternative anesthetics were not totally devoid of hepatotoxicity either. Hence the risk/benefit ratio was still in favor of the drug's staying on the market (Lloyd, *Br Med J* 1986;293:1436). In practice, now that the reaction is well described, should an anesthesiologist observe a posthalothane hepatitis, and if this observation does not add anything to the known risk factors for the reaction, the signaling value of this case of icterus is not strong.

ORAL CONTRACEPTIVES AND THROMBOEMBOLIC PHENOMENA

▶ Patient Surveillance

The Norwegian pharmacovigilance authorities received eight case reports of fatal thromboembolic events in young women (mean age 24) who had taken oral contraceptives over a 6-year period (1978–1984). In half of the women prodromal signs and symptoms of pulmonary emboli were present. The pharmacovigilance authorities thus undertook a preventive measure, reminding physicians to explain the ADRs carefully to users of oral contraceptives with a warning to get emergency medical attention if any of the symptoms occurred (*WHO Drug Information* 1989:3(1)).

▶ Surveillance of the Oral Contraceptives

After the problem that thromboembolic events followed use of oral contraceptives became clear, the dosage of the estrogen was reduced by manufacturers and the incidence of thromboembolic phenomena also dropped, representing a *positive collective dechallenge*.

ORAL HYPOGLYCEMICS

▶ Surveillance of Diabetics

The patient who uses oral hypoglycemic drugs must be informed of the possibility of experiencing syncope, weakness, somnolence, headache, sweating, and hypoglycemia. The prescriber should also be aware that the various hypoglycemic agents have different pharmacokinetic properties and should be customized to the patient to minimize the risk of hypoglycemic episodes. As another example, lactic acidosis is a rare ADR seen with metformin, particularly in patients with renal insufficiency, in whom this drug is contraindicated. The prescriber should follow the patient's renal function periodically.

▶ Surveillance of Oral Hypoglycemics

When it was found that the biguanide phenformin led to an unacceptable risk of lactic acidosis, it was withdrawn from the market.

LITHIUM

▶ **Patient Surveillance**

Patients should be carefully monitored (including measuring blood levels as appropriate) when receiving lithium to guard against signs of intoxication.

▶ **Lithium Surveillance**

Although the safety profile of this drug is well described, the possibility of a drug interaction with newly introduced products is real. Any suspicion of such an event in a patient should be promptly reported to a pharmacovigilance center. "Lithium clinics" are always on the lookout for new interactions.

PARENTERAL BENZODIAZEPINES

▶ **Patient Surveillance**

The use of parenteral benzodiazepines during surgery or invasive procedures (e.g., endoscopy) can produce respiratory depression or even respiratory arrest. Thus during such procedures the following procedures are necessary:

- Prevent this ADR by proper dosing according to weight and age
- Detect this ADR by surveillance of the patient's respiratory status
- Treat this ADR by ventilatory assistance or by pharmacologic reversal of its action (antagonist)

▶ **Product Surveillance**

Since this ADR is well known, only a new new drug interaction or new risk factor merits reporting to a pharmacovigilance center.

SUSPECT DRUG

In a spontaneously reported adverse effect, the suspect drug is a product administered before the AE has begun and is believed by the reporter, the manufacturer, or the health agency to have contributed to its occurrence. It is "suspected" of being the cause of the event and this suspicion makes the *event* a *reaction*. As soon as there is a suspicion in the mind of the reporter the AE becomes an ADR for regulatory reporting purposes. If the suspect drug reaches causality level -1 (i.e., excluded, ruled out), it becomes a *concomitant drug* and the *ADR* becomes an *AE* with nondrug causality.

SUSPECT PRODUCTS: DIVERSITY

The following are among the types of suspect drugs.

▶ **Products of biologic origin: vaccines, blood products**

▶ **Products that are extracted and purified biologics or those totally or partially synthesized by bioengineering:**
Tetanus antitoxin, collagenase, streptokinase, urokinase, purified protein derivative (PPD), alteplase, erythropoietin alpha, interferons alpha-n3, alpha-2a, alpha-2b, interleukin 2

▶ **Products available without prescription over the counter (OTC)**
"Natural" products: medicinal plant/herb products, allopathic, homeopathic, traditional, and alternative products (see PHYTOVIGILANCE).

- Diagnostic products (contrast agents, allergens)
- Blood products

▶ **Replacement drugs: hormones, vitamins, minerals, electrolytes, fluids**

▶ **Nonactive ingredients: excipients**

▶ **Medical, surgical, and dental devices and their interactions with drugs**

SUSPENSION

In regulatory terminology, the temporary or permanent prohibition by the authorities of the right to market a product. Definitive suspension is equivalent to withdrawal of the product. This term is not to be confused with the galenic term *suspension*, which refers to a type of liquid medication for oral use.

SYNDROMES

A certain number of AEs, usually type A, when appearing together can constitute syndromes that are often neurologic or endocrinologic. Unless widely understood by the medical community, syndromes should not be used in product labeling.

NEUROLOGIC SYNDROMES
These syndromes are usually linked to a physiologic modification of neurotransmitters in the central, autonomic, or peripheral nervous system.

▶ **Anticholinergic**

- Central: confusion, memory difficulties, delirium, withdrawal effects
- Peripheral: urinary retention, dry mouth (xerostomia), accommodation problems, increased intraocular pressure (glaucoma), dryness of eyes (xerophthalmia), constipation

▶ **Serotonin**

- At least three of the following: agitation, ataxia, confusion, diarrhea, fever, hypomania, hyperreflexia, myoclonus, sweating, trembling
- Many others such as parkinsonism, toxic malignant hyperthermia with neuroleptics, and Guillain-Barré syndrome (acute polyradiculitis), are neurologic syndromes

ENDOCRINE SYNDROMES
Substitutive hormonal therapy for long periods can produce syndromes ranging from mild to severe. The most well known is hypercorticism (Cushing's syndrome). The example that follows is related to acquired immunodeficiciency syndrome (AIDS):

Lipodystrophy: Lipodystrophy has been observed in AIDS patients receiving antiretroviral therapy (including but not limited to protease inhibitors). This has constituted a new syndrome, sometimes called *pseudo-Cushing's disease* or *fat redistribution syndrome*. A publication of a series of spontaneous cases was an early signal of this syndrome (Massip, *Thérapie* 1997;52 615, English abstract). The signal has been confirmed and must be searched for in patients receiving anti-AIDS therapy (Moyle, *Drug Saf* 1999;4:310).

SYSTEM ORGAN CLASS (SOC)

In the *WHO-ART*, *MedDRA*, and *COSTART* dictionaries of AE/ADR terms, the SOC is the highest level of classification of AEs and covers broad categories (e.g., respiratory system, endocrine system). There are approximately 26 terms in this category (see HIGH-LEVEL TERM, INCLUDED TERM, PREFERRED TERM, *MedDRA*).

TEMAFLOXACIN: MARKET WITHDRAWAL

This quinolone antibiotic was introduced in the United States in mid-February 1992. Within 3 months the Food and Drug Administration had been informed of some 50 serious AEs/ADRs of which 3 were fatal. The product was withdrawn from the market in June 1992 after only 4 months. The AEs/ADRs included hypoglycemia, hemolytic anemia, renal insufficiency, hepatic insufficiency, coagulopathies, and multiple organ failure. Yet the product had been studied in phase III in 4000 patients and had already been on sale in six other industrialized countries (FDA, *Med Bull* 1992;22(2):4; Bakke, *Clin Pharmacol Ther* 1996;58:108; see also the websites www.fda.gov/bbs/topics/NEWS/NEW00279.html and www.fda.gov/medwatch/report/desk/casestud.htm).

This withdrawal illustrates three points:

■ The spontaneous reporting system of pharmacovigilance was very effective (in the United States at least) in discovering these serious ADRs in only 4 months. This speaks to the usefulness of the spontaneous reporting of serious unexpected AE/ADRs.

■ This product did *not* belong to a new class of drugs. Other quinolones were on the market. This illustrates that *class effects* do not always apply. That is, within the same class of drugs, one drug may cause a particular ADR and another one may not.

■ The phase III study of 4000 patients did not reveal these problems. This may reflect the rarity of the ADRs and/or the postmarketing use in types of patients not exposed to the drug in phase III.

TERATOGENICITY

The capability of a substance, when administered to a mother, of producing abnormalities in the offspring.

IN THE ANIMAL

Preclinical animal studies of reproduction and development are required by regulation in most countries. Six segments can be distinguished:

■ Fertility: from mating to conception
■ Preembryonic period: from conception to implantation
■ Embryonic period: from implantation to closure of the palate
■ Fetal period: from closure of the palate to birth
■ Perinatal and postnatal periods: from birth to the end of nursing
■ Late effects: from the end of nursing to the sexual maturity of the animal.

IN THE HUMAN

The use of medications by a pregnant woman can have several types of harmful consequences. The various types of toxicities should be distinguished: inhibition of fertility versus abortive effects (abortifacients); neonatal toxicity before birth due to placental passage of the drug or its metabolites versus that caused by medications taken during nursing and passed to the newborn in the breast milk.

- Segmentation phase (blastogenesis): during the 15 preembryonic days a medication can have a toxic or fatal effect on the blastocyte.
- Embryonic period: teratogenicity is possible if the drug is taken (or persists in the tissues) during the 15th through the 90th day after conception (the first trimester). The period of organogenesis (days 15 to 56) represents the period of the greatest risk for malformations.
- Fetal period: fetal toxicity is possible if the drug is consumed between the 90th day and birth; both structural (bone, brain) and growth abnormalities can occur.

TERATOGENICITY AND FETAL TOXICITY LABELING

There are several scales in use throughout the world and none seems particularly satisfactory.

THE AMERICAN SCALE

This classification has five levels and was proposed in 1979 by the Food and Drug Administration (21CFR201.57).

A: Adequate and well-controlled studies in pregnant women have failed to demonstrate a risk to the fetus in the first trimester of pregnancy (and there is no evidence of risk in the later trimesters).

B: Animal reproduction studies have failed to demonstrate a risk to the fetus, and there are no adequate and well-controlled studies in pregnant women.

C: Animal reproduction studies have shown an effect on the fetus, and there are no adequate and well-controlled studies in humans; the benefits from the use of the drug in pregnant women may be acceptable despite its potential risks.

D: Positive evidence of fetal human risk based on adverse reaction data from investigational or marketing experience or human studies has been found, but the potential benefits from the use of the drug in pregnant women may be acceptable despite its potential risks.

X: Studies in animals or humans have demonstrated fetal abnormalities, or there is positive evidence of fetal risk based on adverse reaction reports from investigational or marketing experience or both, and the risk of the use of the drug in a pregnant woman clearly outweighs any possible benefit.

This scale has been the object of criticism and FDA is indeed reexamining the scales and the entire issue of drug risk and pregnancy (Friedman, *Teratology* 1993;48:5; Teratology Society, *Teratology* 1994;49:446). New initiatives are under way at the FDA to look at pregnancy labeling. See also FDA's draft "Guidance for Industry: Establishing Pregnancy Registries" (www.fda.gov/cder/guidance/2381dft.pdf).

THE SWEDISH SCALE

Sweden was the first country to publish a fetal risk classification (1978). Several other countries followed suit. An X category (absolute contraindication) was not in the original scale but has been proposed as an addition to the Swedish scale (Sannerstedt, *Drug Saf* 1996;14:69). There are four levels:

A: Reliable clinical data indicate no evidence of disturbance of the reproductive process.

B: Data from pregnant women are insufficient.

C: Pharmacologic action of the drug may have undesirable effects on the fetus or the newborn infant.

D: Data indicate an increased incidence of malformations in humans.

THE AUSTRALIAN SCALE

Introduced in 1989, it is based on the four categories used in Sweden and on the X category of the U.S. scale.

TERATOVIGILANCE (BIRTH DEFECT MONITORING)

NARROW DEFINITION

Surveillance of fertile, sexually active women (and occasionally men) with the goal of prevention of congenital malformations. This is done by studying malformations seen with the use of medications (or toxic substances) taken from conception to the end of the embryonic development period.

BROAD DEFINITION

Extended surveillance through the perinatal period, which includes fetal toxicity and neonatal toxicity until the end of weaning. Also called *maternal and neonatal pharmacovigilance.*

This subdomain of pharmacovigilance is quite technical and requires expertise in several fields, including embryology, epidemiology, genetics, neonatology, obstetrics, and pharmacology. Causality determination poses special problems; the use of a universal algorithm is not possible. A pharmacovigilance center wishing to create a particular specialty in this domain must develop a clinical *registry* that includes detailed prospective information on the mothers, fathers, and offspring. Thousands of records must be kept by a dedicated team of experts with the ultimate goal of being able to answer the questions, "I took drug X while pregnant; what will happen to my baby?" and "Can I safely use drug Y during my pregnancy?" Although it may never be possible to give yes or no responses to these questions, it may ultimately be possible to respond with clear probabilities and recommendations backed by solid medical and scientific data. The responses to these questions are obviously quite important since they lead to irreversible decisions and lifelong family consequences for parents and child since a birth defect has consequences for many people, not just one.

PREGNANCY REGISTRIES

Many registries of congenital abnormalities are maintained throughout the world.

▶ Swedish Birth Registry

This registry is unique. It was started in 1973 and contains computerized summaries of maternal, paternal, and offspring antenatal care; delivery records; and results of pediatric examination of the newborn for all pregnancies in Sweden. Data are usually obtained prospectively. To a large degree this is achieved for as many as 80% of pregnancies.

▶ Organization of Teratology Information Services (OTIS)

An umbrella organization of many of the pregnancy and birth registries (http://orpheus.ucsd.edu/otis/).

SPONTANEOUS NOTIFICATION VERSUS REGISTRIES

Retrospective isolated reports of birth defects in which one or more drugs are taken during the pregnancy are not sufficient since some 2% or more of all newborns have some sort of (often minor) birth defect and many women take some medication (including over the counter (OTC) products) during the first trimester of pregnancy. There is significant reporting bias in these retrospective reports: that is, it is likely that women who had a baby with a birth defect and took a medication will report it, whereas a mother who took a medication whose newborn is normal is almost never reported. In addition, there is recall bias, in which women with a baby with a birth defect are more likely to remember having taken a medication than those who had normal offspring. For these reasons, it is generally believed that prospective reporting of pregnancies is the best way to generate solid data with the least bias.

Surveillance is epidemiologic and ideally is conducted by centers that specialize in teratovigilance and maintain registries of exposure and cases. This system allows both a case-control approach for comparison of mothers exposed to drugs who have normal babies with those whose babies are abnormal, as well as cohort studies for comparison of women exposed with women not exposed to the drug whose babies had malformations, all conducted in a prospective manner from conception to delivery.

Although there may not be any further catastrophes of the magnitude of thalidomide and diethylstilbestrol (DES), there are still drugs with teratogenic potential present and on the horizon: thalidomide reintroduced for the treatment of leprosy; retinoic acid, used for the treatment of acne—particularly in young women; as well as other known and unknown teratogens and abortifacients. It is also possible that, in spite of extensive preclinical animal testing, a drug may fail to show teratogenicity until it reaches the human. There is no room for any sense of security in the field of teratovigilance.

TERATOVIGILANCE CENTERS

▶ The Example of *Motherisk*

This well-known center at the Hospital for Sick Children in Toronto, Canada, is dedicated to maternal, fetal, and neonatal surveillance. The unit provides a center for data collection and epidemiologic studies and serves as an information center in pregnancy. Their website (www.motherisk.org) contains the interesting *Motherisk Update* (also published in the *Canadian Family Physician* (www.cfpc.ca)) and their other publications in the medical literature (including *The Motherisk Newsletter)* are full of useful, detailed, and specific information. They are also not hindered by the litigious climate present in the U.S. preventing the dissemination of the information.

REFERENCES

For an introduction try the chapter by Alan Mitchell of the Sloan Epidemiology Unit of Boston University in Strom 2000 and read Gideon Koren (*N Engl J Med* 1998;338:1128).

Teratovigilance centers can subscribe on line to Micromedex's REPRORISK database, which includes *Teris, Reprotox, Reprotext,* and *Shepard's.*

The following are some of the many good references available:

- Briggs G, Freeman R, and Yaffe S. *Drugs in pregnancy and lactation,* 5th edition. Baltimore: Williams & Wilkins, 1998, 1200 pp., also available on CD-ROM; see

the website of the publisher (www.wwilkins.com)
- Koren G. *Maternal-fetal toxicology: a clinician's guide,* 2nd edition. New York: Marcell Dekker, 1994; a new edition is in preparation
- Friedman J and Polifka J. *The effects of drugs on the fetus and nursing infant.* London: Johns Hopkins, 1994 and 1996
- Schardein J. *Chemically induced birth defects.* 3rd edition. New York: Dekker, 2000

TERFENADINE: WITHDRAWAL

Several countries, including the United States in 1998 (*Federal Register* 1997;62(9)1889; *FDA Talk Paper* , 27 February 1998; www.fda.gov/medwatch/safety/1997/seltext.htm.) suspended this H_1 nonsedating antihistamine from the market because of a risk of torsades de pointes discovered through spontaneous AE/ADR reports, noting a drug interaction in most cases. It had been introduced in the early 1980s and only the spontaneous notification system proved capable of detecting this rare ADR. The arrhythmogenic potential was subsequently confirmed by examining all ADR databases available.

CARDIOTOXICITY

The ADR begins with the prolongation of the QT/QTc interval that leads to ventricular tachycardia (of which torsades de pointes is a variant that is often of drug origin), which can degenerate into fatal ventricular fibrillation. Terfenadine is a cardiotoxic prodrug that is normally 99% metabolized to fexofenadine, an active but noncardiotoxic metabolite, during the first pass through the liver by way of the cytochrome P450 isoenzyme CYP3A4. Accumulation in the blood of terfenadine, which is arrhythmogenic at high concentrations, can result from overdose or pharmacokinetic or pharmacodyamic factors.

RISK FACTORS: PHARMACOKINETIC

- Liver disease: hepatitis, cirrhosis, others
- Concomitant medications, some of which are competitively metabolized by the same p450 isoenzyme
- Certain *azole antifungals,* such as ketoconazole, itraconazole, and fluconazole, at high doses
- Certain *macrolide antibiotics,* such as erythromycin, clarithromycin, troleandomycin
- Certain *foods,* such as pineapple juice, which contain flavonoids

RISK FACTORS: PHARMACODYNAMIC

- Electrolyte abnormalities: hypokalemia, hypocalcemia, hypomagnesemia
- Cardiac disease: congenital or acquired QT prolongation, bradycardia
- Concomitant medications: antiarrhythmics of class Ia and III, psychotropics, antimalarials

WHAT ALTERNATIVES?

Even if the risk of fatal arrhythmias is very rare, no fatal or life-threatening reaction is acceptable since the indication is benign (allergic rhinitis, urticaria, etc.) and alternative nonsedating H_1 blockers that do not present this risk are available (Lindquist, *Lancet* 1997;349:1322). Thus terfenadine has been withdrawn from the market, and fexofenidine, the noncardiotoxic metabolite, has recently been marketed.

TEXTBOOK OF ADVERSE DRUG REACTIONS

The excellent textbook by D.M. Davies et al. (5th edition, Chapman & Hall, London, U.K., 1998) aims at presenting the wide range of iatrogenic diseases of drug origin, thus contributing to the clinical knowledge and the differential diagnosis of adverse effect. It is entirely devoted to AEs/ADRs classified by organ systems. It is also useful for clinicians, academic physicians, clinical pharmacologists, and those giving expert medical advice or testimony who wish an expert opinion on the risks of older products used in medical treatment. Pharmacoepidemiologists appreciate in particular the chapters that treat the historic aspects, the epidemiologic characteristics, and mechanisms of action of ADRs as well as later chapters dealing with medical-legal issues, interactions, and excipients.

THALIDOMIDE: TRAGIC TERATOGENICITY

INTRODUCTION

Thalidomide was launched in 1957 and withdrawn from the market in 1961 after the occurrence of the most well-known ADR tragedy since World War II. This episode resulted in the creation of governmental pharmacovigilance structures in many countries that had never had such oversight before and pushed countries that did to tighten their existing systems.

It is estimated that between 7000 and 8000 people were affected. Introduced as a tranquilizer in Europe in 1957, it was unfortunately used by women during pregnancy. It was shown to be teratogenic when taken during the first trimester, producing phocomelia (abnormal development of the arms and/or legs), which was so unusual as to be almost diagnostic for thalidomide use. Between 1946 and 1961 no episodes of phocomelia similar to the thalidomide cases were seen in the 12,000 reports in a pregnancy registry at Columbia Presbyterian Hospital in New York City.

The natural incidence (*reference* or *baseline risk*) is estimated to be around 1/10,000 births (though this seems to be an overestimate). It is interesting to note that chemically related drugs (e.g., chlorthalidone, a diuretic, and glutethimide, a hypnotic) did not produce phocomelia. The drug was never approved by the Food and Drug Administration in the United States, but some samples were distributed. It should also be noted that thalidomide can produce neurotoxicity in the patient taking it quite apart from the teratogenic effects.

The developmental abnormalities are varied and related to a critical period ("the teratogenic window"), as expressed in terms of days of the pregnancy (days since conception):

    34–38 days: absence of the ear

    38–45 days: absence of the thumbs or extremities

    38–50 days: shortening of the arms or dislocation of the hip

    42–46 days: absence of the legs

The preclinical animal toxicology testing did not reveal this effect: the rat and mouse did not show the effect and the rabbit and hamster had only occasional abnormalities. The New Zealand white rabbit appears to be the best model but was not used in the initial animal testing (Mellin, *N Engl J Med* 1962;267:1184; Nowack, *Human-Genetik* 1965;1:516; Griffin, *Adv Drug React Toxicol Rev* 1994;13:65).

IN GERMANY

The drug was first synthesized in Germany in 1954 and commercialized there in 1956 as a sedative-hypnotic. One case of phocomelia was observed in 1959 in a pediatric clinic in Hamburg. No cases had been seen in that clinic from 1949 to 1959, but after 1959 the number increased rapidly. In November 1961 at a pediatrics meeting a presentation of a possible link to thalidomide was made. Also that year several case reports were published (Distillers Company, Biochemicals Ltd., *Lancet* 1961;2:1262; Mcbride, *Lancet* 1961;2:1538).

A case-control study was conducted in the course of the pharmacovigilance investigation (Mellin, *N Engl J Med* 1962;267:1238). The relative risk was clearly shown to be very high: phocomelia occurred in 20% of the exposed women compared to a rate in nonexposed women of 0.01% (1/10,000), resulting in a relative risk of 2000:1.

The increase in the number of cases (154 in one Hamburg clinic alone) correlated with the use of the product. The subsequent withdrawal of the product from the market was followed by a fall in the number of cases. This approach, the linking of records from a case registry with drug use, represented a positive *collective dechallenge* (Taussig, *JAMA* 1962;180:101 and 1106). A retrospective cohort study of 113 pregnancies also served to confirm the causality (Kajii, *Teratology* 1973;8:163).

IN CANADA

Thalidomide was sold briefly for 8 months in Canada even though the problem had already been noted in other countries. At the time there was no national legislation allowing the government to withdraw medications that were judged dangerous from the market; rather, the product labeling carried restrictions for use aimed at physicians. In reaction to the thalidomide tragedy, the Canadian government changed the law in 1962, allowing the authorities to withdraw a medication from the market for safety reasons.

IN SOUTH AMERICA

The product is used against a form of leprosy, the type 2 leprous reaction, present in 10% to 50% of patients. In Brazil, annual production of some 8 million tablets is permitted even though the teratogenic effects are well known (Cutler, *Lancet* 1994;343:795).

NEW INDICATIONS – "A SECOND CAREER" – NEW RISKS

Thalidomide has returned as an immunomodulator. It is now the subject of numerous requests for marketing approval in spite of the teratogenic consequences of its use. In the United States, the Food and Drug Administration authorized its use in 1998 for the cutaneous manifestations of leprosy, 37 years after the phocomelia catastrophe. Additional indications are being studied, including acquired immunodeficiciency syndrome (AIDS), some rare autoimmune diseases, such as Behcet's Syndrome and discoid lupus erythematosus, as well as use in transplant patients.

These new immunomodulatory indications pose the obvious problem: how to prevent women of childbearing potential from being exposed to the drug and giving birth to a baby with a high probability of having phocomelia? In the United States, the labeling has a severe black box warning, and an informed consent must be signed by patients (both male and female) using the drug and by physicians authorizing its use. In the United Kingdom dermatologists are permitted to treat prurigo nodularis with thalidomide in carefully selected patients: men and postmenopausal women. Frequent pregnancy tests are required as well as two means of contraception (Gunzler, *Drug Saf* 1992;7:116; Powell, *Postgrad Med J* 1994;70:901; CSM/MCA, *Curr Probl Phamacovigil* 1994;20:8).

THERAPEUTIC DRUG MONITORING

The expression *therapeutic drug monitoring* is used in two senses:

PLASMA OR SERUM LEVEL BLOOD LEVEL

This measurement is very useful in long-term treatment with a drug whose therapeutic index is very narrow. It fulfills the double objective of determining whether the drug level is sufficiently high to be efficacious and, at the same time, sufficiently low to prevent toxicity. The detection of elevated levels also fulfills the objective of preventing dose-dependent ADRs and aiding causality assessment of an adverse effect: a high blood level is interpreted as a risk factor in favor of a drug cause of an AE.

MEASURE OF THE DRUG'S ACTIVITY

Anesthetics: Patient monitoring during anesthesia represents a particular type of drug monitoring. The anesthesiologist simultaneously monitors the effects of the surgery as well as blood loss and drug effects. Anesthesiologists are often the best pharmacologists in all the medical specialties. They do minute-by-minute, if not second-by-second, verification of beneficial and undesirable pharmacologic effects. They may be the only physicians who truly see the results of their pharmacologic choices of drug, route of administration, doses, and effects since they have the benefit of immediate feedback. In this high-stress area, error is not permitted and death hovers close by. The remarkable development of surveillance techniques and technology for cardiovascular and respiratory functioning has reduced the morbidity and mortality rates surrounding modern-day surgery.

Anticoagulants: The dosing of anticoagulants is not done directly but rather indirectly by use of anticoagulant activity as a surrogate for plasma or serum concentration.

THERAPEUTIC GOODS ADMINISTRATION (TGA)

The Australian drug authority. The counterpart of the Medicines Control Agency in the United Kingdom and the Food and Drug Administration in the United States (www.health.gov.au/tga).

THERAPEUTIC MEASURES; TREATMENT OF THE ADVERSE EFFECT

In pharmacotherapy, the clinician confronted with an AE suspected of being an ADR must decide which measure or measures to take in order to act in the best interests of the patient:

- Cessation
- Dose Reduction: daily dose is reduced if a suspected ADR is dose dependant (type A)
- Change in the method of administration: the treatment is continued with the suspect product but using a different route (a nonsteroidal anti-inflammatory drug (NSAID) by suppository when the oral form causes nausea) or a different dosing schedule (e.g., with food instead of fasting).

- Addition of a (corrective) treatment: the treatment with the suspect product is continued, but a corrective treatment (e.g., a potassium-sparing diuretic to prevent the hypokalemia induced by a potassium-losing diuretic)
- Substitution: replacement of stopped drug with another version of the same active entity, with a different drug from the same class, or with a drug from a different class
- Diagnostic measures to determine the cause of the AE: if the product in question is determined to be necessary for the patient's well-being and not easily substitutable, the clinician may undertake diagnostic measures in the hope of showing the drug is not the cause of the AE

Cessation and (corrective) treatment: there are five categories of corrective treatments:

- Specific antidote (naloxone in respiratory depression induced by a narcotic) Nonspecific antagonist (a beta-blocker for a tachycardia induced by an anti-thyroid medication)
- Treatment to remove the drug (activated charcoal, hemodialysis, other)
- Pharmacologic treatment of the AE (epinephrine for anaphylactic shock)
- Cessation of the drug followed by its reintroduction (the physician may try an intentional rechallenge and, if the AE does not reappear, continue treatment)
- Other examinations and tests: blood levels of the product determined if overdosage is suspected, cutaneous biopsy of skin lesions to obtain a precise diagnosis, allergy tests, response to antagonist, others

It must be noted that when a second drug is given to treat or prevent an ADR caused by the initial drug, this "counterdrug" may produce ADRs itself, making the determination of which drug produced an ADR very difficult indeed. This is particularly true in cases of withdrawal syndromes that occur after both the stopping of the suspect drug and the beginning of the antagonist drug or of an ADR that is labeled for both drugs.

THERAPEUTIC PRODUCTS PROGRAMME (TPP)

In Canada, the name given in 1996 to the Drugs Directorate. This change was adopted after the creation in the United States of the MedWatch program in 1993.

THERAPEUTIC WINDOW; THERAPEUTIC INDEX

This term refers to the difference, the spread, between the toxic blood concentration (or dose) of the drug in question and the therapeutic, effective blood level (or dose). During the phase I trials of the clinical development of a product, one of the objectives is to find the maximal tolerated dose of the product in question. The term *toxic* refers to unacceptable ADRs and the term *therapeutic* refers to pharmacologic activity. A *narrow* therapeutic window or index refers to a situation in which the toxic and the therapeutic levels are very close to each other and the risk of toxicity is greater than that seen with a product that has a wide therapeutic window.

A narrow therapeutic window is accepted when the expected benefit is great and there are no other acceptable alternative therapies (e.g., anticoagulants, lithium in bipolar disorders, certain cancer drugs, antibiotics of last resort).

The monitoring of blood levels of a drug is indicated in the pharmacosurveillance of patients when the therapeutic window is narrow. Although the term *digitalis intoxication* has become hallowed by usage, this is more properly a question of supratherapeutic doses. Clinical toxicologists in poison control centers prefer to reserve the terms *intoxication* or *massive overdose* for those patients who took accidental or suicidal doses of drugs rather than for those who took ostensibly *normal* doses of a drug that produced toxicity as a result of narrow therapeutic windows.

THÉRAPIE

The official journal of the French Society of Pharmacology (Société Française de Pharmacologie). The articles have English abstracts or are written in English. It is indexed in Medline, Embase/Excerpta Medica Drugs and Pharmacology and Current Contents and contains the proceedings of an annual meeting on pharmacovigilance (an example to follow in other countries) and several original ADR case reports. See the website of the society (http://www.pharmacol-fr.org/). It is published by John Libbey & Co Ltd in the United Kingdom.

THIRD PARTY ADVERSE DRUG REACTION

Expression sometimes used to describe ADRs that occur in a sexual partner (see TRANSMISSION, SEXUAL), an embryo/fetus (see TERATOVIGILANCE), a breast-fed infant, or a medical professional (e.g., bronchospasm in a nurse inhaling psyllium while mixing the powder).

TICRYNAFEN: RAPID MARKET WITHDRAWAL

This drug was launched in the United States in May 1979 and withdrawn from the market 8 months later because of fulminant hepatitis (FDA, *Drug Bulletin* 1980;10:3; Zimmerman, *Hepatology* 1984;4:315; Kaitin, *Clin Pharmacol Ther* 1989; 46:121; see also the Food and Drug Administration's website, www.fda.gov/cder/fdama/fedreg/pcwdrawn.pdf).

Rapid withdrawals are the signs of a well-functioning pharmacovigilance system, in which important signals are acted upon in a timely fashion with the interest of public health in mind. Hepatic ADRs represent a frequent cause of drug withdrawal.

TIME HORIZON; TEMPORAL WINDOW

The interval during which an undesirable event is capable of occurring in patients exposed to the product in question. This temporal window is used in the Bayesian model of causality assessment; for further information see Lane (*Drug Inf J* 1986;20:455).

TEMPORAL PLAUSIBILITY
If an AE/ADR occurs outside the reasonable period during which it is likely to occur as a drug effect, then the drug can be considered causally excluded. There are several possibilities:

▶ Occurrence Before the Drug Is Used
The first sign of the AE occurs *before* the patient has taken the first dose of the suspect product. For example, icterus occurs 6 days after the first dose of the product, but, upon careful questioning, the physician elicits the fact that anorexia, asthenia, and malaise occurred 8 days before the first dose. In clinical trials, it is particularly important to elicit and note all problems before starting the study drug, since failure to do so could falsely implicate the drug in the causality of an AE that existed before the trial started.

▶ **Too Short an Interval After the Start of Treatment**

Suppose that corneal deposits ("cat scratches") appeared after only three doses of amiodarone. This is too short a period to implicate amiodarone as a cause.

▶ **Too Long an Interval After a Single Dose**

Anaphylactic shock occurred 3 weeks after a single dose of penicillin. The penicillin cannot be implicated as a cause.

▶ **Too Long an Interval After the Last Dose**

Cholestatic hepatitis that appears more than 2 months after the last dose or a cytolytic hepatitis that occurs more than 1 month after the last dose of a rapidly metabolized drug cannot reasonably be attributed to the drug.

▶ **Occurrence Outside the Teratogenic Window**

In the case of a congenital malformation, the critical teratogenic period in the development of the embryo/fetus in utero must be taken into account. The following is the classic example:

> *Thalidomide:* Thalidomide taken toward the end of the second trimester of pregnancy cannot be implicated in the production of phocomelia. In fact, there are temporal limits in pregnancy for each of the malformations: 34–38 days for the absence of the ear, 38–45 days for the absence of the thumb or limbs, 38–50 days for the shortening of the arms or for dislocation of the hips, 42–46 days for the absence of the legs.

TIME TO IMPROVEMENT OR DISAPPEARANCE

Also called time to offset (Stephens 1999;304) in opposition to time to onset. A critical piece of information in an AE report. It is the interval between the last dose of the suspect drug and either the beginning of the improvement or the complete resolution of the problem. The reliability of the observation is perhaps greater when it is that of the physician or is documented by laboratory examinations rather than by reliance on the patient's memory of the event, which is subject to recall bias. Especially in ADRs of type A, the time to improvement may have more diagnostic value than the time to complete resolution.

TIME TO ONSET

The interval between the *critical dose* of the suspect drug and the first manifestation of the AE. It is the principal chronologic characteristic of the event that is used in the determination of causality.

THE CRITICAL DOSE

The *critical dose* usually is the first dose but not necessarily so.

▶ **The Last Dose**

- In a withdrawal or rebound adverse effect, the time to onset is calculated from the last dose.
- In teratology both the first and the last dose are important; their occurrence must be compared with the fetal developmental period.
- When the period is rather long, we usually speak of latency.
- Cancer of the vagina appeared 20 years after in utero exposure to diethylstilbestrol: a latency period of 20 years after the last exposure; congenital anomalies usually have a built-in latency period since the exposure occurs in utero and the clinical appearance does not occur for several months (at birth) or even later.

■ Acute hepatitis that is thought to be caused by a drug with a very short half-life, might have a different cause if the latency period exceeds 15 days for a cytolytic (necrosis) hepatitis or exceeds 30 days for a mixed or cholestatic hepatitis (Benichou 1994).

▶ **An Erroneous Dose**

An erroneous dose may be the first, last, or only dose.

▶ **The First Dose at a Higher Dosage**

For a dose-dependent ADR that abates with dose reduction, the first higher dose may be the critical dose.

▶ **The First Dose of a Second Drug**

The first dose of the second drug that is suspected of interacting with the first drug may act as a triggering factor for the ADR and thus be the critical dose; an example would be a macrolide antibiotic added to the antihistamine terfenadine producing a severe cardiac arrhythmia taken daily during the hay fever season.

▶ **Every Dose**

Every dose of a drug given at regular and fixed intervals (e.g., daily) and for which the ADR follows with the same time to onset after each dose may constitute the critical dose.

TIME TO ONSET: VARIABILITY MISLEADING TO THE DIAGNOSTICIAN

A time to onset that is variable from patient to patient can lull the clinician into a false sense of security, thinking that the danger period has passed. As eternal vigilance is the price of liberty, it is also the price of good pharmacovigilance.

▶ **Angiotensin Converting Enzyme (ACE) Inhibitor-Induced Angioedema**

This ADR can appear after several years of treatment and can occur one time only or multiple times if the product is not suspected and stopped. In the Australian experience with these products, the reaction appeared during the first week of treatment in 42% of the cases, after 1 month in 32%, and after more than 3 months in 22%. The world's record for time to onset seems to be 7 years in three cases!

At least two patients had the unbelievable record of three dozen positive rechallenges (ADRAC, *Aust ADR Bull* 1996;15:15; Black, *Ausr N Z J Med* 1995;25:746) and a third had 19 emergency room visits with angioedema and respiratory difficulties (Finley, *Am J Emerg Med* 1992;10:550). Once the diagnosis of ACE inhibitor–induced angioedema is made or suspected, it is dangerous to continue the treatment with the suspect drug or with any other ACE inhibitor, since the relative risk of recurrence after the first episode increases 10-fold and it is never clear whether the next episode will produce possibly fatal respiratory compromise.

Fatal cases have been reported with many of the ACE inhibitors that have been widely used. The mechanism is probably a class effect and related to kinin production by inhibition of kininase. The long time to onset is a source of diagnostic confusion since it may falsely lower the physician's level of suspicion of the ACE inhibitor and of a pathologic cause related to the absence of an inhibitor of C1 esterase (C1 INH), which allows an accumulation of kinins by reducing their metabolism (Career, *Eur J Clin Chem Clin Biochem* 1992:30:793).

TIME TO RECURRENCE OR REAPPEARANCE

The interval between a rechallenge and the reappearance of the AE. If the mechanism is immunologic, this time is usually shorter and more severe than that of the original challenge. This shortness and the increase in severity argue in favor of an immunologically mediated ADR. The reappearance of the same undesirable effect after a rechallenge is usually a very strong factor in linking the event to the drug in question.

TIME TO REPORT/PUBLISH

FOR MANUFACTURERS

The term *time to report* can have two meanings. For the pharmaceutical manufacturer it can refer to the legally permissible time between first receipt of an AE and the date it must be reported to health authorities. During this time follow-up may need to begin and the case be written up on the appropriate form (e.g., MedWatch, CIOMS 1 form). The time frames, depending on the drug and the event, may be quite stringent (7 or 15 calendar days for certain serious and unexpected events) or more relaxed (e.g., 3 months, yearly, 5-yearly) for other cases.

FOR CLINICIANS

The second meaning of *time to report* or *time to publish* can refer to the clinician who is aware of a serious unexpected ADR in one of his or her patients. It is not rare for a clinician who intends to report to wait before filling out the notification form and sending it off to the authorities. This may occur for many reasons including a lack of time or a desire to follow the patient to observe the course and outcome of the event. Sometimes a clinician may wait to observe a second, similar case before reporting both.

In a study of five medical journals comprising 297 articles containing 384 cases (i.e., 1.29 cases per article), it could be calculated that as many as 87 of the authors (23%) had waited for a second case before sending in a manuscript (Haramburu, *Lancet* 1985;2:550).

During this study the authors looked at the mean delay between the date of the first observation of an unexpected adverse effect and its appearance in one of the journals studied: *Lancet, British Medical Journal, Journal of the American Medical Association, New England Medical Journal* and *La Presse Médicale.* The mean time for a case that was thought to have a strong signal value was 62 weeks and for all AEs studied, 69 weeks. The authors concluded that clinicians who observe important new AEs/ADRs should report these cases to medical journals more quickly and that the journal editors should also publish the cases more rapidly even if only as letters to the editor. With earlier reporting perhaps fewer people would suffer from ADRs.

TOLRESTAT: RAPID WITHDRAWAL

This aldose-reductase inhibitor used to treat the severe retinal, renal, and neurologic complications of diabetes was launched in Argentina in 1992.

SIGNAL

After 3 years on the market and exposure of about 3000 patients, a 41-year-old female reported with abdominal pain and icterus after 50 days of tolrestat treatment. In spite of a dechallenge, she died 30 days later of massive hepatic necrosis. This signal case was reported in March 1995.

PHARMACOVIGILANCE INVESTIGATION

The Argentine pharmacovigilance authorities conducted a literature search and requested a search for cases in the World Health Organization (WHO) Uppsala database and in the database of the manufacturer.

CALL FOR REPORTS AND SURVEILLANCE

The Argentine authorities sent out a call for reports and had the manufacturer send a Dear Doctor letter to 1200 endocrinologists asking for case reports as well as requesting monthly alanine aminotransferase (ALT) measurements in patients taking the drug. This resulted in two reports in October 1996 of fatal hepatic necrosis, one in Canada and one in Italy.

WITHDRAWAL

Given the limited clinical impact of the product, the three deaths were thought to render the risk/benefit ratio unacceptable and the product was withdrawn from the world market by the manufacturer in October 1996 in a timely manner.

TORSADES DE POINTES

A type of ventricular tachycardia characterized by a cause that is almost always drug-related or at least xenobiotic-related. It is rare but has the potential for evolution into a possibly fatal arrhythmia.

First described by Dessertene (*Presse Med* 1969;77:193; see also Roden, *Heart* 2000;84:235), torsades de pointes (which translates to "twisting around the peaks") is identified by an initial prolongation of the QT/QTc interval on the electrocardiogram followed by cyclical variations in the duration and amplitude of the QRS waves, producing an oscillation ("twisting") around the baseline. This ADR was the cause of the suspension of marketing of the nonsedating antihistamine terfenadine.

In April 2000 the manufacturer and the Food and Drug Administration decided to discontinue general U.S. marketing of cisapride, a gastric motility promoter used for heartburn. The drug was made available only through an investigational limited access program because of 341 cases of arrhythmias (ventricular tachycardia and fibrillation, torsades de pointes and QT prolongation) with 80 deaths. (Janssen, *Dear Doctor Letter*, 12 April 2000). Drug-induced QTc prolongation and torsades de pointes are now under intensive scrutiny by the FDA, EMEA, and other organizations.

TOXIC EPIDERMAL NECROLYSIS (TEN)

A type of bullous skin reaction also designated Lyell's syndrome. It is more severe than Stevens-Johnson syndrome and is often of drug origin. It is a medical emergency for which treatment, similar to that of severely burned patients, is often required at a tertiary care medical center. This important adverse effect is well covered in dermatovigilance literature.

TOXICOLOGY STUDY; ANIMAL TOXICOLOGY STUDY

A study performed in animals to determine the target organs of action by the drug in question or its metabolites. A dose that is sufficiently high must be used in order to produce toxicity. That is, a toxicology study that does not demonstrate toxicity is an inadequate toxicology study, suggesting that an insufficient dose was used or the route of administration that was chosen was inadequate for absorption of enough of the product to produce toxicity. Thus, it is generally not acceptable to say that an animal toxicology study showed no toxicity.

During the course of a pharmacovigilance investigation it is useful to review the animal toxicology studies in order to:

- Reproduce the ADR to confirm its causality in the human
- Identify the molecule responsible for toxicity in a combination product
- Identify the site of concentration of the molecule
- Identify risk factors
- Elucidate the mechanisms of action
- Develop an antidote, a prophylactic treatment or a curative treatment
- Test a modification of the molecule (for example, replacement of terfenadine by its metabolite fexofenadine)

TOXICOVIGILANCE AND CLINICAL TOXICOLOGY

Surveillance of poisoning, both due to medications and due to other causes. The major practitioners of this science are the poison control centers throughout the world. As soon as a new drug arrives on the market it becomes a candidate for accidental and nonaccidental (suicidal) overdosages, which obviously cannot be studied during the clinical trial period. Thus, it is imperative to rapidly develop the diagnostic techniques to identify overdoses (blood and urine levels if appropriate), treatments for the overdoses, and, where applicable, prophylaxis for overdose. This information should be added to the product labeling as soon as it is available. The poison control centers play a major role in elucidating this information.

CLINICAL TOXICOLOGY

This medical specialty applies medical and toxicologic science to the diagnosis and treatment of poisoning by medication overdosage and by nonmedication intoxication as practiced in poison control centers in collaboration with specialists in the pharmaceutical, toxicologic, and environmental professions.

TRANSIT SITE REACTION

This type of ADR is not always evident and the clinician must maintain a level of suspicion to make the diagnosis. It usually occurs in a hollow viscus (e.g., the gastrointestinal (GI) tract) and can be characterized by obstruction, ulceration, perforation, or hemorrhage. Its causality is almost always considered "very probable, definite, certain," corresponding to a causality level of 4.

ESOPHAGEAL RETENTION AND POSSIBLE OBSTRUCTION OR ULCERATION

An esophageal ulcer in situ by local retention of the pharmaceutical product swallowed must be distinguished from a pharmacologic effect of a drug that acts on the esophagus after reaching the circulation. Some products have a topical corrosive action on the esophageal or pharyngeal mucosa if the product remains in contact with these areas for extended periods. This may occur if the patient does not use sufficient fluid in swallowing the drug to lubricate the esophagus (usually at least 180 ml or 6–8 ounces), if the patient has a motility disorder in the esophagus or pharynx (more frequent in the elderly), if the patient has an esophageal stricture (usually due to peptic acid disease), or if the drug has a large size, unusual shape, and/or sticky coating. It has been recommended that patients swallow fluid *before, during,* and *after* taking the pill and that patients should be upright when taking the drug and not lie down for at least a half-hour thereafter; oesophageal motility is reduced in the supine posture. For an example with the product alendronate, see De Groen (*N Engl J Med* 1996;335:1016).

TRANSMISSION, PLACENTAL

A drug administered to a pregnant woman can be transmitted to the fetus via the placenta. There are two types of AE/ADR reports that can be made (ICH E2B): if the ADR affects the fetus but not the mother, this is referred to as a *parent-fetus report* and only a single form (e.g., CIOMS 1, MedWatch) need be filled out. If the mother and the fetus are affected, it is recommended that two separate reports be made, specifying that they are *linked.*

TRANSMISSION, SEXUAL

A medication can be involuntarily transmitted to another person for whom it was not prescribed. This type of transmission is relatively rare but is certainly possible. There are multiple routes of transmission from the sexual organs to other sexual organs and to other orifices.

SPERM-VAGINA

Antibiotic anaphylaxis: Ms. X is allergic to penicillin, when her husband was prescribed oral dicloxacillin she developed a mild anaphylactic reaction 30 minutes after each episode of unprotected sexual intercourse while the husband was taking the antibiotic. The use of a condom prevented this reaction. This published case report is a "gem" of differential diagnosis and case causality assessment by an astute clinician, definitely worth reading (Green, *JAMA* 1985;254:531).

Antibiotic allergy: Ms. Y is allergic to penicillin; when her husband is given mezlocillin injections she experiences an immediate postcoital allergic reaction. The concentration of the antibiotic in the seminal fluid is 42 mg/ml (Burks, *Arch Intern Med* 1989;149:1603).

Phenothiazine urticaria: A 28-year-old female without any previous history of allergy had an urticarial reaction 24 hours after coitus with her husband after he had begun taking 10 mg of thioridazine, a phenothiazine antipsychotic, before bedtime. Her allergy skin test result was positive for this drug. The spermatic concentration of thioridazine was 17 ng/ml. The use of a condom ended this reaction (Sell, *Am J Psychiatry* 1985;142:271).

Chemotherapy vaginitis: A postcoital vaginitis appeared rapidly in a woman after her partner began treatment for Hodgkin's disease with vinblastine (Paladine, *N Engl J Med* 1975;292:52).

VAGINA-PENIS

Estrogen and gynecomastia: A woman whose 60+-year-old husband remained sexually active was using a dienestrol 0.01% cream for vaginal lubrication just before sexual relations. One month later unilateral gynecomastia developed in the husband. This led to surgical treatment with all the risks and costs inherent therein. Ten months later gynecomastia occurred in the remaining breast. At this point the cream became the prime suspect. Three months after stopping of the cream, the gynecomastia in the remaining breast disappeared (Diraimondo, *N Engl J Med* 1980;302:1089). A similar case was reported several years later (Moore, *Lancet* 1988;1:468).

Nitrate headache: A 72-year-old male with coronary artery disease who habitually used a transdermal nitrate patch decided to apply the patch to his penis. Twelve hours later he had sexual intercourse with his wife. Several minutes later she experienced a very severe headache (Talley, *Ann Intern Med* 1985;103:804).

Testosterone hypertrichosis: A man who believed he was suffering from hypogonadism began on his own initiative to apply testosterone cream on various parts of his body. Soon his wife experienced androgenic-type facial hypertrichosis. Dechallenge was positive (Moore, *Lancet* 1988;1:468).

SKIN-TO-SKIN

Vasodilator flushing: A 60-year-old man with coronary artery disease applied isosorbide cream to his precordial chest region. His wife of the same age complained of headache and flushing several minutes after the start of sexual relations. The dechallenge was positive when the husband changed the site of the application of the isosorbide (Lewis, *Lancet* 1983;1:1441).

TRETINOIN: ZERO TOLERANCE

The addition of retinoic acid to cosmetic products was banned in March 1988 in Germany because of its teratogenic potential. The permitted concentration of the product was only 0.001%, but because the benefit was thought to be minimal or nonexistent, and the risk to the fetus theoretically established for other tretinoin-based products, the risk/benefit ratio was judged to be unacceptable. This is an example of zero tolerance of risk (WHO, *Drug Inf* 1988;2(3)).

TROGLITAZONE: MARKET WITHDRAWAL

This first product in a new family of oral diabetes drugs—the thiazolidinediones—showed significant toxicity soon after its launch in the United States and Japan in 1997 (CSM/MCA, *Curr Probl Phamacovigil* 1997;23:13; FDA, *Talk Paper,* December 1, 1997).

SIGNAL
Spontaneous reports of liver toxicity including two severe outcomes (a death and a liver transplant) occurred soon after launch.

PREVENTIVE MEASURE
A Dear Doctor letter was sent to professionals by the manufacturer, suggesting surveillance of liver function.

LITERATURE/DATABASE SEARCH
In less than a year after launch, the worldwide ADR database contained 130 cases of which 6 were fatal. Analysis of these cases revealed the following:

- A mean time to onset of 3 months before the appearance of the hepatotoxicity, with a range of 2 to 32 weeks
- A minimal estimated frequency of 160 cases in 370,000 exposures or 0.04% or 1/2300 subjects treated
- No evident risk factor

REGULATORY MEASURES

The drug was withdrawn from the market in the United Kingdom in December 1997 and in the United States in March 2000 after strengthening of the drug's labeling several times and recommendation of close monitoring of liver function. In March 1999 the Food and Drug Administration Endocrine and Metabolic Drugs Advisory Committee reviewed the status of the drug and recommended its continued availability for a select group of patients—those not well controlled on other diabetes drugs. It was only after two other drugs of the same class were marketed in the United States and showed the same benefits as troglitazone without the same risk that the drug was withdrawn from the market (HHS News. FDA News Release. 21 March 2000; www.fda.gov/bbs/topics/NEWS/NEW00721.html).

TWO-BY-TWO TABLE (ABCD TABLE)

In epidemiology, a contingency table with 4 cells also called an "ABCD Table" used to present the results of a structured study where:

a = exposed patients with a particular adverse effect

b = exposed patients without the AE

c = unexposed patients with the AE

d = unexposed patients without the AE

	Patients with the AE (Cases)	Patients without the AE (Controls)
Exposed (to drug)	*a*	*b*
Unexposed (to drug)	*c*	*d*

IF THE DATA ARE FROM A PROSPECTIVE COHORT STUDY

The *attributable risk* (risk difference, excess risk) is calculated as follows:

$$a/[a+b] - c/[c+d]$$

The *relative risk* is calculated as follows:

$$a/[a+b] \div c/[c+d]$$

IF THE DATA ARE FROM A RETROSPECTIVE CASE-CONTROL STUDY

The approximate relative risk can be calculated from the odds ratio if the cases are rare, for example, less than 2%.

The *odds ratio* can be calculated:

$$[a/c] \div [b/d] \text{ or } ad/bc$$

For further discussion, see any textbook of statistics/epidemiology (e.g., Gardner, M and Altman, D. *Statistics with confidence*, 2nd edition. London: British Medical Journal, 2000; Greenhalgh T. http://www.bmj.com//archive/7107/7017ed.htm and http://www.chestx-ray.com/Statistics/TwobyTwo.html).

U

UNDERREPORTING OF ADVERSE EFFECTS (see REPORTING RATE: SPONTANEOUS)

UNEXPECTED ADVERSE DRUG REACTION

In the regulatory context of an expedited (or alert) report, the definition of an *unexpected ADR* recommended by ICH E2A (www.ifpma.org/pdfifpma/e2a.pdf) is "An adverse reaction, the nature or severity of which is not consistent with the applicable product information."

For a marketed product, the official product information is that which is in the approved monograph or labeling in the country in question. In this situation, the classic definition has been that *unexpected* is equivalent to *unlabeled* meaning that the event does not appear in the official labeling. New usage has been proposed with the advent of the Summary of Product Characteristics and the Company Core Data Sheet (CCDS) and the Company Core Safety Information (CCSI). If an event is the CCDS/CCSI, it is considered *listed;* if the event is the officially approved labeling (which may be different from the CCDS/CCSI), it is considered *labeled.*

An unexpected event, however, is still open to interpretation.

The FDA definition of *unexpected* includes the following (21CFR 310.305):

> Any adverse drug experience that is not listed in the current labeling for the drug product. This includes events that may be symptomatically and pathophysiologically related to an event listed in the labeling, but differ from the event because of greater severity or specificity. For example, under this definition, hepatic necrosis would be unexpected (by virtue of greater severity) if the labeling only referred to elevated hepatic enzymes or hepatitis. Similarly, cerebral thromboembolism and cerebral vasculitis would be unexpected (by virtue of greater specificity) if the labeling only listed cerebral vascular accidents.

The CPMP (CPMP/PhVWP/108/99 corr), as described in the *Notice to Marketing Authorization Holders Pharmacovigilance Guidelines* of January 1999 (www.eudra.org/humandocs/humans/phvwp.htm), defines *unexpected adverse reaction* as follows:

> This is an adverse reaction which is not specifically included as a suspected adverse effect in the SPC. This includes any adverse reaction whose nature, severity or outcome is inconsistent with the information in the SPC. It also includes class-related reactions which are mentioned in the SPC but which are not specifically described as occurring with this product.

Thus there is often debate as to whether a particular adverse reaction is considered expected as the definitions of expectedness cited are often not clear. For example, if dizziness is labeled, would vertigo be considered labeled? A survey indicated that there is considerable disagreement on this issue between pharmacovigilance officers in Europe and those in the United States (Castle, *Drug Inf J* 1996;30:73).

UNEXPECTED BENEFICIAL DRUG REACTION

An advantage of pharmacovigilance after the launch of a new product, both for patients and for the manufacturer, is the occasional observation of new and often unexpected beneficial effects. Sometimes these effects are followed up with controlled clinical trials, the submission of a new New Drug Application (NDA), and the addition of a new indication to the labeling. Sometimes even more satisfying is the turning of an AE into a therapeutic benefit. For example, minoxidil produced abnormal hair growth in patients using the product for hypertension. The drug was studied in a different formulation and was relaunched as a topical product to promote hair growth in male-pattern baldness (see ORPHAN BENEFICIAL DRUG EFFECT).

UNLISTED ADVERSE DRUG REACTION

A regulatory term used in regard to the preparation of Periodic Safety Update Reports (PSURs), as described in ICH E2C. A term is unlisted if it does not appear in the Company Core Safety Information (CCSI) in regard to its nature, severity, specificity, and outcome. It is to be distinguished from *unlabeled* (see UNEXPECTED ADVERSE DRUG REACTION), which refers to whether an AE is included in the SPC.

UNTOWARD EFFECT

This is a loosely defined term that has been used as a synonym for both *AE* and *ADR*. The term *effect* includes a suspicion of causality.

UPPSALA MONITORING CENTRE (UMC)

A collaborating center of the World Health Organization (WHO); it is an international structure that maintains a worldwide registry of spontaneously reported AEs/ADRs transmitted to them from national centers.

HISTORY

After the thalidomide drama of 1961, several countries created national centers to monitor ADRs. By 1968 there were ten. It was at this time that a consensus was reached to collect the data at an international surveillance center. The World Health Organization was charged with this duty and a pilot project was created in 1968 (Program on International Drug Monitoring), temporarily located in the United States. In 1970 it was transferred to Geneva, Switzerland, and finally found its home in the university town of Uppsala, Sweden. In addition to its "passive" role as the world's largest depository of AEs/ADRs it plays a very active role in pharmacovigilance. The center is headed by Professor I. Ralph Edwards.

ACTIVITIES

- The center is encouraging all countries (particularly in the third world) to create, maintain, and improve the standards and functioning of pharmacovigilance centers.
- The center provides consultation and permits querying of its database (which contains data from over 60 pharmacovigilance centers worldwide) for specific information. This consultation is available on demand over the Internet as well as by more classic means at very reasonable costs. Unfortunately, only certain countries (approximately 29) allow their data to be used in queries by

the public. The remaining countries refuse to allow the AEs/ADRs that they have transmitted to the Monitoring Centre to be made public.

- The center organizes yearly National ADR Training Workshops held in a different country each year.
- The center holds an assembly of national pharmacovigilance centers each year, including the WHO Drug Monitoring Annual Program Meeting.
- The center publishes a news bulletin, *Uppsala Report*. It is aimed at national centers and any others interested in pharmacovigilance.
- The center also publishes the bulletin *Adverse Reactions Newsletter* on the Internet at (www.who-umc.org).
- The center maintains and updates an AE coding dictionary, *WHO-ART*; it is available on CD-ROM. The terms have been translated into English, French, Spanish, German, and Portuguese.
- The center maintains and updates the *WHO Drug Dictionary,* which is also available on CD-ROM.
- The center works with the WHO Dictionary Users' Group, which meets annually, usually in conjunction with a major congress. Minutes of the meeting are available on the Internet (www.who-umc.org/meetings.html#WHODRUG).
- In parallel, the WHO Collaborating Centre for Drug Statistics Methodology in Oslo, Norway, coordinates and publishes information for the Anatomic Therapeutic Chemical classification and determines the *defined daily dose* (see DEFINED DAILY DOSE).
- The center coordinates the ADR Signals Analysis Project cross-linking the WHO database and the IMS Health Inc. database of drug usage. Since 1990, the center has published a bulletin aimed at national pharmacovigilance centers, *SIGNAL.*
- The center also works on the Bayesian Confidence Propagation Neural Network (BCPNN) to improve detection of signals in their spontaneous AE database. The center has launched "ADRespherics" as a commercial venture to track AE/ADRs and signals after the launch of a new drug (www.who-umc.org).

The Uppsala Monitoring Centre is located at Stora Torget 3, S-753 20 Uppsala, Sweden (website: www.who-umc.org; e-mail address: info@who-umc.org; telephone: 48.18.65.60.60; Fax: 46.18.65.60.80).

UPPSALA REPORTS

The news bulletin published by the World Health Organization (WHO) Monitoring Centre in Uppsala, Sweden. It is available on the center's website (www.who-umc.org).

URTICARIA AND ANGIOEDEMA

Superficial vasodilatation and edema of the dermis with a red appearance that blanches with pressure and can change site from day to day. It can evolve into angioedema. It is often pruritic. A medication cause should always be considered in patients with urticaria. Drug-induced urticaria disappears rapidly after cessation of the causative agent (dechallenge). The mechanism is immunologic with two possibilities: more frequently the drug stimulates immunoglobulin E (IgE), which acts on mast cells, releasing histamine; less frequently the drug activates complement, which acts on mast cells releasing histamine.

Angioedema (Quinke's edema) is localized to the deep layers of the skin and represents a more severe type of immediate reaction. Its seriousness depends upon the anatomic site affected. Respiratory obstruction (a medical emergency) can occur if the angioedema involves the larynx or glottis. Angioedema can also be seen in the face, on the lips and around the eyes. The example that follows the rare anatomic localization of the event makes the diagnosis difficult:

ACE inhibitors and visceral angioedema: The diagnosis of deep visceral angioedema due to ACE inhibitors is unlikely to be suspected because angioedema is rare at these sites and it has a very variable, and often long, time to appearance. Both the site and the delay become misleading for the clinician (Mullins, *Med J Aust* 1996;165:319; Gregory, *N Engl J Med* 1996;334:1641).

VACCINE ADVERSE EVENT REPORTING SYSTEM (VAERS)

The vaccinovigilance program of the U.S. Food and Drug Administration and of the Center for Disease Control (POB 1100, Rockville, MD 20849-1100; (www.fda.gov/cber/vaers/vaers.htm).

VACCINOVIGILANCE

The surveillance of AEs regarding vaccines. This function is usually the responsibility of a governmental agency separate from that handling drug surveillance (pharmacovigilance). Severe adverse reactions from vaccines are relatively uncommon. The Food and Drug Administration's Vaccine Adverse Event Reporting System (VAERS) reports that 85% of its reports are minor, whereas 15% are serious events, such as seizures, high fevers, life-threatening illnesses, or deaths. The true ratio is hard to know since all AEs are not reported. See the FDA's vaccine reporting website (www.fda.gov/cber/vaers/vaers.htm).

A large series of cases occurred in the United States when the Guillain-Barré syndrome was seen after use of an influenza vaccine of porcine origin. Particular problems arise in the assignment of causality in vaccine reactions as the time to appearance is often long. See the chapter by Chen in Strom 2000.

Most agencies use a data collection form that is different from that used for drug AEs/ADRs. In the United States, the form is VAERS-1, which is very different from the drug and biologic reporting forms (MedWatch 3500/3500A and CIOMS 1 forms). See the FDA's vaccine website on vaccine event reporting (www.fda.gov/cber/vaers/report.htm).

A DIFFERENT RISK/BENEFIT RATIO

In the course of normal clinical practice, a patient seeks out a physician because of a particular problem. After diagnosis, a course of treatment is chosen after comparing risks and benefits applicable to the individual patient. With vaccinations, however, the equation is somewhat different. Vaccinations are usually encouraged or even required (e.g., in children in order to attend school) by the government and are given to healthy rather than sick people. The goal is not just protection of the individual but also of the community at large. Thus it is necessary to consider personal and public health benefits and risks:

- Individual prophylaxis: an infectious disease can be avoided in the future (e.g., hepatitis, whooping cough, tetanus)
- Public health prophylaxis: the propagation of an infectious disease can also be prevented (e.g., influenza, hepatitis)
- Individual risk: short- and long-term local and systemic adverse reactions
- Public health risk: monetary costs of the vaccines, adverse reactions that may prevent people from working (lost productivity), reactions that may occur in the future (latent slow viruses in vaccines, etc.), failure to predict the correct pathogens (e.g., influenza vaccines) that results in ineffective vaccinations, and others

The following example does not change the risk/benefit ratio for the population as a whole but does indeed change it for the individual patient vaccinated:

Encephalitis after smallpox vaccination: Ten days after receiving his first vaccination against smallpox, an Australian man suddenly developed fever, delirium, and nucal rigidity before falling into a coma. He recovered without neurologic deficit a week later with supportive treatment (*Aust Prescriber* 1978;2:82). This type of reaction is well described though very rare. Age is a risk factor. Mortality rate can be as high as 35%, but for those patients who recover, sequelae are rare.

One of the key roles of vaccinovigilance agencies is to provide continued reassurance to the general public and even medical professionals by putting the risk/benefit ratio in perspective and highlighting the individual and public health benefits in contrast to the rare, minimal risks of most vaccines. A clear example of vaccination that has high utility and low risk is the influenza vaccination of elderly people (WHO, *Drug Inf* 1991;5(2) and 1993;7(4)).

Influenza vaccine. A cohort that says yes, a study that says no: An observational study conducted in Canada demonstrated that 49% of those vaccinated complained of various general problems (Scheifel, *Can Med Assoc J* 1990;142:127), but a double-blind, placebo-controlled trial in the Netherlands showed no difference between the groups in regard to general reactions such as fever, malaise, and headache (Govaert, *Br Med J* 1993;307:988). Although this example suggests that vaccines can produce nocebo effects in addition to minor ADRs, it should always be kept in mind that severe adverse reactions, particularly in the geriatric population, can still occur in rare instances.

VAGINAL SPONGE

A medical device that was associated with cases of toxic shock in the United States some of which were fatal. The labeling of the product was changed to indicate this potential. The risk/benefit ratio was definitely at stake when the safety investigation began after the spontaneous reports: the rare adverse reactions were serious and the device was being used by healthy women.

VALIDATION

IN PHARMACOVIGILANCE

This refers to the verification of the correctness of the facts presented in a spontaneous case report. In particular, it can refer to a report made by a consumer that is confirmed by the patient's physician.

IN THE INFORMATION TECHNOLOGY WORLD

This refers to the validation of computer systems (e.g., pharmacovigilance systems, electronic transmission systems) and concerns the testing and verification that the data entered in the system are properly processed and reported outside the system. All computer systems involved in pharmacovigilance must be validated. This is now a component of regulatory agency (e.g., Food and Drug Administration, European Medicinal Evaluation Agency (EMEA)) pharmacovigilance audits.

VALIDITY OF A CASE REPORT

This expression is used in three contexts:

REGULATORY

Pharmaceutical companies and health authorities can receive spontaneous AE/ADR reports that often lack important data elements. Most health authorities' safety regulations require a certain level of information before they are required to be reported.

The Council for International Organizations of Medical Sciences (CIOMS) Working Group considers that four elements (a reporter, a patient, a product, an event) must be identifiable to declare a report *valid*. Let us discuss these elements:

▶ Reporter

By requiring an identifiable reporter (even if his or her name is kept secret), some reports that are malicious, false, or intended to be humorous can be eliminated. A name and a verifiable phone number or address usually suffice for health care professionals and consumers. A new problem has arisen with the reporting of AEs/ADRs over the Internet or by e-mail. An e-mail address does not serve as adequate identification, and usually a return e-mail must be sent to obtain a name, address, and phone number. In some countries the reporter must be a medical professional for a case to be considered valid, whereas in others (notably the United States and Canada) a consumer is considered to be a valid reporter.

In some countries, a case reported by someone who is not a health care professional must be medically substantiated by a medical professional even if all four elements are present. In effect, medical verification of the facts is a fifth validity criterion. In the United States, however, this is not necessary. Unsubstantiated consumer cases are reportable. The pharmaceutical company that receives unsubstantiated reports is expected to make the appropriate due diligence efforts to substantiate the report, including asking the patient for the name of the physician and contacting him or her for medical confirmation of the facts of the case.

▶ Patient

An identifiable patient is necessary. Usually age or sex or initials suffice. There must be sufficient data to warrant the conclusion that the patient truly exists. Usually one of these details is considered sufficient for regulatory reporting purposes.

▶ Suspect Drug or Biologic Product

There must be an identifiable drug product identified by brand, generic, or chemical name.

▶ Adverse Event

There must be an identifiable occurrence of an AE. Medical terms are preferred to lay terms where possible.

Examples of nonvalid reports include "A doctor said that three patients in New York took drug X and had myocardial infarcts" (no identifiable reporter or patient) or "Dr. Jones said that a 53-year-old female in Boston took a nonsteroidal anti-inflammatory and bled from a gastric ulcer" (no identifiable drug).

A special situation: ADRs that are reported in the medical literature must be sought out by the manufacturer and reported to the health authorities when the validity criteria are met. Follow-up from the author is often necessary and appropriate.

See the requirements from the Food and Drug Administration, *Guidance for Industry* published in 1997 (www.fda.gov/cber/gdlns/advexp.pdf). The similar International Conference on Harmonization (ICH) definition of valid case report is found in the E2A document (www.ifpma.org/pdfifpma/e2a.pdf), which was adopted by ICH as a guideline (www.eudra.org/humandocs/humans/ICH.htm). When all of these criteria are met (even minimally) the case is considered valid for regulatory reporting purposes. Cases that do not meet these criteria should not be reported. Due diligence in follow-up and in attempts to get further information is expected and required of pharmaceutical manufacturers when incomplete (invalid) reports are made to them.

CASE CAUSALITY

For causality assessment of a case report, the criteria for *validity* are more rigorous and correspond to quality control as applied to a report.

This usage—validity of causal assessment—refers not just to the regulatory criteria for reporting but also to the quality control, medical facts, and plausibility of the case. When a case is valid in this sense it carries weight in a pharmacovigilance investigation.

A case may be reportable (valid in the regulatory sense) because it contains the four elements but may make little medical sense and thus is not *medically valid.*

Medical validity should not be confused with *causality.* A case may be medically valid (complete, plausible, factual), but the event may prove to be unrelated to the drug in question once the case has been assessed properly.

PHARMACOVIGILANCE INVESTIGATION

The term *validity* may be applied to the aggregate data found in ADR databases, in linked health databases, or in observational studies made during a safety signal investigation. Thus a signal investigation may be said to have been *validated* if the hypothesis has been confirmed by the data mentioned.

VIDAL, DICTIONNAIRE

The drug compendium for medications in France. Its contents are usually taken from the Summaries of Product Characteristics (SPCs) submitted by the manufacturers.The supplement on drug interactions is helpful. It is updated yearly and is the equivalent of the U.S. *Physicians' Desk Reference (PDR)* or the *Rote Liste* in Germany (*Dictionnaire Vidal.* Paris: OVP, Editions du Vidal, 33 ave. de Wagram, F-75854 Paris Cedex 17 France; www.vidal.fr/).

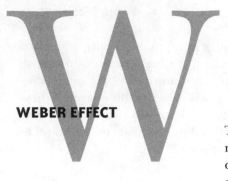

WEBER EFFECT

The Weber effect, also called the "product life cycle effect," describes the phenomenon of increased voluntary reporting after the initial launch of a new drug. "Voluntary reporting of AEs for a new drug within an established drug class does not proceed at a uniform rate and may be much higher in the first year or two of the drug's introduction." (Weber in *Advances in Inflammation Research*, Raven Press, NYC, 1984, pages 1–7). This means that for the period of time after launch (from 6 months to as long as two years) there will be a large number of spontaneously reported AEs/ADRs, which taper down to steady state levels after this effect is over. It is to be distinguished from "Secular Trends" (see SECULAR TRENDS).

WITHDRAWAL

IN PHARMACOTHERAPY
On the individual level, withdrawal refers to the stopping (discontinuation, cessation, "D/C") of a medication in a specific patient.

IN REGULATORY AFFAIRS
On the national and population level, the term refers to the withdrawal (suspension) of the marketing authorization or New Drug Application (NDA). This may be done for safety reasons by the government authority and/or the company. It may also be done for commercial reasons when a drug has become outmoded, as newer and better products are now on sale and the manufacturer chooses to cease commercial production or because the patent has expired.

Thus, in either case, the product will no longer be sold or distributed. Depending upon the individual situation, this may be an emergency with the immediate withdrawal and recall of the drug, or it may be done over time if there is no health issue.

See the website listing drugs not to be compounded (http://www.ijpc.com/chart.html) that originally appeared in the *Federal Register* (63[195]:54083-54087).

WITHDRAWAL: VOLUNTARY

Withdrawal of a drug from the market by the manufacturer may be due to the following:

- Change in risk/benefit ratio. This could be due to an internal company examination of the safety profile and the realization that the risk/benefit ratio is no longer favorable.
- Business considerations (dropping sales, loss of patent, merger with a manufacturer of a competing drug, etc.) may also cause a market withdrawal.
- Pressure from the health authorities may spur withdrawal.
- Pressure from various sources, such as consumer groups (via petitions, adverse publicity, picketing, etc.), the media, or lawsuits (individual or class action) may motivate withdrawal (see BENDECTIN).

Thus a "voluntary withdrawal" is not always voluntary.

WHO DICTIONARY USERS' GROUP

The Uppsala Monitoring Centre in Uppsala, Sweden, and various national pharmacovigilance centers meet annually. This meeting is held to discuss content and to train new users in the centers and in industry in the use of the World Health Organization (WHO) dictionaries for adverse effect terms (*WHO-ART*) and for drugs (*WHO Drug Dictionary*). See the Uppsala Monitoring Centre website (www.who-umc.org).

WHO DRUG INFORMATION

A quarterly journal published since 1987 by the World Health Organization (WHO) covering:

- Newly detected ADRs
- Dangerous drug interactions
- Contraindications in certain groups of patients
- Important changes in labeling of a product
- New information on the preferred treatments for diseases
- New indications for marketed drugs

The journal provides a global view of issues in drug developments and surveillance (WHO, CH-1211, Geneva 27 Switzerland; www.who.int).

WITHDRAWAL EFFECT

The withdrawal effect or syndrome is the manifestation of a pathologic condition that is *qualitatively different* from the indication being treated and occurs after the cessation of the product or drug. Three conditions are required:

- The cessation of the drug or product must be sudden.
- The duration of treatment must have been sufficiently long.
- The half-life of the drug or product must be relatively short.

In causality determination, the time to onset is calculated, paradoxically, from last dose to first symptom. In elderly patients a well-managed withdrawal from a medication may take a long time. Withdrawal syndromes are not limited to substances such as alcohol or benzodiazepines, as the following examples illustrate:

Delivery of a baby: Natural or cesarean birth represents a withdrawal for the baby when the mother has been taking a medication that crosses the placenta.

Serotoninergic antidepressants: An attenuated form of withdrawal, known as a *discontinuation syndrome,* that can produce dependence may explain the difficulties experienced by some patients taking certain antidepressants (with a short half-life) when they stop their treatment after a successful resolution of the depression (Schatzberg, *J Clin Psychiatry* 1997;58(suppl 7):5).

Muscle relaxant: neuropsychiatric problems: Hallucinations, convulsions, and other similar problems can occur with the sudden stopping of baclofen, a derivative of gamma-aminobutyric acid used as a voluntary muscle relaxant.

Corticoid therapy: intracranial hypertension: This rather unusual adverse reaction is one of a number that can complicate the sudden cessation of long-term corticosteroid therapy.

Antidepressant: mania: A 49-year-old male who was taking a serotoninergic antidepressant suddenly decided not to renew his prescription. In less than 2 weeks he had symptoms of mania. Two days after he recommended treatment the symptoms began to disappear: an orphan ADR (Propost, *Can J Clin Pharmacol* 1997;4:115).

WITHDRAWALS FROM THE MARKET FOR SAFETY PROBLEMS

For a list of withdrawals over the years, see Stephens 1999:422. The main sources are Bakke (*Clin Pharmacol Ther* 1984;35:559 and 1995;58:108) and C. Spriet-Pourra and M. Auriche (*Drug withdrawal from sale.* Scrip Report/PJB Publications, Richmond, Surrey, U.K. 1988 and 1994). There is a lot to be learned from any safety withdrawal story.

WORLD HEALTH ORGANIZATION ADVERSE REACTION TERMINOLOGY (WHO-ART)

A thesaurus of AE/ADR terms and synonyms produced by the Monitoring Centre in Uppsala, Sweden. It is one of the standard coding dictionaries in use in the industry and in health agencies. There are four levels of terminology. The first or lowest level contains *included terms,* which provide the most specific descriptions of signs and symptoms. The next higher level contains *preferred terms,* under which the included terms are found. The next ascending level is *high-level terms,* which number about 150. Finally the terms all fall into one or more of the 30 highest-level body system organ classes (SOCs). The dictionary is revised periodically to incorporate new terms and concepts. See the Uppsala Monitoring Centre's product website (www.who-umc.org).

WORLD HEALTH ORGANIZATION DATABASE OF ADVERSE REACTIONS

A database of some 2 million spontaneous reports of AEs/ADRs maintained by the Uppsala Monitoring Center. It receives these reports from national health organizations. It may be queried on-line for a small fee, though not all of the national health organizations allow their data to be released. Information is available at the Uppsala Monitoring Centre's product website (www.who-umc.org).

WORLD HEALTH ORGANIZATION DRUG DICTIONARY (WHODD; WHO DRUG DICTIONARY)

A dictionary of drug products begun in 1968 that is updated quarterly by the World Health Organization (WHO). It is widely used by the pharmaceutical industry and national pharmacovigilance centers. Information is available at the Uppsala Monitoring Centre's product website (www.who-umc.org).

WORST PILLS BEST PILLS; WPBP NEWS

A book published by Dr. Sidney Wolfe and the Public Citizen/Health Research Group (PC/HRG), an American consumer association. It is subtitled, *A Consumer's Guide to Avoiding Drug-Induced Death or Illness* (www.worstpills.org). The bulletin *WPBP News* is also published by Public Citizen (1200 20th Street NW, Washington, DC 20009; www.citizen.org/hrg).

XYZ

YELLOW CARD SYSTEM

The first national spontaneous reporting scheme was introduced in 1964 in the United Kingdom in the wake of the thalidomide disaster in 1961. Its first director, Professor W. H. W. Inman, used yellow cards to distribute the reporting forms to physicians. Equivalent to *national pharmacovigilance program, system,* or *scheme.*

ZIMELDINE: WITHDRAWAL

After the launch of this molecule, one of the first of the new class of serotonin uptake inhibitors, cases of Guillain-Barré syndrome were reported. A pharmacovigilance investigation was done and an attributable risk of 560 cases per million patient-years was calculated. This risk of 1 case per 1785 patient-years was judged unacceptable as other treatments were available, and the drug was withdrawn from the market (Kaitin, *Clin Pharmacol Ther* 1989;46:121).

ZOMEPIRAC: WITHDRAWAL

This nonsteroidal anti-inflammatory drug (NSAID) was first marketed in the United States in 1980 and in the United Kingdom in 1981. Severe and fatal anaphylactoid reactions were soon reported to the Food and Drug Administration and published in the medical literature. The drug was withdrawn from the market in 1981 after several deaths. The risk was evaluated to be between 0.9 and 2.7 reported deaths per million prescriptions written. The decision to withdraw the product was made because other NSAIDs were available on the market without this risk (Samuel, *N Engl J Med* 1981;304:978; Strom, *Arthritis Rheum* 1987;30:1142; Corre, *Ann Emerg Med* 1988;17:145; Kaitin, *Clin Pharmacol Ther* 1989;46:121; Ross-Degnan, *JAMA* 1993;270:1937).